Case Files™
Neurology

NOTICE

Medicine is an ever-changing science. As new research and clinical experience broaden our knowledge, changes in treatment and drug therapy are required. The authors and the publisher of this work have checked with sources believed to be reliable in their efforts to provide information that is complete and generally in accord with the standard accepted at the time of publication. However, in view of the possibility of human error or changes in medical sciences, neither the editors nor the publisher nor any other party who has been involved in the preparation or publication of this work warrants that the information contained herein is in every respect accurate or complete, and they disclaim all responsibility for any errors or omissions or for the results obtained from use of the information contained in this work. Readers are encouraged to confirm the information contained herein with other sources. For example and in particular, readers are advised to check the product information sheet included in the package of each drug they plan to administer to be certain that the information contained in this work is accurate and that changes have not been made in the recommended dose or in the contraindications for administration. This recommendation is of particular importance in connection with new or infrequently used drugs.

Case Files™
Neurology

EUGENE C. TOY, MD
The John S. Dunn, Senior Academic Chief and Program Director
The Methodist Hospital-Houston Ob/Gyn Residency
Clerkship Director, Clinical Associate Professor
Department of Obstetrics and Gynecology
University of Texas—Houston Medical School
Houston, Texas

ERICKA SIMPSON, MD
Assistant Professor, Neurology
Weill-Cornell Medical College, New York
Co-Director MDA Neuromuscular Clinics and
Director of ALS Clinical Research Division
Methodist Neurological Institute
Program Director
The Methodist Hospital Neurology Residency
Houston, Texas

MILVIA PLEITEZ, MD
Assistant Professor, Neurology
Weill-Cornell Medical College, New York
Methodist Neurological Institute
Houston, Texas

DAVID ROSENFIELD, MD
Professor, Neurology
Weill-Cornell Medical College, New York
Director EMG and Motor Control Laboratory
Methodist Neurological Institute
Houston, Texas

RON TINTNER, MD
Associate Professor, Neurology
Weill-Cornell Medical College, New York
Co-Director Movement Disorders and Rehabilitation Center
Methodist Neurological Institute
Houston, Texas

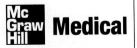

New York Chicago San Francisco
Lisbon London Madrid Mexico City
Milan New Delhi San Juan Seoul
Singapore Sydney Toronto

The McGraw·Hill Companies

Case Files™: Neurology

1 2 3 4 5 6 7 8 9 0   DOC/DOC   0 9 8 7

ISBN: 978-0-07-148287-5
MHID: 0-07-148287-3

This book was set in Times Roman by International Typesetting and Composition.
The editors were Catherine Johnson and Penny Linskey.
The production supervisor was Catherine Saggese.
Project management was provided by International Typesetting and Composition
The cover designer was Aimee Davis.
The index was prepared by Ken Hassman.
RR Donnelly was printer and binder.

This book is printed on acid-free paper.

Library of Congress Cataloging-in-Publication Data

Case files. Neurology / Eugene C. Toy ... [et al.].
    p. ; cm.
    Includes index.
    ISBN-13: 978-0-07-148287-5 (pbk. : alk. paper)
    ISBN-10:   0-07-148287-3
    1. Neurology—Case studies.   2. Nervous system—Diseases—Case studies.   I. Toy, Eugene C.   II. Title: Neurology.
    [DNLM: 1. Nervous System Diseases—Case Reports.   2. Nervous System Diseases—Problems and Exercises.   3. Neurology—methods—Case Reports.   4. Neurology—methods—Problems and Exercises. WL 18.2 C337 2008]
RC359.C33 2008
616.8—dc22

2007034864

*To Dr. Alan L. Kaplan, whose generosity, clinical and educational
excellence, and impeccable character have set a high standard for
so many of us.*

—ECT

*To my eternal source of peace and strength, Jesus Christ;
to my son, Christopher, who is my daily inspiration and joy;
to my Mentor and Chair, Stanley H. Appel for setting a standard of
excellence and leadership—I thank you.*

—EPS

❖ CONTENTS

❖ CONTRIBUTORS

David Chiu, MD
Associate Professor
Director, Eddy Scurlock Stroke Center
Methodist Neurological Institute
Weill-Cornell Medical College
Houston, Texas
Acute Cerebral Infarction
Stroke in Young Person

Lance Davis, MS IV
University of Texas Southwestern Medical School
Dallas, Texas
Student reviewer

Howard Derman, MD
Professor, Neurology
Methodist Neurological Institute
Weill-Cornell Medical College
Houston, Texas
Chronic Progressive Headache
Episodic Headache (Migraine)

Stanley Fisher, MD
Assistant Professor, Neurology
Co-Director of Movement Disorder and Neurorehabilitation
Methodist Neurological Institute
Weill-Cornell Medical College
Houston, Texas
Syncope versus Seizure
Tourette Syndrome

Paul Gidley, MD
Associate Professor,
Head and Neck Center
The University of Texas M. D. Anderson Cancer Center
Houston, Texas
Facial Paralysis
Meningioma & Glioblastoma
Vertigo

James Ling, MD
Assistant Professor, Neurology
Methodist Neurological Institute
Weill-Cornell Medical College
Houston, Texas
Lissencephaly
New Onset Seizure, Child
Subarachnoid hemorrhage

Jeetha Nair, MD
Research Post-doctoral Fellow
Cain Foundation Laboratories
Department of Pediatrics
Baylor College of Medicine
Houston, Texas
Acute Spinal Injury

James W. Owens, MD, PhD
Assistant Professor of Child Neurology
Director, Medical Student Neurology Education
Departments of Neurology and Pediatric Neurology
Baylor College of Medicine
Houston, Texas
Acute Spinal Injury
Autism/Developmental Delay
Benign Rolandic Epilepsy
Cerebral Contusion
Febrile Seizure
Headache, Child

Martin Paukert, MS IV
University of Texas Medical School at Houston
Houston, Texas
Tourette Syndrome
also Principal Student Reviewer

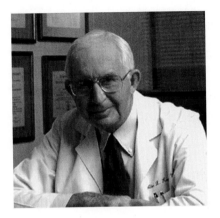

This is the first Case Files book that has originated from The Methodist Hospital-Houston. It is dedicated to **DR. ALAN L. KAPLAN,** the excellent, insightful, and compassionate chairman of the Department of Obstetrics and Gynecology at The Methodist Hospital and professor of Obstetrics and Gynecology at the Weill Medical College of Cornell University. He received his medical degree in 1955 from Columbia University of Physicians and Surgeons in New York. He completed his residency at Columbia Presbyterian Medical Center in 1959. He then served two years in the Army, following which he returned to Columbia Presbyterian Medical Center for fellowship training, which he completed in 1963. He joined Baylor College of Medicine in 1963 and was with the Department of Obstetrics and Gynecology for 42 years. He served as Professor and Director of the Division of Gynecologic Oncology. Dr. Kaplan became a certified Diplomate of the American Board of Obstetrics and Gynecology in 1966, and earned his certification in Gynecologic Oncology in 1974. Dr. Kaplan is a member of numerous professional societies, many of which relate to his specialty field—female cancers. He has served on various editorial boards and is active on committees of both the professional organizations and the hospitals at which he practices. In his clinical practice, he cares for women with gynecologic surgical problems and female cancers. He enjoys jogging, swimming, reading, and tennis.

❖ ACKNOWLEDGMENTS

The curriculum that evolved into the ideas for this series was inspired by two talented and forthright students, Philbert Yau and Chuck Rosipal, who have since graduated from medical school. It has been a pleasure to work with Dr. Ericka Simpson, a brilliant, compassionate and dedicated teacher and the other talented neurologists. I am greatly indebted to my editor, Catherine Johnson, whose exuberance, experience, and vision helped to shape this series. Likewise, Penny Linsky has been a dream with whom to collaborate. I appreciate McGraw-Hill's believing in the concept of teaching through clinical cases. My "family" at McGraw-Hill have been most gracious, particularly recently giving my entire family a royal tour at the New York facility. At Methodist Hospital, I thank our excellent administrators Drs. Mark Boom, Karin Larsen-Pollock, H. Dirk Sostman, and Judy Paukert, and Mr. John Lyle and Mr. Reggie Abraham. Likewise, I am indebted to the numerous excellent physicians in the Obstetrics/Gynecology department, among whom I particularly appreciate Drs. Tri Dinh, Eric Haufrect, Raymond Kaufman, Sam Law II, Waverly Peakes, Keith Reeves, and David Zepeda. At St. Joseph Medical Center, I applaud the excellent administrators: Phil Robinson, Pat Mathews, Laura Fortin, Dori Upton, Janet Matthews, and Drs. John Bertini and Thomas V. Taylor for their commitment to medical education, and Marla Buffington for her sage advice and support. I owe a huge debt to gratitude to Martin Paukert, probably the most brilliant medical student who has walked through our hospital doors, for agreeing to meticulously review the manuscript on such a short timeline. Most of all, I appreciate my ever-loving wife Terri, and four wonderful children, Andy, Michael, Allison, and Christina for their patience, encouragement, understanding, and "sharing their father" with my students and writing.

Eugene C. Toy

❖ INTRODUCTION

Mastering the cognitive knowledge within a field such as neurology is a formidable task. It is even more difficult to draw on that knowledge, procure and filter through the clinical and laboratory data, develop a differential diagnosis, and finally to form a rational treatment plan. To gain these skills, the student often learns best at the bedside, guided and instructed by experienced teachers, and inspired toward self-directed, diligent reading. Clearly, there is no replacement for education at the bedside. Unfortunately, clinical situations usually do not encompass the breadth of the specialty. Perhaps the best alternative is a carefully crafted patient case designed to stimulate the clinical approach and decision-making. In an attempt to achieve that goal, we have constructed a collection of clinical vignettes to teach diagnostic or therapeutic approaches relevant to the discipline of neurology. Most importantly, the explanations for the cases emphasize the mechanisms and underlying principles, rather than merely rote questions and answers.

This book is organized for versatility: it allows the student "in a rush" to go quickly through the scenarios and check the corresponding answers, as well as the student with more time to have thought-provoking explanations. The answers are arranged from simple to complex: a summary of the pertinent points, the bare answers, an analysis of the case, an approach to the topic, a comprehension test at the end for reinforcement and emphasis, and a list of resources for further reading. The clinical vignettes are purposely placed in random order to simulate the way that real patients present to the practitioner. A listing of cases is included in Section III to aid the student who desires to test his or her knowledge of a certain area, or to review a topic including basic definitions. Finally, we intentionally did not primarily use a multiple choice question (MCQ) format because clues (or distractions) are not available in the real world. Nevertheless, several MCQs are included at the end of each scenario to reinforce concepts or introduce related topics.

HOW TO GET THE MOST OUT OF THIS BOOK

Each case is designed to simulate a patient encounter with open-ended questions. At times, the patient's complaint is different from the most concerning issue, and sometimes extraneous information is given. The answers are organized with four different parts:

PART I

1. Summary—the salient aspects of the case are identified, filtering out the extraneous information. The student should formulate his or her summary from the case before looking at the answers. A comparison to the summation in the answer will help to improve one's ability to focus on the important data, while appropriately discarding the irrelevant information, a fundamental skill in clinical problem solving.

2. A straightforward answer is given to each open-ended question.

3. The Analysis of the Case, which is comprised of two parts:
    a. Objectives of the Case—a listing of the two or three main principles that are crucial for a practitioner to manage the patient. Again, the student is challenged to make educated "guesses" about the objectives of the case on initial review of the case scenario, which help to sharpen his or her clinical and analytical skills.
    b. Considerations—A discussion of the relevant points and brief approach to the specific patient.

PART II

Approach to the Disease Process—This has two distinct parts:
    a. Definitions or neurophysiology—terminology or neuroanatomy correlates pertinent to the disease process.
    b. Clinical approach—a discussion of the approach to the clinical problem in general, including tables, figures, and algorithms.

PART III

Comprehension Questions—Each case contains several multiple-choice questions that reinforce the material, or introduce new and related concepts. Questions about material not found in the text will have explanations in the answers.

PART IV

Clinical Pearls—A listing of several clinically important points that are reiterated as a summation of the text and to allow for easy review such as before an examination.

How to Approach Clinical Problems

PART 1. APPROACH TO THE PATIENT

Applying "book learning" to a specific clinical situation is one of the most challenging tasks in medicine. To do so, the clinician must not only retain information, organize facts, and recall large amounts of data but also apply all of this to the patient. The purpose of this text is to facilitate this process.

The first step involves gathering information, also known as establishing the database. This includes taking the history, performing the physical examination, and obtaining selective laboratory examinations, special studies, and/or imaging tests. Sensitivity and respect should always be exercised during the interview of patients. A good clinician also knows how to ask the same question in several different ways, using different terminology. For example, patients may deny having "tremulousness" but will answer affirmatively to feeling "shaky."

CLINICAL PEARL

❖ The history is usually the single most important tool in obtaining a diagnosis. The art of seeking this information in a nonjudgmental, sensitive, and thorough manner cannot be overemphasized.

---

1. Basic Information:
   a. Age: Some conditions are more common at certain ages; for instance, forgetfulness is more likely to be caused by dementia in an elderly patient than the same complaint in a teenager.
   b. Gender: Some disorders are more common in men such as cluster headaches. In contrast, women more commonly have migraine headaches. Also, the possibility of pregnancy must be considered in any woman of child-bearing age.
   c. Ethnicity: Some disease processes are more common in certain ethnic groups (such as type 2 diabetes mellitus in Hispanic patients).

CLINICAL PEARL

❖ The discipline of neurology illustrates the importance of understanding how to correlate the neuroanatomical defect to the clinical manifestation.

---

2. Chief complaint: What is it that brought the patient into the hospital? Has there been a change in a chronic or recurring condition or is this a

completely new problem? The duration and character of the complaint, associated symptoms, and exacerbating/relieving factors should be recorded. The chief complaint engenders a differential diagnosis, and the possible etiologies should be explored by further inquiry.

CLINICAL PEARL

❖ The first line of any presentation should include *age, gender, marital status, handedness, and chief complaint.* Example: A 32-year-old married white right-handed male complains of left arm weakness and numbness.

---

4. Past Medical History:
   a. Major illnesses such as hypertension, diabetes, reactive airway disease, congestive heart failure, angina, or stroke should be detailed.
      i. Age of onset, severity, end-organ involvement.
      ii. Medications taken for the particular illness including any recent changes to medications and reason for the change(s).
      iii. Last evaluation of the condition (example: when was the last stress test or cardiac catheterization performed in the patient with angina?)
      iv. Which physician or clinic is following the patient for the disorder?
   b. Minor illnesses such as recent upper respiratory infections should be noted.
   c. Hospitalizations no matter how trivial should be queried.

5. Past Surgical History: Note the date and type of procedure performed, indication, and outcome. Surgeon and hospital name/location should be listed. This information should be correlated with the surgical scars on the patient's body. Any complications should be delineated including anesthetic complications, difficult intubations, and so forth.

6. Allergies: Reactions to medications should be recorded, including severity and temporal relationship to medication. Immediate hypersensitivity should be distinguished from an adverse reaction.

7. Medications: A list of medications, dosage, route of administration and frequency, and duration of use should be developed. Prescription, over-the-counter, and herbal remedies are all relevant. If the patient is currently taking antibiotics, it is important to note what type of infection is being treated.

8. Immunization History: Vaccination and prevention of disease is one of the principal goals of the family physician; however, recording the immunizations received including dates, age, route, and adverse reactions if any is critical in evaluating the neurology patient as well.

9. Social History: Occupation, marital status, family support, and tendencies toward depression or anxiety are important. Use or abuse of illicit drugs, tobacco, or alcohol should also be recorded.

10. Family History: Many major medical problems are genetically transmitted (e.g., hemophilia, sickle cell disease). In addition, a family history of conditions such as breast cancer and ischemic heart disease can be a risk factor for the development of these diseases. Social history including marital stressors, sexual dysfunction, and sexual preference are of importance.

11. Review of Systems: A systematic review should be performed but focused on the life-threatening and the more common diseases. For example, in a young man with a testicular mass, trauma to the area, weight loss, and infectious symptoms are important to note. In an elderly woman with generalized weakness, symptoms suggestive of cardiac disease should be elicited, such as chest pain, shortness of breath, fatigue, or palpitations.

Physical Examination

1. General appearance: Note mental status, alert versus obtunded, anxious, in pain, in distress, interaction with other family members and with examiner. Note any dysmorphic features of the head and body may also be important for many inherited or congenital disorders.

2. Vital signs: Record the temperature, blood pressure, heart rate, and respiratory rate. An oxygen saturation is useful in patients with respiratory symptoms. Height and weight are often placed here with a body mass index (BMI) calculated (BMI $= kg/m^2$ or lb/in^2).

3. Head and neck examination: Evidence of trauma, tumors, facial edema, goiter and thyroid nodules, and carotid bruits should be sought. In patients with altered mental status or a head injury, pupillary size, symmetry, and reactivity are important. Mucous membranes should be inspected for pallor, jaundice, and evidence of dehydration. Cervical and supraclavicular nodes should be palpated.

4. Breast examination: Inspection for symmetry and skin or nipple retraction as well as palpation for masses. The nipple should be assessed for discharge, and the axillary and supraclavicular regions should be examined.

5. Cardiac examination: The point of maximal intensity (PMI) should be ascertained, and the heart auscultated at the apex as well as base. It is important to note whether the auscultated rhythm is regular or irregular. Heart sounds (including S_3 and S_4), murmurs, clicks, and rubs should be characterized. Systolic flow murmurs are fairly common as a result of the increased cardiac output, but significant diastolic murmurs are unusual.

6. Pulmonary examination: The lung fields should be examined systematically and thoroughly. Stridor, wheezes, rales, and rhonchi should be recorded. The clinician should also search for evidence of consolidation (bronchial breath sounds, egophony) and increased work of breathing (retractions, abdominal breathing, accessory muscle use).

7. Abdominal examination: The abdomen should be inspected for scars, distension, masses, and discoloration. For instance, the Grey-Turner sign of bruising at the flank areas can indicate intraabdominal or retroperitoneal hemorrhage. Auscultation should identify normal versus high-pitched and hyperactive versus hypoactive bowel sounds. The abdomen should be percussed for the presence of shifting dullness (indicating ascites). Then careful palpation should begin away from the area of pain and progress to include the whole abdomen to assess for tenderness, masses, organomegaly (i.e., spleen or liver), and peritoneal signs. Guarding and whether it is voluntary or involuntary should be noted.

8. Back and spine examination: The back should be assessed for symmetry, tenderness, or masses. The flank regions particularly are important to assess for pain on percussion that may indicate renal disease.

9. Perform genital examination and rectal examination as needed.

10. Extremities/Skin: The presence of joint effusions, tenderness, rashes, edema, and cyanosis should be recorded. It is also important to note capillary refill and peripheral pulses.

11. Neurologic examination: Patients who present with neurologic complaints require a thorough assessment including mental status, cranial nerves, muscle tone, and strength, sensation, reflexes, and cerebellar function, and gait to determine where the *lesion* or problem is located in the nervous system. *Locating the lesion* is the first step to generating a differential of possible diagnoses and implementing a plan for management.
    a. Cranial nerves need to be assessed: ptosis (III), facial droop (VII), hoarse voice (X), speaking and articulation (V, VII, X, XII), eye position (III, IV, VI), pupils (II, III), smell (I); visual acuity and visual fields, pupillary reflexes to light and accommodation; hearing

acuity and Weber and Rinne test, sensation of three branches of V of face; shrug shoulders (XI), protrude tongue (VII).

b. Motor: Observe for involuntary movements, muscle symmetry (right vs. left, proximal vs. distal), muscle atrophy, gait. Have patient move against resistance (isolate muscle group, compare one side vs. another, and use 0–5 scale).

c. Coordination and gait: Rapid alternating movements, point-to-point movements, Romberg test, and gait (walk, heel-to-toe in straight line, walk on toes and heels, shallow bend and get up from sitting).

d. Reflexes: biceps (C5,6), triceps (C6,7), brachioradialis (C5,6), patellar (L2–4), ankle (S1–2).

e. Clonus and plantar reflex.

f. Sensory: Patient's eyes should be closed, compare both sides of body, distal versus proximal; vibratory sense (low pitched tuning fork); subjective light touch; position sense, dermatome testing, pain, temperature.

g. Discrimination: Graphesthesia (identify number "drawn" on hand), stereognosis (place familiar object in patient's hand), and two-point discrimination.

12. Mental status examination: A thorough neurologic examination requires a mental status examination. The Mini-Mental Status examination is a series of verbal and non-verbal tasks that serves to detect impairments in memory, concentration, language, and spatial orientation.

CLINICAL PEARL

❖ A thorough understanding of functional anatomy is important to optimally interpret the physical examination findings.

13. Laboratory assessment depends on the circumstances

a. Complete blood count (CBC) can assess for anemia, leukocytosis (infection), and thrombocytopenia.

b. Basic metabolic panel: electrolytes, glucose, blood urea nitrogen (BUN) and creatinine (renal function).

c. Urinalysis and/or urine culture to assess for hematuria, pyuria, or bacteruria. A pregnancy test is important in women of child-bearing age.

d. Aspartate aminotransferase (AST), alanine aminotransferase (ALT), bilirubin, alkaline phosphatase for liver function; amylase and lipase to evaluate the pancreas.

e. Cardiac markers (creatine kinase myocardial band [CK-MB], troponin, myoglobin) if coronary artery disease or other cardiac dysfunction is suspected.

    f. Drug levels such as acetaminophen level in possible overdoses.

    g. Arterial blood gas measurements give information about oxygenation, but also carbon dioxide and pH readings.

14. Diagnostic adjuncts

    a. Electroencephalogram (EEG) if focal or gross central nervous system pathology is suspected.

    b. Computed tomography (CT) is useful in assessing the brain for masses, bleeding, strokes, skull fractures.

    c. Magnetic resonance imaging helps to identifies soft tissue planes very well.

    d. Lumbar puncture is indicated to assess any inflammatory, infectious, or neoplastic processes that can affect the brain, spinal cord, or nerve roots.

PART 2. APPROACH TO CLINICAL PROBLEM-SOLVING

Classic Clinical Problem-Solving

There are typically four distinct steps that the family physician undertakes to systematically solve most clinical problems:

1. Making the diagnosis
2. Assessing the severity of the disease
3. Treating based on the stage of the disease
4. Following the patient's response to the treatment

Making the Diagnosis   This is achieved by carefully evaluating the patient, analyzing the information, assessing risk factors, and developing a list of possible diagnoses (the differential). Usually a long list of possible diagnoses can be pared down to a few of the most likely or most serious ones, based on the clinician's knowledge, experience, and selective testing. For example, a 30-year-old patient who complains of acute onset of right facial weakness and drooling from the right side probably has a cranial nerve VII palsy. Yet another individual who is a 60-year-old man with right sided facial weakness and left arm numbness likely has an ischemic stroke.

CLINICAL PEARL

The first step in clinical problem solving is making the diagnosis.

Assessing the Severity of the Disease   After establishing the diagnosis, the next step is to characterize the severity of the disease process; in other words, to describe "how bad" the disease is. This can be as simple as determining whether a patient is "sick" or "not sick." Is the patient with a hemorrhagic stroke comatose or with a "blown pupil"? In other cases, a more formal staging can be used. For example, cancer staging is used for the strict assessment of extent of malignancy.

CLINICAL PEARL

❖   The second step is to establish the severity or stage of disease. This usually impacts the treatment and/or prognosis.

Treating based on Stage   Many illnesses are characterized by stage or severity because this affects prognosis and treatment. As an example, a patient with mild lower extremity weakness and areflexia that develops over 2 weeks may be carefully observed; however once respiratory depression occurs, then respiratory support must be given.

CLINICAL PEARL

❖   The third step is tailoring the treatment to fit the severity or "stage" of the disease.

Following the Response to Treatment   The final step in the approach to disease is to follow the patient's response to the therapy. Some responses are clinical such as improvement (or lack of improvement) in a patient's strength; a standardized method of assessment is important. Other responses can be followed by testing (e.g., visual field testing). The clinician must be prepared to know what to do if the patient does not respond as expected. Is the next step to treat again, to reassess the diagnosis, or to follow up with another more specific test?

CLINICAL PEARL

❖   The fourth step is to monitor treatment response or efficacy. This can be measured in different ways–symptomatically or based on physical examination or other testing.

PART 3. APPROACH TO READING

The clinical problem-oriented approach to reading is different from the classic "systematic" research of a disease. Patients rarely present with a clear diagnosis; hence, the student must become skilled in applying textbook information to the clinical scenario. Because reading with a purpose improves the retention of information, the student should read with the goal of answering specific questions. There are several fundamental questions that facilitate clinical thinking. These are:

1. What is the most likely diagnosis?
2. How would you confirm the diagnosis?
3. What should be your next step?
4. What is likely neuroanatomical defect?
5. What are the risk factors for this condition?
6. What are the complications associated with the disease process?
7. What is the best therapy?

> ### CLINICAL PEARL
>
> ❖ Reading with the purpose of answering the seven fundamental clinical questions improves retention of information and facilitates the application of "book knowledge" to "clinical knowledge."

What Is the Most Likely Diagnosis?

The method of establishing the diagnosis has been covered in the previous section. One way of attacking this problem is to develop standard approaches to common clinical problems. It is helpful to understand the most common causes of various presentations (see the Clinical Pearls at the end of each case), such as "the worst headache of the patient's life is worrisome for a subarachnoid hemorrhage."

The clinical scenario would be something such as:

"A 38-year-old woman is noted to have a 2-day history of a unilateral, throbbing headache and photophobia. What is the most likely diagnosis?"

With no other information to go on, the student would note that this woman has a unilateral headache and photophobia. Using the "most common cause" information, the student would make an educated guess that the patient has a migraine headache. If instead the patient is noted to have "the worst headache of her life," the student would use the clinical pearl: "The worst headache of the patient's life is worrisome for a subarachnoid hemorrhage."

> ### CLINICAL PEARL
> ❖ The more common cause of a unilateral, throbbing headache with
> photophobia is a migraine, but the main concern is subarachnoid
> hemorrhage. If the patient describes this as "the worst headache of
> his or her life," the concern for a subarachnoid bleed is increased.

How Would You Confirm the Diagnosis?

In the scenario above, the woman with "the worst headache" is suspected of having a subarachnoid hemorrhage. This diagnosis could be confirmed by a CT scan of the head and/or lumbar puncture (LP). The student should learn the limitations of various diagnostic tests, especially when used early in a disease process. The LP showing xanthochromia (red blood cells) is the gold standard test for diagnosing subarachnoid hemorrhage, but it can be negative early in the disease course.

What Should Be Your Next Step?

This question is difficult because the next step has many possibilities; the answer can be to obtain more diagnostic information, stage the illness, or introduce therapy. It is often a more challenging question than "What is the most likely diagnosis?" because there may be insufficient information to make a diagnosis, and the next step may be to pursue more diagnostic information. Another possibility is that there is enough information for a probable diagnosis, and the next step is to stage the disease. Finally, the most appropriate answer may be to treat. Hence, from clinical data, a judgment needs to be rendered regarding how far along one is on the road of:

1. Make a diagnosis → 2. Stage the disease → 3. Treat based on stage → 4. Follow response

Frequently, the student is taught "to regurgitate" the same information that someone has written about a particular disease but is not skilled at identifying the next step. This talent is learned optimally at the bedside, in a supportive environment, with freedom to take educated guesses and with constructive feedback. A sample scenario can describe a student's thought process as follows:

1. **Make the diagnosis:** "Based on the information I have, I believe that Mr. Smith has a left-sided cerebrovascular accident."
2. **Stage the disease:** "I don't believe that this is severe disease because his Glasgow score is 12, and he is alert."
3. **Treat based on stage:** "Therefore, my next step is to treat with oxygenation, monitor his mental status and blood pressure, and obtain a CT scan of the head."
4. **Follow response:** "I want to follow the treatment by assessing his weakness, mental status, and speech.

> ### CLINICAL PEARL
>
> ❖ Usually, the vague query, "What is your next step?" is the most difficult question because the answer can be diagnostic, staging, or therapeutic.

What Is Likely Neuroanatomical Defect?

Because the field of neurology seeks to correlate the neuroanatomy with the defect in function, the student of neurology should constantly be learning the function of the various brain centers and the neural conduits to the end organ. Conveniently, neurology can be subdivided into compartments such as movement disorders, stroke, tumor, and metabolic disorders for the purpose of reading; yet, the patient can have a disease process that affects more than one central nervous function.

What Are the Risk Factors for This Process?

Understanding the risk factors helps the practitioner to establish a diagnosis and to determine how to interpret tests. For example, understanding risk factor analysis may help in the management of a 55-year-old woman with carotid insufficiency. If the patient has risk factors for a carotid arterial plaque (such as diabetes, hypertension, and hyperlipidemia) and complains of transient episodes of extremity weakness or numbness, she may have either embolic or thrombotic insufficiency.

> ### CLINICAL PEARL
>
> ❖ Being able to assess risk factors helps to guide testing and develop the differential diagnosis.

What Are the Complications to This Process?

Clinicians must be cognizant of the complications of a disease, so that they will understand how to follow and monitor the patient. Sometimes the student will have to make the diagnosis from clinical clues and then apply his or her knowledge of the consequences of the pathologic process. For example, "A 26-year-old male complains of severe throbbing headache with clear nasal drainage." If the patient has had similar episodes, this is likely a cluster headache. However, if the phrase is added, "The patient is noted to have dilated pupils and tachycardia," then he is likely a user of cocaine. Understanding the types of consequences also helps the clinician to be aware of the dangers to a patient. Cocaine intoxication has far different consequences such as myocardial infarction, stroke, and malignant hypertension.

What Is The Best Therapy?

To answer this question, not only do clinicians need to reach the correct diagnosis and assess the severity of the condition, but they must also weigh the situation to determine the appropriate intervention. For the student, knowing exact dosages is not as important as understanding the best medication, route of delivery, mechanism of action, and possible complications. It is important for the student to be able to verbalize the diagnosis and the rationale for the therapy.

CLINICAL PEARL

❖ Therapy should be logically based on the severity of disease and the specific diagnosis. An exception to this rule is in an emergent situation such as respiratory failure or shock when the patient needs treatment even as the etiology is being investigated.

SUMMARY

1. There is no replacement for a meticulous history and physical examination.
2. There are four steps in the clinical approach to the neurology patient: making the diagnosis, assessing severity, treating based on severity, and following response.
3. There are seven questions that help to bridge the gap between the textbook and the clinical arena.

REFERENCES

Folstein MF, Folstein SE, McHugh PR. Mini-Mental State: a practical method for grading the state of patients for the clinician. J Psychiatr Res 1975;12:189–198.

SECTION II

Clinical Cases

❖ CASE 1

A 65-year-old right-handed man is being evaluated for a tremor that has been present for approximately 20 years. It began insidiously and has progressed gradually. It involves both hands and affects his handwriting, drinking coffee and other liquids with a cup, and general work that requires manual dexterity. Other people occasionally notice a tremor in his head. He is otherwise healthy, although he feels his balance is not quite as good as it used to be. A glass of beer or wine markedly decreases the tremor severity. His mother and daughter also have tremor. On examination he has a rather regular tremor of approximately 8 cycles per second (Hz) with his hands extended and also on finger-nose-finger maneuver. Mild regular "waviness" is seen when writing or drawing spirals. His tone is normal although, when performing voluntary movements with one hand there is a "ratchety" quality felt in the tone of the contralateral arm. Occasional tremor is also noted in the head and voice.

◆ **What is the most likely diagnosis?**

◆ **What is the next diagnostic step?**

◆ **What is the next step in therapy?**

ANSWERS TO CASE 1: Essential Tremor

Summary: A 65-year-old right-handed gentleman has a 20-year-history of tremor predominantly limited to activities, such as writing, drawing, or holding objects. There is also head tremor. The history is significant for similar signs and symptoms in his family members. Alcohol use decreases its severity.

◆   **Most likely diagnosis:** Essential tremor (ET)

◆   **Next diagnostic step:** MRI of brain and spine

◆   **Next step in therapy:** Primidone or propranolol

Analysis

Objectives

1.   Understand the differential diagnosis of tremor.
2.   Describe the clinical manifestations of ET.
3.   Be aware of the different modes of treatment of ET.

Considerations

This case is typical for ET, although at this age, Parkinson disease (PD) is a consideration. ET is the most common of the many movement disorders, and more common than PD. Also, ET does not have dangerous sequelae, although it can be very debilitating. The cogwheel effect when testing muscle tone (especially in the arms) without increased tone (i.e., rigidity) is known as Froment sign and is seen in many tremulous disorders. **Parkinson disease is associated with cogwheel rigidity** not just *cogwheel effect*. In addition, sustention tremor seen in the outstretched arms can be seen in ET and PD. The diagnosis of ET is clinical, and several aspects help to distinguish between these two disorders. The tremor with PD usually appears after a latent period of several seconds, not immediately (as in ET). Although PD patients can have jaw and tongue tremor (usually at rest), head tremor is very rare. Essential tremor of the hands typically occurs when the hands are in use. Tremors from PD are most prominent when the hands are at the sides or resting in the lap. This type of tremor usually decreases with movement of the hands. In addition, ET does not cause other health problems, whereas PD is associated with a stooped posture, slow movement, a shuffling gait, speech problems other than tremor, and sometimes memory loss (Table 1–1).

Table 1–1
ESSENTIAL TREMOR VERSUS PARKINSON DISEASE

	ESSENTIAL TREMOR (ET)	PARKINSON DISEASE (PD)
Onset of disease	Bilateral arm involvement	Unilateral tremor, associated with stooped posture, shuffling gait, memory loss
Body affected by tremor	Arms most commonly then head, legs, larynx, trunk	Stooped posture, shuffling gait
Tremor characteristics	Associated with purposeful movement	Tremor in arms at side
Latency period	Immediate	Longer (several seconds)

Source: DeLong MR, Luncos JL. Parkinson's disease and other movement disorders. In: Kasper DL, Fauci AS, Longo DL, et al, eds. Harrison's Principles of Internal Medicine. Vol 2. 16th ed. New York: McGraw-Hill. 2005:2406–2418.

APPROACH TO TREMOR

Definitions

Cogwheel rigidity—The feeling of periodic resistance to passive movement felt by the examiner in a limb.

Bradykinesia—Slowed ability to start and continue movements and impaired ability to adjust the body's position.

Lead-pipe rigidity—The hypertonicity felt in a parkinsonian limb throughout the range of movements of a joint. It is indicative of increased tone in all the sets of muscles around a joint.

Physiological tremor—This is a very-low-amplitude fine tremor (between 6 Hz and 12 Hz) that is barely visible to the naked eye. It is present in every normal individual during maintaining a posture or movement. Neurologic examination results of patients with physiologic tremor are usually normal.

Enhanced physiological tremor—This is a high-frequency, low-amplitude, visible tremor that occurs primarily when a specific posture is maintained. Drugs and toxins induce this form of tremor.

Clinical Approach

Essential tremor is the most common of the many movement disorders. It is far more common than PD. Unlike PD, ET does not lead to serious complications. It is considered a *monosymptomatic* disease; that is, it causes tremor and nothing else. Essential tremor often begins gradually, and sometimes it appears during adolescence. More often, though, tremors begin in mid to late life. The most common sign is a trembling, up-and-down movement of the hands, although the arms, legs, head, and even the tongue and voice box (larynx) can also be affected. Most affected individuals have tremors in **both hands**, and although some have tremors in only one hand initially, there is often progression to include both hands.

Tremors usually occur only when the patient engages in a voluntary movement, such as drinking a glass of water, writing, or threading a needle. Actions requiring fine-motor skills—using utensils or small tools, for example—can be especially difficult. Fatigue, anxiety, and temperature extremes make the signs worse, but tremors usually disappear asleep or at rest. **Low doses of alcohol,** such as a glass of beer or wine, can dramatically decrease the tremor in approximately one-half of the cases. Besides the tremor, there can be mild impairment of balance. There is **no objective test to definitively diagnose the disorder,** and **diagnosis is by clinical judgment.**

Etiopathogenesis

Approximately **one-half of all cases of ET appear to occur because of an autosomal dominant genetic mutation, associated with a disorder referred to as benign familial tremor.** Exactly what causes ET in people without a known genetic mutation is not clear. Positron emission tomography (PET) scanning shows that certain parts of the brain—including the thalamus—have increased activity in people with ET. More research is needed to understand the precise mechanism behind the disease.

Diagnosis

In addition to ET and PD, other etiologies for tremors should be considered. Tremor as part of **dystonic conditions** is typically more asymmetric than ET and has a jerky quality, as opposed to the more sinusoidal movement in ET. **Purely kinetic or *intention* tremors** are seen with disruption of the output from the neo-cerebellum (most commonly noted in multiple sclerosis patients) or red nucleus (commonly after closed-head injury). **Hyperthyroidism,** and other conditions associated with increased adrenergic activity can cause tremors that resemble ET.

Essential tremor is a clinical diagnosis; however, laboratory studies can be indicated to rule out thyroid disease, heavy metal poisoning, or other conditions. Neuroimaging can also be indicated if degenerative or structural changes of the nervous system are suspected. Common types of tremor include **resting tremor** that occurs when a body part is at complete rest against gravity, seen in PD. Tremor amplitude decreases with voluntary activity, such as in **postural tremor** that occurs during maintenance of a position against gravity and increases with action; action or **kinetic tremor** that occurs during voluntary movement; **task-specific tremor that** emerges during specific activity (e.g., writing tremor); and **intention or terminal tremor** that manifests as a marked increase in tremor amplitude during a terminal portion of targeted movement (seen in tremor of multiple sclerosis or cerebellar disease).

Management

For some people, ET may be distressing but not debilitating. Others may find that their tremors make it difficult to work, perform everyday tasks that require fine-motor skills, or do the things they enjoy. Severe tremors can lead to social withdrawal and isolation. Fortunately, a variety of treatments exist that may help bring the tremors under control.

Medications provide relief from tremors roughly half the time. **The mainstay of ET treatment are beta-blockers and primidone.**

Beta-blockers. Normally used to treat high blood pressure, beta-blockers, such as propranolol (Inderal), help relieve tremors in some people. Because beta-blockers are especially likely to cause dizziness, confusion, and memory loss in older adults, they may be a better choice for younger people. They may also not be an option for patients with asthma, diabetes, or certain heart problems.

Other medications include anti-seizure medications such as primidone (Mysoline), which may be effective in patients who do not respond to beta-blockers; they are usually given at much lower doses than in epilepsy, typically 50 to 700 mg per day. The main side effects are drowsiness and flu-like symptoms, which usually disappear within a short time. **Tranquilizers such as** diazepam (Valium) and alprazolam (Xanax) are sometimes used to treat people whose tremors are made much worse by tension or anxiety. Side effects can include confusion and memory loss. **Botulinum toxin type A (Botox) injections** can also be useful in treating some types of tremors, especially of the head and voice. Botox injections can improve problems for up to 3 months at a time. When used to treat hand tremors, Botox can sometimes cause weakness in the fingers. For severe disabling tremor, **surgery** may be an option for patients who do not respond to medications. Deep brain stimulation (DBS) is a treatment involving a brain implant device called a *thalamic stimulator* that may be appropriate if the patient has severe tremors and if medications are not effective.

Comprehension Questions

[1.1]   A 59-year-old man is diagnosed with a probable ET. A PET scan is performed on the brain. Which of the following is most likely to be highlighted on the imaging?

     A. Cerebellum
     B. Cerebral cortex
     C. Pituitary gland
     D. Thalamus

[1.2]   A 45-year-old woman is noted to have a distinct tremor with voluntary activity. Multiple family members also are noted to have tremors. If ET is diagnosed, what pattern of inheritance is most likely?

     A. Autosomal dominant
     B. Autosomal recessive
     C. X-linked dominant
     D. X-linked recessive
     E. Y-linked

[1.3]   A 58-year-old man is noted to have a noticeable tremor that has pro-
         gressed over 5 years. The tremor occurs in the hands, there are some prob-
         lems with his gait, and there is also presence of tremor of the head. Which
         of the following helps to support of the diagnosis of ET rather than PD?

   A. Gait disturbance
   B. Male gender
   C. Slow progression of the tremor over 5 years
   D. Tremor in the head

Answers

[1.1]   **D.** The thalamus tends to be highlighted on PET imaging in individu-
         als with ET. It should be noted however, that no imaging studies have
         a definitive positive predictive value.

[1.2]   **A.** An apparently autosomal dominant history of tremor is often seen
         in ET. A familial tendency may also be seen in PD.

[1.3]   **D.** The tremor involving the head is more typical of ET. There can be
         gait problems and also slow onset of tremor in both ET and PD.

CLINICAL PEARLS

❖ Essential tremor is the most common movement disorder and
     affects up to 10 million adults.
❖ The latency (time of onset) for the tremor to appear in PD is signi-
     ficantly longer than the latency for ET (9 seconds vs. 1–2 seconds)
     and helps to distinguish the two disorders.
❖ There is a familial predisposition to both ET and PD.
❖ Essential tremor is often relieved with low doses of alcohol.
❖ The mainstay of treatment of ET is beta-blockers.
❖ Severe cases of ET may require surgery, such as placement of a
     deep brain stimulator.

REFERENCES

Louis ED. Essential tremor. Lancet Neurol 2005;4:100–110.
Lyons K, Pahwa R, Comella C, et al. Benefits and risks of pharmacological treat-
     ments for essential tremor. Drug Saf 2003;26:461–481.
Pahwa R, Lyons KE, Wilkinson SB, et al. Comparison of thalamotomy to deep brain
     stimulation of the thalamus in essential tremor. Mov Disord 2001;16:140–143.
Zesiewicz TA, Elble R, Louis ED, et al and the Quality Standards Subcommittee of
     the American Academy of Neurology. Practice parameter: therapies for essential
     tremor: report of the Quality Standards Subcommittee of the American Academy
     of Neurology. Neurology 2005;64:2008–2020.

A 40-year-old man presents to the psychiatry emergency room for inappropriate behavior and confusion. He works as a janitor and has had reasonably good work attendance. His coworkers say that he has appeared "fidgety" for several years. They specifically mention jerky movements that seem to affect his entire body more recently. His mother is alive and well, although his father died at age 28 in an auto accident. On examination, he is alert but easily distracted. His speech is fluent without paraphasias but is noted to be tangential. He has trouble with spelling the word "world" backwards and serial seven's, but recalls three objects at 3 minutes. His constructions are good. When he walks, there is a lot of distal hand movement, and his balance is precarious, although he can stand with both feet together. His reflexes are increased bilaterally, and there is bilateral ankle clonus. A urine drug screen is negative.

◆ **What is the most likely diagnosis?**

◆ **What is the next diagnostic step?**

◆ **Molecular or genetic basis of this disorder?**

ANSWERS TO CASE 2: Huntington Disease

Summary: A 40-year-old man is seen in the emergency room for inappropriate behavior and confusion. He has appeared "fidgety" for several years and, more recently, has choreiform movements. He is alert, but easily distracted, and tangential. With ambulation, distal chorea is present, and his balance is altered. He also has evidence of pyramidal tract involvement with symmetrically increased reflexes.

◆ **Most likely diagnosis:** Huntington disease.

◆ **Next diagnostic step:** Genetic counseling and genetic testing for Huntington disease. Review the history very carefully with patient and his relatives and assess medications—either illicit or licit that could be responsible.

◆ **Molecular or genetic basis:** Repeat CAG triplets present in a gene called *huntingtin* located on chromosome 4p16.3. Repeat lengths greater than 40 are nearly always associated with clinical Huntington disease.

Analysis

Objectives

1. Understand the differential diagnosis of chorea.
2. Describe the basis for genetic confirmation of Huntington disease testing.
3. Be aware of the limitations of pharmacotherapy and the benefits of "lifestyle" manipulations for family members with Huntington disease.

Considerations

Huntington disease is a progressive degenerative disorder affecting both men and women, most prominently associated with *dance-like* choreiform movements. Early on, personality changes or cognitive difficulties are present, balance is disturbed, and then progresses to dementia, chorea, and difficulty with speech. This is a 40-year-old man who has had a history of fidgeting for several years, and now has confusion, difficulty with calculations but has intact short-term memory. He has more recently developed "jerky movements affecting his entire body." He has difficulty with balance and has brisk reflexes. The distal hand movements and long history of fidgeting are typical for Huntington disease. The long slow onset is typical. Delirium and medication or illicit drug effects should be ruled out. Laboratory testing should be aimed at the differential diagnosis such as antinuclear antibody (ANA), electrolytes, glucose level, creatinine level, rapid plasma reagin (RPR), thyroid stimulating hormone level, HIV antibody, and vitamin B_{12} level. Imaging such as with MRI scan is often done. Lumbar puncture may be considered. Genetic testing is the best diagnostic test for Huntington disease.

APPROACH TO HUNTINGTON DISEASE

Definitions

Chorea—Sudden jerky irregular movements with muscle contractions that are not repetitive or rhythmic but appear to flow from one muscle to the next.

Athetosis—Twisting and writhing movements often associated with chorea.

Dystonia—Sustained muscle contractions cause twisting and repetitive movements or abnormal postures.

Tardive dyskinesia—Neurologic disorder caused by the long-term and/or high-dose use of dopamine antagonists, usually antipsychotics and among them especially the typical antipsychotics. It is an impairment of voluntary movement that continues or appears even after the drugs are no longer taken.

Clinical Approach

Huntington disease is inherited in an **autosomal dominant fashion.** The disease is associated with increases in the length of a **CAG triplet repeat** present in a gene called *huntingtin* located on chromosome 4p16.3. Repeat lengths greater than 40 are nearly always associated with clinical Huntington disease. Less than 25 repeat lengths almost never, and between 26–30 repeats sometimes is associated with Huntington disease. There is a rough correlation between the size of the excess expansion and the size and onset of clinical symptoms. The average age of onset is approximately 40 years old. **The repeat length can increase from generation, particularly with paternal transmission**, often resulting in a phenomenon known as *anticipation* in which the age of onset gets progressively earlier. If one parent has 39 repeats and the child has 42, the parent may show symptoms late in life or never, while the child has onset at age 40, and a confusing inheritance pattern emerges in the family history.

Huntington disease is manifested by motor, cognitive, and behavioral problems. The most well-known feature is *chorea* (from the Greek word for *dance*) and consists of graceful, random movements involving the limbs, trunk, and face. Problems with coordination, dexterity, and balance can occur, and ultimately problems with swallowing and choking occur. Slowing of saccades (smooth, slow and fast eye movements) is an early sign, and increased reflexes with disinhibition of primitive reflexes may be seen. Problems with executive function are relatively frequent, and patients can develop a subcortical dementia. Behavioral disinhibition, depression, and anxiety are often seen. The balance between different types of signs and symptoms varies greatly from patient to patient.

When Huntington's Disease develops in childhood (~5% of patients) it is more severe and can be of the **Westphal variant,** which looks more like parkinsonism with bradykinesia and rigidity. Dystonia, myoclonus, and seizures can occur. Diagnosis has been greatly aided by the ability to test for the number of repeats in the huntingtin gene. Anatomically, the predominant involvement is of the neostriatum, with atrophy of the head of caudate nucleus and putamen (Fig. 2–1).

There is a large differential diagnosis for chorea including other inherited conditions, autoimmune, metabolic, and drug or toxin induced. (Table 2–1), but in the context of an adult with insidious onset and slow progression over several years, the likelihood is that this is a degenerative disease. Another form of chorea is Sydenham chorea, which is an acute, usually self-limited disorder of early life, usually between ages 5 and 15, or during pregnancy, and closely linked with rheumatic fever. It is characterized by involuntary movements that gradually become severe, affecting all motor activities including gait, arm movements, and speech.

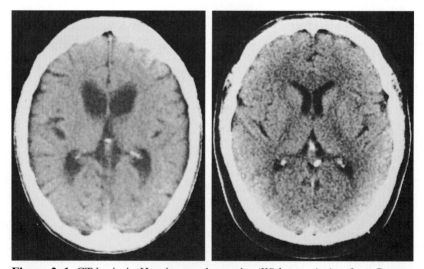

Figure 2–1. CT brain in Huntington dementia. *(With permission from Ropper AH, Brown RH. Adams and Victor's principles of neurology, 8th ed. New York: McGraw-Hill; 2005.)*

Table 2–1
DIFFERENTIAL DIAGNOSIS OF CHOREA IN ADULTS

Hereditary
  Huntington disease *
  Spinocerebellar ataxia 1–3 *
  Pseudohypoparathyroidism/pseudopseudohypoparathyroidism
  Dentatorubropallidoluysian atrophy
  Fahr disease
  Neuroferritinopathy

Autoimmune
  Systemic lupus erythematosus *
  Polyarteritis nodosa *
  Behçet disease *
  Sjögren syndrome *
  Sydenham chorea
  Antiphospholipid syndrome *
  Multiple sclerosis *
  Celiac disease

Neoplasia
  Directly involving striatum
  Paraneoplastic syndrome *

Vascular
  Infarct
  Arteriovenous malformation
  Subdural hematoma

Infectious

Metabolic
  Hyponatremia/hypernatremia
  Hypocalcemia
  Hypoglycemia/hyperglycemia
  Hyperthyroidism *
  Hepatocerebral degeneration
  Renal failure
  Thiamine deficiency
  Niacin deficiency
  Hypoparathyroidism
  Polycythemia
  Chorea gravidarum

Toxins
  Alcohol (intoxication and withdrawal)
  Carbon monoxide
  Mercury
  Manganese
  Post-anoxia

(Continued)

Table 2–1

DIFFERENTIAL DIAGNOSIS OF CHOREA IN ADULTS *(Continued)*

Drugs
    Neuroleptics (tardive) *
    Antiparkinsonian medications
    Anticonvulsants *
    Amphetamines *
    Steroids
    Opiates

* Those entities that merit consideration in this case.

Management

Currently, there are no drugs that appear to affect the course of Huntington disease. Although experiments on transgenic mice with the huntingtin gene have suggested certain compounds exerting a neuroprotective effect, this remains to be confirmed in human beings with Huntington disease. The motor and psychiatric symptoms are usually treated symptomatically.

1. **Chorea** is typically improved with drugs that interfere with dopaminergic function. High potency neuroleptics such as **haloperidol** are typically used. These do carry the risk of tardive dyskinesia, and this has rarely been reported in this condition. Tetrabenazine is a dopamine-depleting agent that is awaiting approval in the United States and has not been associated with tardive dyskinesia. As Huntington disease progresses, bradykinesia is a problem and is exacerbated by neuroleptics. It is not uncommon for these agents to be discontinued as the disease progresses.
2. Depression is very common as is irritability and anxiety and usually treated with selective serotonin reuptake inhibitors (SSRIs).
3. Problems with swallowing and aspiration are apparent late in the course. Discussion in consideration of percutaneous gastric (PEG) tube is advised especially early in the course of the disease to provide adequate nutrition and decrease aspiration.
4. Genetic counseling of the patient's relatives is extremely important.
5. Care should be extended to help to prevent falling and injury.

Comprehension Questions

[2.1]   A 24-year-old man is noted to have dance like movements of his arms and head. The best test to confirm the diagnosis of Huntington disease is:

   A. Cerebral positron emission tomography (PET) scanning
   B. Genetic testing
   C. MRI scan
   D. Rectal biopsy

[2.2]   The same patient noted in question 2.1 is noted to have disabling chorea. Which of the following is most likely to be helpful for the choreiform movements?

   A. Haloperidol 1 mg 1 to 3 times per day.
   B. Carbidopa/levodopa 3 times per day
   C. Deep brain stimulation of the subthalamus
   D. Fluoxetine 10 mg daily

[2.3]   Which of the following clinical features are associated with juvenile or childhood Huntington disease?

   A. Seizures
   B. Myoclonus
   C. Rigidity
   D. Dystonia
   E. All of the above

Answers

[2.1]   **B.** Greater than 40 CAG repeats in the *huntingtin* gene confirms the diagnosis of Huntington disease.

[2.2]   **A.** Judicious use of dopamine-blocking agents are effective in many patients with chorea. These need to monitored for side effects, particularly parkinsonism and tardive dyskinesia. Levodopa can worsen chorea, although in Huntington disease patients with significant bradykinesia, this can be helpful.

[2.3]   **E.** Onset of Huntington disease in childhood (~5% of patients) is more severe and can be of the Westphal variant, which looks more like parkinsonism with bradykinesia and rigidity. Dystonia, myoclonus, and seizures are additional clinical features that may occur.

CLINICAL PEARLS

❖ Huntington disease is a classical autosomal dominantly inherited disease, yet the family history can be negative. However, the diagnosis can be *ruled in* with genetic testing.

❖ Medications are rarely a complete answer to treatment of Huntington disease.

❖ Abnormal *triplet repeat* nucleotides such as the three nucleotides cytosine, adenine, and guanine (CAG) in the huntingtin gene located on chromosome 4p 16.3 is associated with HD.

❖ In huntington's disease the CAG sequence is repeated between 40 and 100 times and as the repetition grows, the disease becomes more severe (anticipation).

❖ Paternal inheritance (from the father) is more strongly associated with earlier onset (anticipation) and worse disease.

REFERENCES

Anderson KE, Marshall FJ. Behavioral symptoms associated with Huntington's disease. Adv Neurol 2005;96:197–208.

Bates GP. History of genetic disease: the molecular genetics of Huntington disease—a history. Nat Rev Genet 2005;6:766–773.

Handley OJ, Naji JJ, Dunnett SB, et al. Pharmaceutical, cellular and genetic therapies for Huntington's disease. Clin Sci (Lond) 2006;110:73–88.

Semaka A, Creighton S, Warby S, et al. Predictive testing for Huntington disease: interpretation and significance of intermediate alleles. Clin Genet 2006;70:283–294.

A 21-year-old man is referred for evaluation and treatment of abnormal movements. He was doing well until the age of 8 when he developed problems with supination of the left arm. He later developed tremor of the left hand, abnormal sustained movements of the left leg; in particular, inversion of the left foot, and back spasms such that he could not walk. His ability to walk improved somewhat, and he was able to ambulate after age 15. Currently he is attending college and doing well. He writes and operates a computer keyboard exclusively with his right hand because of the rhythmic spasms on the left. His voice has been involved for the past 4 years. He has been tried on trihexyphenidyl, carbidopa/levodopa, carbamazepine, and diazepam with very modest improvement. His examination was remarkable for abnormal involuntary movements of his upper extremities, left more than right, consisting of a rhythmic, tremor with arm sustention, associated with wrist flexion/extension as well as a pinching motion of the thumb and index finger. In addition, there are rhythmic, rostral trunk movements associated with his movements, and his voice is affected by significant tremor. The patient also has rapid, nonstereotyped movements of distal and proximal muscles that suggest multifocal myoclonus in combination with sustained, stereotypic muscle contractions of the left wrist, arm extensors, and finger flexors. His head assumes opisthotonic postures with walking but is extended to the right during much of the examination. His mental status exam, sensation, tendon reflexes, muscle bulk, and strength is normal. Gait is impaired because of the involuntary movements described above. There is no postural stability, and Romberg test is negative. There is also scoliosis to the left.

◆ **What is the most likely diagnosis?**

◆ **What is the next diagnostic step?**

◆ **What is the next step in therapy?**

ANSWERS TO CASE 3: Dystonia

Summary: This is a 21-year-old man with a history of progressive dystonia beginning in his left upper extremity and spreading to back and left lower extremity. His abnormal movements are complex, involving dystonia, myoclonus, and tremor that limit his posture, gait, and extremity use.

◆ **Most likely diagnosis:** Primary generalized dystonia–DYT-1

◆ **Next diagnostic step:** MRI of brain

◆ **Next step in therapy:** Deep brain stimulation of the globus pallidus, pars interna

Analysis

Objectives

1. Describe the classification of dystonia.
2. Understand the differential diagnosis of dystonia.
3. Describe the diagnostic modalities that are useful in the evaluation of patients with dystonia.
4. Be aware of the therapeutic modalities that are useful in the treatment of patients with dystonia.

Considerations

This is a case of childhood onset of generalized torsion dystonia. Dystonia is a syndrome characterized by sustained muscle contraction, which provokes twisting and repetitive movements or abnormal postures. A key differentiation is to identify primary versus secondary dystonia. Secondary dystonia has an underlying etiology such as drug effect, and can be amenable to therapy, whereas primary dystonia has no discernible cause. After searching for secondary causes including laboratory testing and brain imaging, primary dystonia is concluded. In this case, with the early onset, two types (of the 15 types of primary dystonia) would be considered: DYT-1, early-onset torsion dystonia, caused by mutation in the torsin A gene at chromosome 9q34; and DYT-5, dopa-responsive dystonia. See Table 3–1 for differential diagnosis of dystonia.

Table 3–1
DIFFERENTIAL DIAGNOSIS OF DYSTONIA

Secondary dystonias
  Drug-induced tardive dystonias
  Antipsychotic drugs: dopamine receptor–blocking older typical and newer atypical drugs
  Anxiolytic drug: buspirone
  Antidepressant agents: selective serotonin-reuptake inhibitors
  Dopaminergic drugs: levodopa and dopamine agonists
  Antiemetic drugs: metoclopramide
  Antiseizure drugs: phenytoin, carbamazepine, gabapentin
  Cerebral palsy
  Wilson disease
  Mitochondrial encephalopathies
  Neuroacanthocytosis
  Pantothenate kinase–associated neurodegeneration (Hallervorden–Spatz disease)
  Fahr disease

APPROACH TO DYSTONIA

Definitions

Dystonia—Sustained muscle contractions cause twisting and repetitive movements or abnormal postures.
Myoclonus—Sudden, involuntary jerking of a muscle or group of muscles.
Opisthotonos—Great rigid spasm of the body with the back fully arched and the heels and head bent back.

Clinical Approach

Dystonia is classified according to etiology, as idiopathic or symptomatic. **Primary dystonia** is defined as a condition with no etiology that can be identified, and dystonia is the sole or major symptom. Primary dystonias are further subdivided by criteria such as age of onset, distribution of affected body parts, presence of diurnal variation of symptoms, responsiveness to drugs, and genetic markers. **Secondary dystonia** refers to dystonia in the context of a neurologic disease in which dystonia is only one of several symptoms or in which dystonia is the result of an environmental insult. There are at least 15 genetic causes of dystonia. Generalized dystonia tends to have its onset in childhood. A three--base-pair guanine–adenine–guanine (GAG) deletion in exon 5 of DYT1 (TOR1A) is the most frequent cause of early onset, generalized dystonia starting in a limb and is known as DYT-1 dystonia. However, there is a large phenotypic variability even within families with an identical mutation. Primary generalized torsion dystonia is a progressive, disabling disorder that usually begins in childhood and is linked to several genetic loci. Many cases are inherited as autosomal dominant traits caused by a deletion in the torsin A gene (DYT1 locus), resulting in the deletion of glutamate in torsin A, a brain protein of unknown function with highest concentrations in the substantia nigra.

Penetrance is 30–40%, and clinical expression varies from generalized dystonia to occasional adult-onset focal dystonias. It begins as a focal action dystonia before the middle of the third decade of life with most cases beginning in childhood. Because of its rarity and unfamiliar features, it is sometimes misdiagnosed a psychogenic disorder. Approximately 65% of cases progress to a generalized or multifocal distribution, 10% become segmental, and 25% remain focal. Childhood-onset cases commonly evolve to generalized dystonia, which produces severe disability owing to serious gait and posture abnormalities (Fig. 3–1). This can result in a life-threatening condition called status dystonicus. The diagnosis of DYT-1 can be made by commercially available testing.

Most primary dystonias have normal routine neuroimaging studies. [18F]-fluorodeoxyglucose and positron emission tomography (PET) has been used with a novel regional network analytical approach to identify a reproducible pattern of abnormal regional glucose metabolism in primary torsion dystonia. This pattern is not specific for the DYT1 genotype, can be present in other primary dystonia genotypes, and is not routinely available.

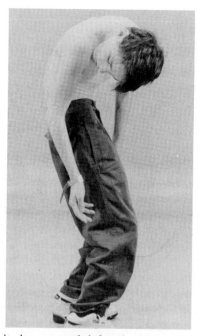

Figure 3–1. Incapacitating postural deformity in a young man with **dystonia.** (*With permission from Ropper AH, Brown RH. Adams and Victor's principles of neurology, 8th ed. New York: McGraw-Hill; 2005: Fig. 4–5c.*)

In any given case, the first consideration is whether this represents a secondary dystonia, particularly one which is amenable to effective treatment, including discontinuation of offending agents. Some clues that dystonia is secondary include:

- History of trauma or exposure to drugs, infections, cerebral anoxia
- Dystonia at rest, rather than with action, at its onset
- Atypical site for age of onset—for example, leg onset in an adult, cranial onset in a child
- Early onset of speech abnormality
- Hemidystonia
- Presence of abnormalities other than dystonia on neurologic examination or general medical examination
- Nonphysiologic findings suggesting a psychogenic basis
- Abnormal brain imaging
- Abnormal laboratory tests

Table 3–2 summarizes common etiologies of secondary dystonia. The current functional model of basal ganglia suggests that dystonia results from abnormally low or generally abnormal pattern of activity of basal ganglia output structures: the internal segment of globus pallidus (GPi) and substantia nigra pars reticulata.

Table 3–2
CAUSES OF SECONDARY DYSTONIA

Hereditary disorders associated with
Neurodegeneration (Huntington disease, juvenile Parkinson disease (parkin), Wilson disease, lysosomal storage disorders, Rett syndrome)

Dystonia-plus syndromes (dopa-responsive dystonia, myoclonus-dystonia, rapid-onset dystonia-parkinsonism)

Acquired/exogenous causes (*Medication:* dopamine receptor-blocking agents, Antiepileptic agents, levodopa, dopamine agonists, calcium-channel blockers; *Toxins:* manganese, carbon monoxide, carbon disulphide, methanol, wasp sting; *Perinatal cerebral injuries:* cerebral palsy, kernicterus; *Vascular lesions:* stroke, arteriovenous malformation, antiphospholipid syndrome ; *Infection:* encephalitis, subacute sclerosing panencephalitis, HIV/AIDS, abscess; *Brain tumors; paraneoplastic syndromes; demyelination:* multiple sclerosis, pontine myelinolysis; *Trauma:* head trauma, cervical cord injury; *Structural:* atlanto-axial subluxation, Klippel-Feil syndrome, Arnold-Chiari malformation)

Parkinson disease and other parkinsonian disorders (progressive supranuclear palsy, corticobasal degeneration, multiple system atrophy)

Other movement disorders (tic disorders, familial paroxysmal kinesigenic dyskinesias, familial paroxysmal non-kinesigenic dyskinesias, episodic ataxia syndromes)

This low activity consequently disinhibits the motor thalamus and cortex, giving rise to abnormal movements. In addition, drugs that inhibit the action of dopamine (through type 2 dopamine [D2] receptors) can cause acute or chronic dystonia. This seems to be mediated by disinhibition of cholinergic neurons.

Symptomatic treatment of dystonia in the past has employed primarily pharmacologic agents. These include systemic agents such as levodopa, blockers of central muscarinic cholinergic receptors, benzodiazepines, and baclofen. Anatomically targeted administration of agents is also feasible including botulinum toxin and intrathecal administration of baclofen. There is mounting evidence that the most effective treatment for generalized dystonia is high-frequency stimulation of the GPi, through the surgical placement of a deep brain stimulator.

Comprehension Questions

[3.1] The drug most likely to help dystonic symptoms in a patient with DYT-1 dystonia is:

A. Haloperidol
B. Trihexyphenidyl (Artane)
C. Phenytoin
D. Chlorpromazine

[3.2] A 12-year-old boy has the acute onset of sustained contractions of the left leg and right arm as well as loss of sensation above the neck. The severity of the symptoms is highly variable. The most likely diagnosis is:

A. DYT-1 dystonia
B. Acute dystonia from a medication
C. Bilateral ischemic infarction of the globus pallidi
D. Psychogenic disorder
E. A right spinal cord hemisection syndrome

[3.3] A 32-year-old woman is seen in the emergency department. She has no medical problems nor allergies to medications. She receives a medication intravenously and has an acute dystonic reaction with muscle spasm of the neck. Which of the following drugs is most likely responsible for this reaction?

A. Haloperidol
B. Trihexyphenidyl (Artane)
C. Phenytoin
D. Levodopa

Answers

[3.1]   **B.** Trihexyphenidyl (Artane) is an antimuscarinics anticholinergic.

[3.2]   **D.** This is likely psychogenic because there is a physiologically incongruent examination.

[3.3]   **A.** Haloperidol is a potent blocker of dopamine D2 receptors and is a common agent responsible for dystonic reactions in otherwise healthy individuals.

CLINICAL PEARLS

❖ DYT-1 dystonia is an autosomal dominant disease, which can be confirmed with genetic testing.

❖ DYT-1 and other primary dystonias usually have the abnormal movements in association with action early in the course of the disease.

❖ In mild cases of DYT-1 and other primary generalized dystonias, systemic drugs, such as anticholinergics, benzodiazepines, and baclofen may control symptoms, in severe cases, deep brain stimulation of the globus pallidi may be required.

REFERENCES

Albanese A. The clinical expression of primary dystonia. J Neurol 2003;250:1145–1151.

Albanese A, Barnes MP, Bhatia KP, et al. A systematic review on the diagnosis and treatment of primary (idiopathic) dystonia and dystonia plus syndromes: report of an EFNS/MDS-ES Task Force. Eur J Neurol 2006;13(5):433–444.

Geyer HL, Bressman SB. The diagnosis of dystonia. Lancet Neurol 2006;5:780–790.

Krauss JK, Yianni J, Loher TJ, et al. Deep brain stimulation for dystonia. J Clin Neurophysiol 2004;21(1):18–30.

Manji H, Howard RS, Miller DH, et al. Status dystonicus: the syndrome and its management. Brain 1998;121:243–252.

Tarsy D, Simon DK. Dystonia. N Engl J Med 2006;355:818–829.

The patient is a 55-year-old man in good health until about 6 months ago. At that time he noticed development of a tremor. He has no other complaints. On examination, there is a tremor in the right arm at rest and while he walks, he has a sustained tremor in both arms, and to some degree during finger-nose-finger maneuver (fairly fine and without an obvious rhythm). He has a poker face and a slow, deliberate gait. Tone is increased in the right arm and leg. The physical examination is otherwise unremarkable. He and his wife deny his use of alcohol or any other medications.

◆ **What is the most likely diagnosis?**

◆ **What is the next diagnostic step?**

◆ **What is the next step in therapy?**

ANSWERS TO CASE 4: Parkinson Disease

Summary: This is a middle-aged man with asymmetric onset of tremor. In addition he has mild poverty of movement (otherwise known as akinesia of the face and body), tremor at rest, as well as increased tone.

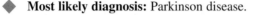 **Most likely diagnosis:** Parkinson disease.

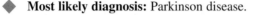 **Next diagnostic step:** Do an MRI of the brain to evaluate other disorders in the differential diagnosis.

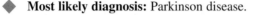 **Next step in therapy:** If the current symptoms are causing the patient disability, initiate therapy with either dopamine agonist or monoamine oxidase type B (MAO-B) inhibitor.

Analysis

Objectives

1. Understand the differential diagnosis of parkinsonism.
2. Know the clinical characteristics of Parkinson disease.
3. Describe the usefulness of different imaging modalities for evaluating spinal cord injury and the importance of patient age.
4. Be aware of the different treatment options for Parkinson disease and their role and liabilities.

Considerations

The patient described in the case above has tremor at rest, rigidity, and hypokinesia, which are the three cardinal features of Parkinson disease–and constitute the syndrome of parkinsonism. The fourth of the cardinal features is postural instability, which in idiopathic Parkinson disease typically has onset several years later. The most common cause of parkinsonism is idiopathic Parkinson disease. A careful search for secondary causes of parkinsonism should be undertaken such as a history of medication use (antipsychotic agents), metabolic or structural diseases of the brain (hydrocephalus), and infectious etiologies. MRI of the brain is typically performed. Levodopa is a standard agent used to treat the symptoms of Parkinson disease; unfortunately, no agent has been shown to slow the progress of the disease.

APPROACH TO SUSPECTED PARKINSON DISEASE

Definitions

Substantia nigra—(Latin for "black substance") or locus niger is a heterogeneous portion of the midbrain, and a major element of the basal ganglia system. It consists of the *pars compacta, pars reticulata,* and the *pars lateralis.*

Lewy body—an eosinophilic, round inclusion found in the cell cytoplasm of substantia nigra, the nucleus basalis of Meynert, locus ceruleus, dorsal raphe, and the dorsal motor nucleus of cranial nerve X. They contain alpha-synuclein, a presynaptic protein, the function of which is unknown. Neurofilament proteins and ubiquitin are other important constituents of Lewy bodies.

Clinical Approach

Parkinson disease is a disorder that gets its name from the *Essay on the Shaking Palsy* by James Parkinson. Features of Parkinson disease can be expressed in other ways including: difficulty arising from a chair, difficulty turning in bed, micrographia, masked face, stooped, shuffling gait with decreased arm swing; and sialorrhea. Although Parkinson disease is thought of as a *motor* disorder, sensory systems are also affected. Loss of sense of smell is almost universal. Pain is very common. Other system involvement can result in autonomic disturbance, depression, a variety of speech disturbances including dysarthria, palilalia, and stuttering. In Parkinson's monograph, he specifically stated "the senses and intellect are preserved." Research has shown that isolated cognitive deficits are extremely common in Parkinson disease, especially executive dysfunction. In addition approximately 50% of patients develop dementia.

The most obvious pathologic feature of Parkinson disease is **loss of pigment in the substantia nigra** caused by loss of neurons in this region. The remaining neurons may show an intra-cytoplasmic eosinophilic inclusion called a **Lewy body** (Fig. 4–1). These neurons project rostrally in the brain to innervate the striatum as well as the cerebral cortex. Parkinson disease is associated with marked striatal dopamine (DA) depletion and is considered by many to be a striatal dopamine deficiency syndrome. At death, DA loss is greater than 90%, and approximately 70% DA loss results in symptom expression. Severity of DA loss best correlates with bradykinesia in Parkinson disease—the correlation with tremor is very poor. In recent years, we have seen a much more comprehensive picture of the pathologic destruction by Parkinson disease, which helps us to understand the wide variety of signs and symptoms besides bradykinesia. Other morphologic and chemical deficits have also been demonstrated in the brains of patients with Parkinson disease in the cholinergic pedunculopontine nucleus, noradrenergic locus coeruleus, serotonergic raphe nuclei, and glutamatergic centromedian/parafascicularis complex of the thalamus. Still, there are many signs and symptoms that are atypical for Parkinson disease and should raise our level of vigilance that another disorder is present. These include:

- Early onset of, or rapidly progressing, dementia
- Rapidly progressive course

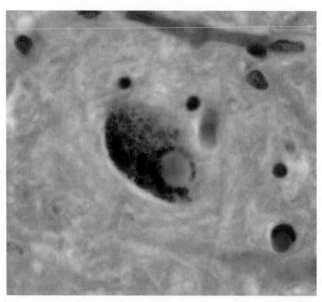

Figure 4–1. Lewy body on microscopy. *(With permission from Ropper AH, Brown RH. Adams and Victor's principles of neurology, 8th ed. New York: McGraw-Hill; 2005: Fig. 39–5.)*

- Supranuclear gaze palsy
- Upper motor neuron signs
- Cerebellar signs—dysmetria, ataxia
- Urinary incontinence
- Early symptomatic postural hypotension
- Early falls

The majority of cases of Parkinson disease are unknown. Familial Parkinson disease, while rare, does occur, and is most commonly associated with a mutation of the *parkin* gene, which is inherited in an autosomal recessive pattern. This mutation is the most common cause of early onset Parkinson disease, without Lewy bodies. Routine neuroimaging is usually normal in Parkinson disease. Functional imaging designed to visualize the dopamine innervation of the striatum, especially in combination with other imaging techniques may provide a way to positively identify the disease, however these techniques are still under investigation and are not available under routine clinical circumstances. Imaging is useful, however, to identify some of the other entities in the differential diagnosis.

The **differential diagnosis** of parkinsonism includes the following categories:

- Drug-induced (antipsychotics, metoclopramide)
- Toxin-induced
- Metabolic
- Structural lesions (vascular parkinsonism, etc.)
- Hydrocephalus (normal-pressure hydrocephalus [NPH])
- Infections

Differential Diagnosis

Parkinson disease is most often mimicked by other neurodegenerative disorders, most commonly by **multiple system atrophy** (MSA). This comes in two major clinical forms: MSA–P, resembles Parkinson disease except that tremor is less prominent, and the disorder tends to be quite symmetric. MSA–C, also called olivopontocerebellar atrophy, presents as a cerebellar syndrome. Both forms may have prominent autonomic insufficiency—including orthostatic hypotension and impotence. Conventional MRI usually show abnormalities.

Dementia with Lewy bodies is a disorder with prominent cognitive dysfunction as well as parkinsonism. The typical clinical hallmarks include early onset dementia, delusions and hallucinations, fluctuations in consciousness and myoclonus. Although listed as a separate entity, there is much controversy about whether this is Parkinson disease or represents parts of the clinical spectrum of the same pathologic entity. Although parkinsonism can be seen in **Alzheimer disease**, it is a rare finding, and dementia is usually the primary clinical syndrome.

Corticobasalganglionic degeneration typically has unilateral, coarse tremor, rigidity, increased reflexes as well as limb apraxia/limb dystonia/alien limb phenomenon. This disorder is the only one that typically has the asymmetric appearance of Parkinson disease. **Progressive supranuclear palsy** is characterized by supranuclear downgaze palsy (inability to voluntarily look down) and square wave jerks on extraocular motion testing. These patients typically have an upright rather than flexed posture. Also frequent falls can be an early finding. Tremor is not common, and there is a pseudobulbar emotionality. As mentioned, several drugs, especially dopamine antagonists (typical neuroleptics, anti-nauseants) can cause drug-induced parkinsonism.

Treatment Options

Treatment is initiated when the patient's quality of life is affected and usually consists of either **levodopa or a dopamine agonist**. Because no treatment currently arrests the degenerative process, symptomatic treatment is the mainstay of therapy. This includes pharmacologic and surgical interventions. Physical measures such as physical therapy, speech therapy, and exercise are important and have a major impact on the lives of patients with Parkinson disease.

Pharmacologic therapy:

- **Dopaminergic agents are the mainstay of treatment for the cardinal features of Parkinson disease.**
  - **Levodopa crosses the blood–brain barrier, whereas dopamine does not; levodopa** is converted to dopamine in the brain. Peripheral breakdown in the gut is inhibited by the addition of inhibitors of aromatic amino acid decarboxylase (dichloroisoprenaline [DCI]), carbidopa. Thus, a Carbidopa/Levodopa formulation is popularly prescribed. Levodopa can also be broken down peripherally by the enzyme catechol-O-methyltransferase (COMT) so COMT inhibitors such as entacapone and tolcapone are often employed. A therapeutic trial of levodopa can confirm Parkinson disease because more than 90% of patients with pathologically proven Parkinson disease have a good to excellent response to adequate doses of levodopa (at least 600 mg/d levodopa with DCI).
  - **Dopamine agonists** cross the blood–brain barrier and act directly as primarily D2-type receptors without requiring conversion. These agents include pramipexole, ropinirole, and bromocriptine.
- **MAO-B inhibitors** such as selegiline and rasagiline can improve symptoms in both patients with mild disease (as monotherapy) and patients already on levodopa therapy. Anticholinergics such as trihexyphenidyl or diphenhydramine (Benadryl) are used primarily to combat tremor, but have many side effects especially in older individuals.
- **Amantadine** is felt to act primarily by blocking glutamate N-methyl-D-aspartate (NMDA) receptors and has a mild attenuation of the cardinal symptoms of resting tremor and dystonia. Recently, amantadine has been shown to help **alleviate levodopa induced dyskinesias**.

Although no treatment slows the degeneration of Parkinson disease, disease mortality been reduced by levodopa therapy. Over time, the response to levodopa becomes unstable, resulting in **motor fluctuations, which are exaggerated clinical manifestations**; also, patients can develop troublesome abnormal involuntary choreiform and dystonic movements called **dyskinesias**. There is good evidence that starting treatment with a dopamine agonist rather than levodopa delays the onset of dyskinesias. Thus, those patients at high risk for developing dyskinesia probably should be treated initially with dopamine agonists.

Younger patients are more at risk for dyskinesia and are likely to be treated for long periods of time (the average age of onset of Parkinson disease is approximately 59 years). Although levodopa is the most efficacious agent for the treatment of Parkinson disease, for mild Parkinson disease, dopamine agonists have comparable benefit. In patients that still have an excellent response to levodopa except for motor fluctuations and dyskinesias, surgical treatment that inhibits the subthalamic nucleus with high-frequency stimulation can provide excellent relief of the cardinal symptoms of disease. **However, placement of a deep brain stimulation (DBS) appears to be the preferable surgical therapy.** It is less invasive, more reversible, and can be adjusted to the individual patient, and remarkable results can be seen. In addition, inhibition of the ventrolateral thalamus can be very effective for treatment of tremor.

Comprehension Questions

[4.1] Which of the following signs is most suggestive of Parkinson disease rather than the other neurodegenerative diseases?

   A. Unilateral resting tremor
   B. Supranuclear downed gaze palsy
   C. Orthostatic hypotension early in the course of the disease
   D. Early falls
   E. Abnormal cerebral MRI

[4.2] Which of the following medications is most likely to be able to help both relieve cardinal features of Parkinson disease as well as reduce drug-induced dyskinesias?

   A. Levodopa
   B. Dopamine agonists
   C. Amantadine
   D. Anticholinergics
   E. Haloperidol

[4.3] Which of the following medications would be most likely to cause drug-induced parkinsonism?

   A. Trihexyphenidyl
   B. Metoclopramide
   C. Diazepam
   D. Carbidopa
   E. Levodopa

Answers

[4.1] **A.** Resting tremor is an early manifestation of Parkinson disease.

[4.2] **C.** Amantadine can decrease the incidence of levodopa induced dyskinesia.

[4.3] **B.** Antiemetic agents such as prochlorperazine (Compazine) and metoclopramide can cause a drug-induced parkinsonism.

CLINICAL PEARLS

❖ The cardinal features of Parkinson disease are resting tremor, rigidity, bradykinesia, and postural instability.

❖ Parkinson disease is usually an asymmetric disorder.

❖ Postural instability leading to falls occurs relatively late in the clinical course of Parkinson disease.

❖ Failure to respond clinically to even large doses of levodopa is relatively strong evidence that the patient does not have idiopathic Parkinson disease.

❖ The mainstay of therapy for Parkinson disease is levodopa, which can lead to dyskinesia.

REFERENCES

Hardy J, Cai H, Cookson MR, et al. Genetics of Parkinson's disease and parkinsonism. Ann Neurol 2006;60:389–398.

Horstink M, Tolosa E, Bonuccelli U, et al. European Federation of Neurological Societies; Movement Disorder Society—European Section. Review of the therapeutic management of Parkinson's disease. Report of a joint task force of the European Federation of Neurological Societies and the Movement Disorder Society-European Section. Part I: early (uncomplicated) Parkinson's disease. Eur J Neurol 2006;13:1170–1185.

de Lau LM, Breteler MM. Epidemiology of Parkinson's disease. Lancet Neurol 2006;5:525–535.

Pahwa R, Factor SA, Lyons KE, et al; Quality Standards Subcommittee of the American Academy of Neurology. Practice parameter: treatment of Parkinson disease with motor fluctuations and dyskinesia (an evidence-based review): report of the Quality Standards Subcommittee of the American Academy of Neurology. Neurology 2006;66:983–995.

Tolosa E, Wenning G, Poewe W. The diagnosis of Parkinson's disease. Lancet Neurol 2006;5:75–86.

❖ CASE 5

This 57-year-old man of Portuguese descent noticed that he had difficulty marching in line as a soldier. From age 20 until the age of 40 he had a slow progression of symptoms. Since then he experienced a rapidly progressing gait disturbance, diplopia, dyssynergia, and paraesthesia in the limbs. At age 45 he was confined to a wheelchair. On examination, he was intellectually normal but had severe dysarthria and constant drooling. He had bulging eyes, slow saccades, and impaired voluntary up- and down-gaze but no nystagmus. He had fasciculations and dyscoordination of the tongue but no facial fasciculations. A general moderate muscle weakness and atrophy were revealed, but muscle tone was normal. Tendon reflexes were absent, but there were bilateral Babinski signs. Deep senses were impaired, and coordination was impaired by severe ataxia, dysmetria, and dysdiadochokinesia. A constant static tremor was seen in the hands. His mother and paternal grandfather as well as his sister and her son also had problems with gait, which were progressive and began during adulthood. MRI of the brain revealed cerebellar folial atrophy.

◆ **What is the most likely diagnosis?**

◆ **What is the next diagnostic step?**

◆ **What is the next step in therapy?**

ANSWERS TO CASE 5: Ataxia, Spinocerebellar

Summary: This is a case of an essentially healthy man who had the insidious onset and gradual progression of the syndrome heralded by gait difficulties, which were later characterized as ataxia.

◆ **Most likely diagnosis:** Autosomal dominant cerebellar degeneration with additional neurologic features with normal cognition–most likely spinocerebellar ataxia type 3 (SCA-3).

◆ **Next diagnostic step:** DNA confirmation of diagnosis.

◆ **Next step in management:** Supportive care, genetic counseling, rehabilitation.

Analysis

Objectives

1.   Describe the movement disorder of ataxia.
2.   List the differential diagnosis of ataxia including genetic and non-genetic etiologies.

Considerations

As stated, this essentially healthy man had an insidious onset and gradual progression of a syndrome heralded by gait difficulties, which were later characterized as ataxia. It later caused dysarthria, abnormal saccades, probable lower motor neuron findings, neuropathy, and upper motor neuron deficits. This clinical picture suggests a multiple system degeneration with the most prominent feature being ataxia, and poor coordination on voluntary movements. These are typically caused by problems either with a motor control as a result of pathology of the cerebellum or its connections or pathologic proprioception because of pathology in sensory pathways. Ataxias can either be isolated or seen as part of the syndrome in conjunction with other neurologic abnormalities or abnormalities in other body systems. This patient has other neurologic abnormalities but no evidence at least at this time of other body system involvement. In addition, there is strong familial involvement; specifically, there are four successive generations affected in his family, and both sexes are affected. Although familial disorders are not necessarily genetic, this extensive involvement actually suggests an autosomal dominant disorder. This is reinforced by the fact that autosomal recessive ataxias tend to have other body systems involved, whereas this is not the case with adult-onset autosomal dominant disease.

It is worth considering some nongenetic causes of ataxia as they would suggest other management issues, although most present over a much shorter time course. Recognizable causes including trauma, toxic and metabolic factors, neoplasms, and autoimmune mechanisms. Paraneoplastic cerebellar degenerations (PCD) associated with specific tumor type antineuronal antibodies are a relatively frequent cause of late-onset ataxia and are characterized by a subacute progressive course and would prompt discovery and treatment of the underlying neoplasm. More rarely (and controversially), subacute spinocerebellar degeneration is associated with nonparaneoplastic immune diseases such as gluten intolerance. In addition, hormonal abnormalities, such as thyroid hormone deficiency can cause ataxia.

APPROACH TO AUTOSOMAL DOMINANT CEREBELLAR ATAXIA

Definitions

Ataxia—an unsteady and clumsy motion of the limbs or torso caused by a failure of the gross coordination of muscle movements.

Trinucleotide repeat expansion disease—caused by stretches of DNA in a gene that contain the same trinucleotide sequence repeated many times. These repeats are a subset of unstable microsatellite repeats that occur throughout all genomic sequences. If the repeat is present in a gene, an expansion of the repeat results in a defective gene product and often disease.

Clinical Approach

Harding (1983) proposed a useful clinical classification for *late onset* autosomal dominant cerebellar ataxias. In addition, sporadic cerebellar syndromes include idiopathic forms of obscure etiology characterized by progressive ataxia, autonomic failure, and extrapyramidal features, such as multiple system atrophy (MSA). In Harding's system autosomal dominant cerebellar ataxia I (ADCA I), cerebellar ataxia is associated with additional features related to the optic nerve (extra) pyramidal system, cerebral cortex, and peripheral nerves. ADCA II is associated with pigmentary macular dystrophy, and ADCA III is a pure late onset cerebellar syndrome.

Since 1993 autosomal dominant cerebellar ataxias have been increasingly characterized in terms of their genetic locus and are referred to as spinocerebellar ataxia. At this point there are more than 25 such disorders, and the number is increasing. The most common types are listed in Table 5–1. Many of these can be definitively diagnosed by DNA testing. Clinical characterization however is helpful in limiting the number of tests required.

There are several gene mutations on different chromosomes that cause spinocerebellar ataxia, and the gene frequency within different populations varies considerably. In general, the incidence is thought to be approximately 1.5 per 100,000 people, with equal gender distribution. Most of the ADCAs are caused by a genetic defect that involves an expansion in the DNA sequence, and most of these are trinucleotide repeat expansions (SCA types 1–3, 6–10, 12, and 17).

Table 5-1

SELECT LIST OF AUTOSOMAL DOMINANT SPINOCEREBELLAR ATAXIAS

DISEASE	INCIDENCE (%)	LOCUS PROTEIN	MUTATION	CLINICAL FEATURES	OCULOMOTOR ABNORMALITIES
SCA-1	6	6p23 Ataxin-1	CAG repeats (38–83)	Ataxia, dysarthria, pyramidal signs, peripheral neuropathy, hyperreflexia, cognitive impairment	Nystagmus, hypermetric saccades, slow saccades, ophthalmoparesis
SCA-2	14	12q24 Ataxin-2	CAG repeats (35–64)	Ataxia, dysarthria, peripheral neuropathy, hyporeflexia, dementia, myoclonus	Slow saccades, ophthalmoplegia
SCA-3	21	14q32 Ataxin-3	CAG repeats (61–84)	Ataxia, dysarthria, spasticity, parkinsonism, amyotrophy	Lid retraction, nystagmus, saccade dysmetria, ophthalmoparesis, square-wave jerks
SCA-6	15	19p13 CACNA1A	CAG repeats (20–33)	Ataxia, dysarthria, sometimes episodic ataxia, very slow progression, lack of family history	Nystagmus (60% down-beating), saccadic pursuit

SCA-7	5	3p14 Ataxin-7	CAG repeats (37- > 300)	Ataxia, dysarthria, retinopathy, peripheral neuropathy, pyramidal signs, infantile phenotypes	Saccadic smooth pursuit, slow saccades
SCA-8	2–5	13q21	CTG (3'UTR) (100–250)	Ataxia, dysarthria, mild sensory neuropathy	Nystagmus, saccadic pursuit

Source: C Mariotti, R Fancellu, S Di Donato. An overview of the patient with ataxia. J Neurol 2005;252:511–518.

Other types of repeat expansions that cause SCA have been discovered. For example, SCA-10 involves an ATTCT repeat expansion of the SCA10 gene, and SCA-8 involves an expansion in the SCA8 gene with the nucleotides CTG repeated. Finally, SCA-4 involves a mutation in a gene that does not involve a trinucleotide repeat expansion.

The average age of onset for all of these types is from 20 to 30 years of age except for SCA-6, which usually occurs between the ages of 40 and 50. People with SCA-8 usually develop symptoms in their late 30s. SCA-2 patients usually develop dementia and slow eye movements. SCA-8 patients, who have normal life spans, and SCA-1 patients generally both have very active reflexes. SCA-7 patients develop visual loss. In SCA types 1–3 and 7, there can be an earlier age of onset with increased severity (called **anticipation**) from one generation to the next. The size of the repeat expansion zone in the affected genes roughly correlates with the severity and age of onset. Penetrance is quite high; however, there are rare cases in which people do not develop symptoms. The reason for the lack of complete penetrance is currently unknown.

The diagnosis of spinocerebellar ataxia is initially suspected by the adult-onset of symptoms. An MRI or CT of the brain can detect atrophy (wasting) of the cerebellum, and a variety of other subcortical structures (Fig. 5–1). A molecular genetic test to determine the gene that has the trinucleotide repeat expansion

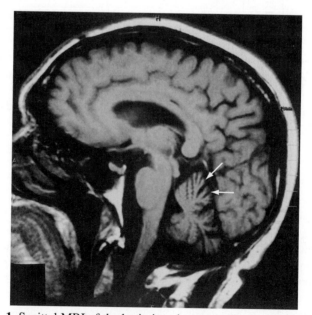

Figure 5–1. Sagittal MRI of the brain in spinocerebellar ataxia. *(With permission from Kasper DL, Braunwal E, Fauci A, et al. Harrison's principles of internal medicine, 16th ed. New York: McGraw-Hill; 2004: Fig. 352–1.)*

can be helpful in quickly identifying other carriers in the family. Many of these disorders can now be confirmed by DNA testing. Rather than just ordering all available DNA tests (which can be quite expensive) there are algorithms that can focus the testing by use of clinical signs; especially retinal degeneration, prominent involvement of noncerebellar symptoms, age of onset, eye-movement disorders, reduced stochastic velocity, and pyramidal signs. The clinical features of these disorders are listed in the accompanying table (see Table 5–1).

Once the genetic defect is characterized, family members can also be tested. Unfortunately, genetic testing is not always 100% informative. There are rare cases of spinocerebellar ataxia diagnosed clinically that cannot be explained by any of the known genetic defects. It is estimated that in approximately 50–60% of white persons with a dominant familial form of cerebellar ataxia, DNA testing can provide a definitive diagnosis.

SCA-3 or Machado-Joseph disease (MJD) is the most common SCA subtype in most populations. The phenotype is one of the most variable among SCAs. The presenting syndromes for SCA-3 include *pure* cerebellar ataxia, familial parkinsonism, hereditary spastic paraplegia, hereditary neuropathy, and restless legs syndrome (RLS). A rarely recognized but common and rather specific sign of SCA-3 is impaired temperature discrimination in all limbs and even trunk and face. Pseudoexophthalmos (bulging eyes caused by lid retraction), faciolingual myokymia, and dystonia have been thought to be characteristic, but not specific, signs of SCA-3.

SCA-3 MJD is an autosomal dominantly inherited disorder with variable expression first described by Nakano and coworkers (1972) in an American family of Portuguese-Azorean descent. Since then more families with MJD have been reported worldwide. Three different clinical subtypes are described: Type I with an early onset (20–30 years of age), pyramidal and extrapyramidal signs, progressive external ophthalmoplegia (PEO), and minor cerebellar deficits; type II with an intermediate age of onset. At neuropathological examination, degeneration of the cerebellum and the thoracic cord is always present in SCA-3, but degeneration of the striatum, substantia nigra, basis pons, oculomotor nuclei, and peripheral nerves is variable.

Treatment

There is **no cure for ADCA and no treatment to slow the progression of the disease**. Nevertheless, supportive treatment is important. Drugs that help control tremors are not effective for treating cerebellar tremors, but can be effective for parkinsonism, dystonia, RLS (restless leg syndrome) and a variety of other neurologic symptoms. Physical therapy does not likely slow the progression of loss of coordination or muscle wasting, but affected patients should be encouraged to be active. Occupational therapy can be helpful in developing ways to accommodate the patient in performing daily activities. Walkers and other devices can assist the patient to have mobility. Other modifications such as ramps for a wheelchair, heavy eating utensils, and raised toilet seats can make patients more independent. Speech therapy and computer-based communication aids often help as the person loses his or her ability to speak.

Although the nature of the specific mutations can help determine the prognosis, the exact age of onset and the specific symptoms are difficult to determine, especially for carriers with no symptoms. Ultimately, as with all progressive degenerative disorders, the disease is fatal. Persons with SCA usually die one to two decades after symptoms develop. The prognosis for SCA-11 and SCA-6 is typically less severe, with a very slow worsening of symptoms, and persons with SCA-8 and SCA-11 have a normal lifespan.

Comprehension Questions

[5.1] A patient with SCA-3, besides having ataxia is very slow with rigidity and rest tremor. Which of the following drugs is most likely to be helpful for these latter symptoms?

A. Carbidopa/Levodopa
B. Haloperidol
C. Diazepam
D. Phenytoin

[5.2] What radiological feature is most characteristic of SCAs:

A. Cerebellar atrophy
B. High T2 signal in the cerebellar cortex
C. High signal lateral to the striatum
D. A high signal "hot cross bun" sign in the brainstem

[5.3] Which familial occurrence pattern would be most suspicious of not being an ADCA.

A. 4/4 siblings (2 male, 2 female ages 4–12) and father in the same household with onset within 1 week of each other, but no other first or second-degree relatives in a large kindred.
B. Male prospectus (affected), father, 1/2 brothers, 0/2 sister, paternal grandfather and uncle.
C. Male prospectus, neither parent, 1/2 brothers, 1/2 sister, paternal great-grandfather. [poor penetrance]
D. Male prospectus, neither parent, 0/2 brothers, 0/2 sister, paternal grandfather and uncle. [poor penetrance]

Answers

[5.1] **A**–the parkinsonism of SCA is often responsive to levodopa

[5.2] **B** is characteristic of neoplastic cerebellar degeneration. C and D are seen with MSA.

[5.3] **A** is suggestive of a toxic or infectious exposure–B is typical; C and D might be seen with poor penetrance.

CLINICAL PEARLS

❖ Spinocerebellar ataxias present in adulthood, generally as cerebellar ataxias, often with other neurologic signs but rarely with non-neurologic system involvement.

❖ DNA testing can be diagnostic, but clinical correlation is helpful in focused ordering of tests

❖ Pharmacologic therapy does not alter the natural course of cerebellar ataxia but can help to relieve neurological symptoms.

REFERENCES

Bataller L, Dalmau J. Paraneoplastic neurologic syndromes: approaches to diagnosis and treatment. Semin Neurol 2003 Jun;23(2):215–224.

Duen AM, Goold R, Giunti P. Molecular pathogenesis of spinocerebellar ataxias. Brain 2006;129:1357–1370.

Hadjivassiliou M, Grunewald R, Sharrack B, et al. Gluten ataxia in perspective: epidemiology, genetic susceptibility and clinical characteristics. Brain 2003; 126:685–691.

Harding AE. Hereditary spastic paraplegias. Seminar Neurol 1993;13:333–336.

Løkkegaard T, Nielsen JE, Hasholt L, et al. Machado–Joseph disease in three Scandinavian families. J Neurol Sci 1998;156:152–157.

Mariotti C, Fancellu R, Di Donato S. An overview of the patient with ataxia. J Neurol 2005;252:511–518.

Schelhaasa HJ, Ippel PF, Beemerb FA, et al. Similarities and differences in the phenotype, genotype and pathogenesis of different spinocerebellar ataxias. Eur J Neurol 2000;7:309–314.

Schöls L, Bauer P, Schmidt T, et al. Autosomal dominant cerebellar ataxias: clinical features, genetics, and pathogenesis. Lancet Neurol 2004;3:291–304.

A 65-year-old woman was referred for problems with abnormal involuntary movements of the mouth and face. She has had good health until 3 years ago when she developed problems with nausea and constipation. She was placed on metoclopramide with some relief of symptoms. A complete gastrointestinal (GI) workup was negative, although it was hypothesized she had decreased gastric motility. These abnormal movements began approximately 1 year ago. They have been getting progressively worse. The movements do not interfere with speech but do interfere with eating. She also occasionally has arching spasms of the back and neck. Her examination is remarkable for stereotypical repetitive movements of the tongue and jaw and the sustained arching.

◆ **What is the most likely diagnosis?**

◆ **What is the next step in therapy?**

ANSWERS TO CASE 6: Tardive Dyskinesia

Summary: A 65-year-old woman was referred for problems with abnormal involuntary movements of the mouth and face. She was placed on metoclopramide, and developed these movements, which were getting progressively worse. The movements do not interfere with speech but do interfere with eating. She also occasionally has arching spasms of the back and neck. Her examination is remarkable for stereotypical repetitive movements of the tongue and jaw and the sustained arching.

◆ **Most likely diagnosis:** Tardive dyskinesia

◆ **Next step in therapy:** Discontinuation of metoclopramide. Treatment with a benzodiazepine or baclofen.

Analysis

Objectives

1. Understand the differential diagnosis of involuntary oral movements.
2. Describe the motor complications of dopamine receptor blocking drugs.
3. Know the modalities available for the treatment of tardive dyskinesia.
4. Be aware of the role of steroids, surgical intervention, and rehabilitation in spinal cord injury.

Considerations

This is an older woman who has developed abnormal involuntary movements involving primarily the oral–buccal–lingual muscles. This has come about rather insidiously and progressed gradually. Her examination is remarkable primarily for these movements. In addition, she has been treated with a medication to help with her gastrointestinal system, but it is also a very potent blocker of dopamine receptors. The two leading candidates for the cause of her disorder would be an idiopathic or genetic dystonia or tardive dyskinesia. The latter is a disorder that develops relatively late after the initiation of medications that block dopamine receptors. There are a variety of disorders caused by these medications (Table 6–1).

APPROACH TO TARDIVE DYSKINESIA

The most common cause of tardive dyskinesia (TD) is chronic exposure to central dopamine blocking agents, such as neuroleptic therapy. The actual cause for TD is unknown. It is thought that the cascade of responses develop in response to blockade of the receptors by dopamine antagonists. Receptor upregulation is a relatively acute event, and the time course is not what is

Table 6–1
CLASSIFICATION OF DYSKINETIC DISORDERS

I. Acute
   Acute dystonia
   Acute akathisia
   Drug-induced parkinsonism

II. Chronic
Common:
   Tardive dyskinesia
   Tardive dystonia
   Tardive akathisia
   Perioral tremor (rabbit syndrome)
Uncommon:
   Tardive myoclonus
   Tardive tics
   Tardive tremor

III. Miscellaneous
   Neuroleptic malignant syndrome

typically seen clinically. The disorder has been operationally defined to require at least 3 months onset, although there have been cases that suggest shorter latency is possible. Stopping medication can ultimately result in cessation of these movements, the frequency of this actually occurring is somewhere between 25% and 50% of cases; however, the data supporting this estimate is not very strong, and there is much controversy about it. It has been estimated that approximately **one-third of patients that are treated with dopamine receptor antagonists develop product dyskinesia eventually.**

The **strongest risk factors** for TD include **advanced age, female gender, and coexistent brain damage.** Treatment with typical antipsychotic agents can be associated with permanent TD in these individuals. Whereas many times these abnormal movements are more distressing to family than patients, they can be quite debilitating and result in significant damage to dentition and interference with oral intake of nutrition. Treatment options include **benzodiazepines, baclofen,** and vitamin E, but these are seldom useful in all but the mildest cases. Treatment with increased doses of dopamine receptor blocking agents is sometimes undertaken, but most clinicians believe that this results in increased risk of ultimate worsening of the condition. Drugs that deplete dopamine do not seem to cause this disorder but can be very beneficial in its treatment. Alpha methyl-p-tyrosine inhibits the formation of catecholamines by blockade of the enzyme tyrosine hydroxylase, and reserpine depletes catecholamines synaptic vesicles. These agents are sometimes useful but have a high incidence of side effects including orthostatic hypotension, depression, and parkinsonism.

Tetrabenazine, another selective depleter of catecholamine vesicles, appears to be more effective with fewer side effects. Although this has been available for many years around the world, it is not currently available in the United States. Botulinum toxin injections into the relevant muscles can be useful also. The best treatment is prevention, and care should be instituted to avoid using dopamine receptor blocking agents unless absolutely necessary.

The incidence of TD appears to have decreased with the use of the so-called atypical antipsychotics that do not cause such complete dopamine receptor blockade. Metoclopramide is used in the treatment of nausea and gastroparesis. There are other agents for nausea that have much less risk for the development of TD. The approved agents for gastroparesis are much more limited in the United States. Domperidone is an excellent alternative for metoclopramide but must be obtained from outside the United States. It is a potent dopamine receptor blocking agent but does not cross the blood–brain barrier.

Differentiation from idiopathic dystonia syndromes is sometimes difficult. Dystonia can occur as a focal manifestation around the mouth, as well as in a so-called *segmental* form involving the muscles of the face and neck. However, **arching spasms of the back and neck are characteristic of the tardive condition.** Whereas, the former disorder responds to anticholinergics or dopaminergic medications, anticholinergic medications often make the typical TD symptoms worse.

TD is sometimes associated with more appendicular involuntary movements. As such, it can be confused with Huntington disease. The chorea of Huntington disease drifts in a random fashion around the musculature, whereas TD tends to be more stereotypic. Patients with Huntington disease, however, can have behavioral problems that are treated with neuroleptics, and neuroleptics are the usual treatment for chorea, so the two conditions can coexist.

Comprehension Questions

[6.3] Which of the following drugs has the highest risk of causing tardive dyskinesia?

A. Haloperidol
B. Trihexyphenidyl
C. Levodopa
D. Diazepam

[6.2] Which one of the following agents results in decreased severity of oral dyskinesias caused by tardive dyskinesia?

A. Fluphenazine
B. Trihexyphenidyl
C. Levodopa
D. Dexedrine

[6.3]   A 25-year-old man that began treatment for schizophrenia 1 week ago
        presents to the emergency room for forceful sustained twisting movements
        of the neck. Which of the following conditions is the likely diagnosis?

    A. Tardive dyskinesia
    B. Huntington disease
    C. Acute dystonic reaction caused by dopamine receptor blocking
        drug
    D. DYT1 dystonia

Answers

[6.1]   **A.** Haloperidol is a dopamine receptor blocker. Although levodopa can
        be associated with dyskinesia in patients with Parkinson disease, this
        does not occur in association with other disorders.
[6.2]   **A.** Further and more complete dopamine receptor blockade will often
        decrease the manifestations of TD, but is felt by many to represent
        increased risk for long-term continuation.
[6.3]   **C.** The acute onset, soon after the initiation of antipsychotic medica-
        tions as well as these clinical manifestations, are typical of acute dys-
        tonic reactions.

CLINICAL PEARLS

❖   The most common cause of tardive dyskinesia is generally the use
    of chronic dopamine blocking agents such as typical antipsy-
    chotic agents.

❖   Tardive dyskinesia generally develops months after beginning
    dopamine receptor blocking drugs and most frequently causes
    stereotypical movements of the mouth and surrounding regions.

❖   Treatment of tardive dyskinesia is generally less than optimal and
    so the best course is to avoid development of this disorder by
    constant reassessment of the need for and the amount of
    dopamine receptor blocking drugs.

❖   Backward arching movements of the neck, sometimes called retro-
    collis, are believed to strongly suggest tardive dyskinesia as
    opposed to other causes of dystonia as their ultimate etiology.

❖   Dopamine depleting agents, such as reserpine or tetrabenazine, that
    do not block receptors have not been shown to cause tardive
    dyskinesia.

REFERENCES

Chou KL, Friedman JH. Tardive syndromes in the elderly. Clin Geriatr Med 2006 Nov;22(4):915–933.

Fernandez HH, Friedman JH. Classification and treatment of tardive syndromes. Neurologist 2003 Jan;9(1):16–27.

Kenney C, Jankovic J. Tetrabenazine in the treatment of hyperkinetic movement disorders. Expert Rev Neurother 2006 Jan;6(1):7–17.

Soares-Weiser K, Rathbone J. Neuroleptic reduction and/or cessation and neuroleptics as specific treatments for tardive dyskinesia. Cochrane Database Syst Rev 2006 Jan 25;(1):CD000459.

Tarsy D, Baldessarini RJ. Epidemiology of tardive dyskinesia: is risk declining with modern antipsychotics? Mov Disord 2006 May;21(5):589–598.

A 13-year-old right-handed male is brought to the emergency room (ER) following a moderate speed motor vehicle accident (MVA). The patient was an unrestrained front-seat passenger but was not ejected during the head-on collision (approximately 35 to 40 mph). According to the paramedics accompanying the patient there was significant front-end damage to the car, and the patient's head appears to have impacted the windshield. On arrival at the scene approximately 4 minutes after the accident, the patient was found to be unresponsive with flaccid muscle tone, bradycardia, and inadequate respiratory effort. His cervical spine was immobilized, he was intubated to maintain adequate ventilation, and he was transported to the ER secured to a rigid backboard. On examination he is afebrile with irregular respiratory effort over the ventilator. Noxious stimulation of his face produces some grimacing, but there is no response to such stimulation of the extremities. There is a large contusion over his forehead but no other external signs of trauma. On neurologic examination his pupils are equally reactive to light, and he has a brisk corneal reflex bilaterally, but there is no gag reflex. His muscle tone is significantly decreased in all four extremities, and he is areflexic throughout including his superficial abdominal reflexes. His rectal sphincter is patulous, and there is no anal wink. According to the patient's father the child was healthy and neurodevelopmentally normal prior to this accident. He is on no medications and has no known allergies.

◆ **What is the most likely diagnosis?**

◆ **What is the next diagnostic step?**

◆ **What is the next step in therapy?**

ANSWERS TO CASE 7: Spinal Cord Injury, Traumatic

Summary: This 13-year-old presents to the ER significantly obtunded with flaccid quadriparesis and agonal respirations following a head-on MVA in which he was an unrestrained passenger. He is now intubated, and his cervical spine is immobilized. He was previously healthy and is on no medications.

 Most likely diagnosis: High cervical spine injury and traumatic brain injury.

 Next diagnostic step: MRI of brain and spine.

 Next step in therapy: Maintain oxygenation and perfusion pressure in a critical care setting.

Analysis

Objectives

1. Understand the initial management of acute spinal cord injury.
2. Know the different types of spinal cord syndromes.
3. Describe the usefulness of different imaging modalities for evaluating spinal cord injury and the importance of patient age.
4. Be aware of the role of steroids, surgical intervention, and rehabilitation in spinal cord injury.

Considerations

This 13-year-old brought to the ER following a significant MVA has findings worrisome for traumatic injury to both his brain and his spinal cord. This chapter will focus on considerations for evaluating and managing the latter. Significant findings on the patient's examination include flaccid quadriparesis (suggesting interruption of the corticospinal tracts in the upper cervical region), failure to grimace or otherwise respond to painful stimulation of any of his four extremities (suggesting interruption of ascending sensory tracts in the upper cervical region), preservation of pupillary light reflex and corneal reflex (indicating that the brainstem is intact above the pontomedullary junction), but poor respiratory function and absence of gag (indicative of injury to the upper cervical cord as well as the lower brain stem). These findings point to a complete or nearly complete acute spinal cord injury at a high cervical level, with ascending spinal shock, and affecting the lower brainstem.

APPROACH TO TRAUMATIC SPINAL CORD INJURY

Epidemiology

There are approximately 10,000 new cases per year of traumatic spinal cord injury in the United States. The peak age-related incidence occurs between 15 to 25 years of age and males outnumber females by 4:1. Approximately 5% of all spinal injuries occur between birth and 16 years of age, and these pediatric patients require special consideration as discussed below. Neonatal (birth-related) spinal cord injury complicates approximately 1 of every 60,000 births and carries a 50% mortality rate. In childhood, the most common causes of spinal cord injury prior to 10 years of age are motor vehicle accidents and falls, whereas in individuals older than 10 years of age, motor vehicle accidents and sports-related injuries are the most common. With regards to motor vehicle accidents, children younger than 13 years of age should be restrained passengers in the backseat only in order to avoid potential injury from airbag deployment. Younger children can sustain significant and often fatal cervical spinal cord injuries from passenger side airbags. The rate of nontraumatic spinal cord injury is at least threefold higher than traumatic cases although the epidemiologic data is not as complete in this regard.

Types of Spinal Cord Injuries

Patients can also present with incomplete lesions of the spinal cord. For example, **hemisection** produces the classic *Brown-Sequard syndrome* with ipsilateral weakness and loss of fine touch and vibration sensation but contralateral loss of pain and temperature below the level of the lesion. This is a result of fibers in the dorsal column remaining ipsilateral to the brainstem while fibers in the spinothalamic tract synapse and cross within one or two spinal levels then travel contralaterally. Trauma would be the most common cause of the Brown-Sequard syndrome, which rarely presents as a pure unilateral injury. *Anterior cord syndrome* is usually caused by either a traumatic or a vascular insult to the anterior two-thirds of the spinal cord. This results in a bilateral loss of spinothalamic tract function (pain and temperature) as well as bilateral weakness (interruption of corticospinal tract) with preservation of dorsal column function (fine touch, proprioception, and vibration). *Central cord syndrome* is caused by injury to the structures around the spinal central canal. Although this can occur acutely with trauma, it more commonly occurs with chronic processes such as intra-axial neoplasms or dilation of the central canal (referred to as syringomyelia). Clinically this typically presents with a bilateral loss of pain and temperature sensation in the upper extremities as well as weakness in the same distribution but with preservation of fine touch. Anatomically this is because the spinothalamic tract decussates immediately anterior to the central canal. Also, motor fibers traveling to the legs tend to run more laterally in the spinal cord and are therefore relatively spared.

Once the patient has been stabilized and an expedited neurologic examination has been performed, the appropriate imaging modality must be selected. In blunt trauma of patients older than 9 years of age, no spine imaging is necessary if they are alert, conversant, nonintoxicated, and have a normal neurologic examination without cervical tenderness. If patients are younger than 9 years of age then imaging is recommended and should be interpreted by a radiologist accustomed to reviewing spine studies from young children. Bony structures can also be well imaged using a helical CT scanner. Visualizing the spinal cord itself is best accomplished using an MRI scan. Children younger than 9 years can develop spinal cord injury without radiographic abnormality (SCIWORA). Given the greater mobility and flexibility of the pediatric spine relative to that found in adults, bony elements can be displaced into the spinal cord and then revert to their normal position. When this occurs, the patient will clinically appear to have a traumatic myelopathy (spinal cord injury) on neurologic examination, but no bony or ligamentous damage is seen with plain films or CT scans. An MRI, however, can demonstrate damage to the spinal ligaments, injury to the spinal cord, or both.

Initial Management of Spinal Cord Injuries

Management of acute spinal cord injury is focused on preventing additional damage. This begins in the field with first responders **immobilizing the spine in a neutral position** using rigid collars and backboards. Further injury can occur because of impingement of bony matter onto the cord, excessive movement of the cord as a result of spinal instability, compression of the cord by hemorrhage, or cord ischemia caused by hypotension. Given the disproportionately large head size in children relative to the trunk, it is often necessary to elevate the torso to achieve a neutral position for the neck. In addition to appropriate positioning, it is vital that an adequate airway is maintained and that respiration is not diminished by tape and restraints over the torso.

In the ER, once stabilization of airway, breathing, and circulation has been achieved, a neurologic examination is performed to assess the clinical level of injury. In this patient there are several findings pointing to an extensive and likely complete high cervical spinal cord injury. The complete loss of motor and sensory function of the upper and lower extremities as well as respiratory difficulties but with preservation of reflexes mediated by cranial nerves would be consistent with this localization (because the upper extremity is innervated by spinal nerves from C5 to T1 and the phrenic nerve arises from C3–C5). In addition to loss of motor and sensory function below the level of the lesion, spinal cord transection also results in loss of autonomic function, which can produce spinal shock. The acute loss of descending sympathetic tone produces decreased systemic vascular resistance, which can result in hypotension. If vagal output is intact then its unopposed influence can further lower vascular resistance and also result in a paradoxical bradycardia. In the context of spinal shock, aggressive fluid resuscitation is necessary to maintain perfusion pressure and prevent cord ischemia. The complete absence of deep tendon reflexes, superficial cutaneous reflexes, and rectal tone also suggests the presence of spinal shock. It is important to remember that, as the inflammatory response to the injury develops and edema occurs the apparent clinical level of the injury can rise to higher spinal levels or into the brainstem. Finally, it is vital to remember to place an indwelling Foley catheter to empty the bladder because the patient will otherwise develop significant urinary retention and stasis.

The Role of Surgery and Steroids

As mentioned above, the principal goal in managing acute spinal cord injury is to prevent secondary injury. Although the initial traumatic event can produce major damage, subsequent inflammation, edema, and ischemia can lead to significant worsening of this primary insult. Surgical intervention to stabilize the spine, remove bony matter, evacuate hemorrhage, and decompress the spinal canal has been evaluated, particularly in adult patients, and remains controversial with little data available in children. Animal work has supported the use of early decompression in order to improve outcome, but surgery is performed sooner after the trauma than may be practical clinically. Significant compromise of the spinal canal and fixation of a very unstable spine are considered the principal indications for early surgery in traumatic spinal cord injury at this point.

Given that inflammation plays a major role in mediating secondary injury, administration of **corticosteroids** has been studied in acute spinal cord injury. Certainly the benefits of steroids in subacute spinal cord injury, such as cord compression by tumor, are well established. However, clinical trials in acutely injured adults have shown little benefit in terms of long-term neurological outcome and an increased rate of complications such as wound infections. Recent evidence indicates that intravenous methylprednisolone is beneficial for adult patients with *incomplete* acute spinal cord injury if administered within 8 hours of injury. Use of steroids in the setting of traumatic spinal cord injury should therefore be considered controversial, particularly in patients with complete spinal cord lesions and in children.

Long-Term Care and Rehabilitation

Maximizing long-term neurologic outcome for survivors of acute spinal cord injury requires an intensive team-based approach to rehabilitation. Important issues to be addressed include development of an appropriate bowel and bladder care program, maintenance of skin integrity, and management of persistent autonomic dysreflexia. As spinal shock subsides and spasticity begins to develop over the course of 1 to 6 weeks, prevention of contractures with preservation of functional position of the joints becomes crucial. Psychological and cognitive rehabilitation is also vital, both in terms of adjusting to life after the injury and also in terms of dealing with concurrent head trauma. In general, patients will spend a significant period of time in an inpatient rehabilitation setting, followed by a transitional outpatient program. Even after this period, however, the patient should continue to be evaluated by a physical medicine and rehabilitation specialist at least yearly to maximize adaptation and function.

Comprehension Questions

[7.1]   Currently, the best strategy for preventing further damage in patients with acute spinal cord injury is:

A. High dose corticosteroids
B. Immediate exploratory surgery
C. Maintenance of oxygenation and spinal cord perfusion
D. Intravenous diuretic therapy

[7.2]   A patient is brought to the ER following an MVA. On examination he has weakness of his left arm and leg and loss of fine touch on the left with loss of pain and temperature sensation on the right. This clinical picture is most consistent with:

A. A complete cord syndrome
B. A central cord syndrome
C. An anterior spinal cord syndrome
D. A left spinal cord hemisection syndrome
E. A right spinal cord hemisection syndrome

[7.3]   A 5-year-old child is brought to the ER following a fall from approximately 4 feet. He is now alert, moving all his extremities, and responding to touch on all four extremities, but he is somewhat irritable and has a large laceration on his chin. Which of the following is true regarding evaluating the child's spine:

A. Since he is moving all extremities and appears to have intact sensation, no further spinal evaluation needs to be performed.
B. Given the child's age, spinal imaging should be performed.
C. Imaging should only be performed if cervical spine tenderness can be demonstrated.
D. Spinal imaging should be arranged as an outpatient.

Answers

[7.1]   **C.** The most important aspect of initial management is to avoid spinal cord ischemia.

[7.2]   **D.** This patient has the classic findings of a left cord hemisection (Brown-Sequard) syndrome with ipsilateral weakness, ipsilateral loss of fine touch, and contralateral loss of pain and temperature sensation.

[7.3]   **B.** Children younger than 9 years of age who experience blunt trauma or falls should have their spine imaged because clinical criteria can still miss injuries. Even if this child were older, the presence of a distracting injury (the large chin laceration) can mask cervical tenderness.

CLINICAL PEARLS

❖ The most important step in the emergency care of children with spinal cord injury is stabilization of the spine. The next step is to maintain spinal cord perfusion pressure.

❖ The most common cause of spinal cord injury in the pediatric population is motor vehicle accidents (MVA).

❖ Traumatic brain injury commonly accompanies traumatic spinal cord injury, including hemorrhage, ischemia, or diffuse axonal injury.

❖ Superficial abdominal reflexes are elicited by scratching the skin in all four quadrants around the umbilicus and watching for contraction of the underlying abdominal musculature. Stimulating above the umbilicus tests spinal levels T8 to T10, whereas stimulating below the umbilicus tests approximately T10 to T12.

REFERENCES

Congress of Neurological Surgeons. Management of pediatric cervical spine and spinal cord injuries. Neurosurgery 2002 March;50(3 suppl):S85–S99.

Eleraky M, Theodore N, Adams M, et al. Pediatric cervical spine injuries: report of 102 cases and review of the literature. J Neurosurg Spine 2000;92(1 suppl):12–17.

McDonald J, Sadowsky C. Spinal cord injury. Lancet 2002;359:417–425.

Saveika J, Thorogood C. Airbag-mediated pediatric atlanto-occipital dislocation. Am J Phys Med Rehabil 2006;85:1007–1010.

Thuret S, Moon L, Gage F. Therapeutic interventions after spinal cord injury. Nat Rev Neurosci 2006;7:628–643.

Tsutsumi S, Ueta T, Shiba K, et al. Effects of the Second National Acute Spinal Cord Injury Study of high-dose methylprednisolone therapy on acute cervical spinal cord injury-results in spinal injuries center. Spine 2006;31(26):2992–2996.

An 18-year-old football player was covering a kickoff when he crashed into an opposing player after losing his helmet, hitting the right side of his head against the opponent's knee. He fell to the ground and was unconscious for 20 to 30 seconds. He was then immediately transported to the nearest hospital. Twenty minutes after the accident, he was alert and conscious without neurologic deficit, but he had amnesia for the event. He had a superficial bruise to the scalp on the right. Approximately 1 hour after the trauma the patient developed a generalized motor seizure. Lorazepam 4 mg IV stopped the seizure. A CT scan, performed 100 minutes after the trauma, was unremarkable. He was then transferred to a larger hospital. On admission, neurologic examination showed a slight psychomotor slowing and slurred speech, which was thought to have been caused by lorazepam administration, in the absence of other neurologic deficits. The Glasgow Coma Scale score was 15 of 15. Routine laboratory investigations and electrocardiography were normal. Eight hours after the trauma, he had nausea, vomiting, and a headache.

◆ **What is the most likely diagnosis?**

◆ **What is the next diagnostic step?**

◆ **What is the next step in therapy?**

ANSWERS TO CASE 8: Epidural/Subdural Hematoma

Summary: This is a case of an 18-year-old athlete with an acute brain injury related to a sports-related trauma. The injury is associated with transient loss of consciousness and a subsequent seizure. Although his examination is relatively nonfocal and imaging of his brain is normal, his condition continues to worsen with nausea, headache, and vomiting.

◆ **Most likely diagnosis:** Intracerebral bleed—epidural hematoma most likely.

◆ **Next diagnostic step:** Repeat noncontrast CT scan of the cranium.

◆ **Next step in therapy:** Careful observation and neurosurgical consultation. Careful evaluation for other signs of trauma.

Analysis

Objectives

1. Understand the mechanism of induction and progression of epidural hematomas.
2. Know the hallmarks that require urgent intervention.
3. Understand the symptoms and signs associated with expanding epidural hematomas.

Considerations

The key feature of this case is that this was a healthy individual who had a closed injury. It was loss of consciousness, but then a normal lucent period. He then had a seizure and later a downward course with cognitive deficit and more fundamental neurologic problems. But, history suggests a delay consequence of head injury. In this case one has to decide whether this suggests an underlying abnormality or one completely caused by the trauma. The lucent period prior to his deterioration is a classical presentation of epidural hematoma, however, less than one-third of patients with this entity have this presentation. Other presentations include headache, vomiting, and seizure. Subarachnoid hemorrhage and subdural hematoma are also strong contenders in this case, as are cerebral contusion and diffuse axonal injury, although a lucent period would not be expected. The clinical picture can develop into one of a rapidly expanding intracranial mass. In particular, patients with posterior fossa epidural hematoma (EDH) can have a dramatic delayed deterioration. The patient can be conscious and talking and a minute later apneic, comatose, and minutes from death.

APPROACH TO EPIDURAL HEMATOMA

EDH is an accumulation of blood between the inner table of the skull and the outer dural membrane. The inciting event often is usually traumatic, often with a "blunt instrument." In 85–95% of patients, this type of trauma results in an overlying fracture of the skull. Blood vessels in close proximity to the fracture are the sources of the hemorrhage in the formation of an EDH. Because the underlying brain has usually been minimally injured, prognosis is excellent if treated aggressively. Outcome from surgical decompression and repair is related directly to patient's preoperative neurologic condition. EDHs are about half as common as subdural hematomas. Males outnumber females 4 to 1. EDHs usually occur in young adults, and are rare in persons younger than 2 years of age or older than 60 years of age (in elderly patients because the dura is strongly adhered to the inner table of the skull). Also, association of hematoma and skull fracture is less common in young children because of the plasticity of the calvariae. EDH also occurs in the spine (SEDH).

Epidural hematomas can be divided into acute (58%) from arterial bleeding, subacute (31%), and, chronic (11%) from venous bleeding. Two-thirds of the cases of cranial EDH are in the temporoparietal area and result from a tear of the middle meningeal artery or its dural branches. Frontal and occipital EDHs each constitute approximately 10%, with the latter occasionally extending above and below the tentorium. The rapid bleeding associated with arterial tears is one of the reasons why these lesions require rapid evaluation. Occasionally, torn venous sinuses cause EDH, particularly in the parietal-occipital region or posterior fossa. These injuries tend to be smaller and associated with a more benign course. Usually, venous EDHs only form with a depressed skull fracture, which strips the dura from the bone and, thus, creates a space for blood to accumulate.

Reported mortality rates range from 5–43%. Higher rates are associated with both ends of the age spectrum (i.e., younger than 5 years of age and older than 55 years of age) and signs of more extensive anatomical (intradural lesions, increased hematoma volume) or clinical (rapid clinical progression, pupillary abnormalities, increased intracranial pressure [ICP], lower Glasgow Coma Scale [GCS]) involvement as well as temporal location. Mortality rates are essentially nil for patients not in coma preoperatively and approximately 10% for obtunded patients and 20% for patients in deep coma.

Evaluation

History and Physical Examination

Symptoms of epidural hematoma include the following:

- Headache.
- Nausea/vomiting.
- Seizures.

- Focal neurologic deficits (e.g., visual field cuts, aphasia, weakness, numbness).
- SEDH typically causes severe localized back pain with delayed radicular radiation that can mimic disk herniation. Associated symptoms can include: weakness, numbness, urinary incontinence, and fecal incontinence.

The physical examination is focused to determine the localization of the deficit as well as looking for signs of increasing ICP and/or herniation.
Physical signs of expanding intracranial mass include:

- Cushing response, (caused by increased ICP)
  - Hypertension, bradycardia, bradypnea
- Decreased or fluctuating level of consciousness/GCS
- Dilated, sluggish, or fixed pupil(s), bilateral or ipsilateral to injury
- Coma
- Decerebrate posturing
- Hemiplegia contralateral to injury
- Other focal neurologic deficits (e.g., aphasia, visual field defects, numbness, ataxia)

In addition, the physical examination should include a thorough evaluation for evidence of traumatic sequelae:

- Skull fractures, hematomas, or lacerations
- Contusion, laceration, or bony step-off in the area of injury
- Cerebrospinal fluid (CSF) otorrhea or rhinorrhea resulting from skull fracture with disruption of the dura
- Hemotympanum
- Instability of the vertebral column

Diagnostic Studies

Laboratory Studies

- Complete blood count (CBC) with platelets
  - To monitor for infection and assess hematocrit and platelets for further hemorrhagic risk, including underlying predisposing disorders
- Prothrombin time (PT)/activated partial thromboplastin time (aPTT): to identify bleeding diathesis
  - Coagulation abnormalities are a marker of severe head injury. Breakdown of the blood-brain barrier with exposed brain tissue is a potent cause of disseminated intravascular coagulation (DIC)
- Serum chemistries, including electrolytes, blood urea nitrogen (BUN), creatinine, and glucose
  - To characterize metabolic derangements that can complicate clinical course

- Toxicology screen and serum alcohol level
  - To identify associated causes of head trauma and establish need for surveillance with regard to withdrawal symptoms
- Type and hold an appropriate amount of blood
  - To prepare for necessary transfusions needed because of blood loss or anemia

Imaging Studies

Immediate unenhanced head CT scan is the procedure of choice for diagnosis. The CT scan shows location, volume, effect, and other potential intracranial injuries. Cervical spine evaluation usually is necessary because of the risk of neck injury associated with EDH. Clinical deterioration should prompt repeat imaging with CT scanning.

On CT scan the typical EDH (Fig. 8–1) is as follows:

- Mass that displaces the brain away from the skull.
- Extra axial.
- Smoothly marginated.
- Lenticular or biconvex homogenous density.
- Most of these masses are high density on the CT scan.

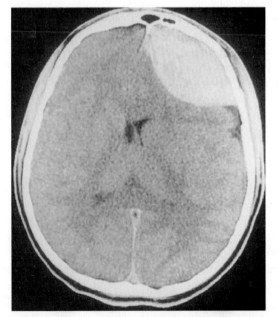

Figure 8–1. CT scan of the brain shows a biconvex hypodensity indicating an epidural hematoma. *(With permission from Kasper DL, Braunwal E, Fauci A, et al. Harrison's principles of internal medicine, 16th ed. New York: McGraw-Hill; 2005, p 2397.)*

- Focal isodense or hypodense zones within EDH indicate active bleeding.
- Rarely crosses the suture line because the dura is attached more firmly to the skull at sutures.
- Air in acute EDH suggests fracture of sinuses or mastoid air cells.

Treatment

Prior to definitive treatment with surgery, or knowing the extent of the situation the most important considerations are to stabilize acute life-threatening conditions, initiate supportive therapy and try to reduce ICP. Airway control and blood-pressure support are vital as is careful observation. A discussion of exact procedures is beyond the scope of this chapter. However, elevation of the head of the bed 30 degrees after the spine is cleared or reverse Trendelenburg position will reduce ICP and increase venous drainage.

Consult a neurosurgeon immediately for evaluation for EDH evacuation and repair.

Consult a trauma surgeon for other life-threatening injuries. Although surgical treatment has been viewed as definitive, under certain conditions these can be treated conservatively with careful observation.

Outcome

The most important factors influencing outcome after evacuation of an epidural hematoma are the initial GCS, pupillary response, motor examination, and associated intracranial injuries seen on the CT scan. In noncomatose individuals, a favorable outcome occurs in 90–100% of patients whereas mortality ranges from 0–5%. For patients in coma, a favorable outcome occurs between 35 and 75% of the time with a mortality rate of between 10 and 40%. Of interest, normally reacting pupils prior to surgery result in a favorable outcome in 84–100% of patients, although the great majority of individuals with bilaterally abnormal pupillary reactions have a poor outcome or death. Associated intracranial injuries such as cerebral contusions also impact adversely on outcome. Rapid diagnosis and timely evacuation of the hematoma are crucial in optimizing outcome.

Comprehension Questions

[8.1] Blunt trauma to the skull followed by brief loss of consciousness, then a period of relative normalcy, then a cranial to caudal pattern of deterioration without stiff neck is most characteristic of which clinical entity?

A. Acute epidural hematoma
B. Chronic subarachnoid hemorrhage
C. Bacterial meningitis
D. Cerebral contusion

[8.2]   Homogeneous high density throughout the ventricular system on an unenhanced CT scan is most characteristic of which clinical entity?

    A. Acute epidural hematoma

    B. Subarachnoid hemorrhage because of a burst proximal middle cerebral artery aneurysm

    C. Basal ganglia hematoma

    D. Ruptured cavernous angioma

[8.3]   Select **T** (true) or **F** (false) for the following statement. A normal brain CT scan performed 1 hour after a closed head injury in the context of a relatively normal neurologic examination precludes development of epidural hematoma.

Answers

[8.1]   **A**

[8.2]   **B**

[8.3]   **False.** An evolving epidural hematoma can occur any time after the immediate injury. Repeat CT brain imaging is indicated if there is any change in the neurologic status of the patient.

CLINICAL PEARLS

❖ The historical hallmark of epidural hematomas is injury followed by a lucent relatively asymptomatic period, followed by deterioration, although the lack of this clinical history is by no means exclusionary.

❖ With suspected epidural hematoma, deterioration can be quite rapid so close observation is necessary.

❖ Epidural hematomas require urgent surgical intervention a large percentage of the time, so neurosurgical consultation early is important.

❖ Noncontrast CT scan of the cranium is the recommended radiologic test for initial evaluation.

REFERENCES

Bullock MR, Chesnut R, Ghajar J, et al. Surgical Management of Traumatic Brain Injury Author Group. Surgical management of acute epidural hematomas. Neurosurgery 2006 Mar;58(3 suppl):S7–15; discussion Si-iv.

Lee EJ, Hung YC, Wang LC, et al. Factors influencing the functional outcome of patients with acute epidural hematomas: analysis of 200 patients undergoing surgery. J Trauma 1998;45:946–952.

Liebeskind DS. Epidural hematoma. Available at: http://www.emedicine.com/NEURO/ topic574.htm. Accessed April 17, 2006.

Offner PJ, Pham B, Hawkes A. Nonoperative management of acute epidural hematomas: a "no-brainer." Am J Surg 2006;192:801–805.

Toyama Y, Kobayashi T, Nishiyama Y, et al. CT for acute stage of closed head injury. Radiat Med 2005 Aug;23(5):309–316.

A 23-year-old female construction worker is brought in to the emergency room (ER) after falling off a beam at work 24 hours ago. The beam was approximately 10 feet off the ground and slippery. Witnesses who reported the fall saw the patient land on her back, hit her head, and sustain a brief period of loss of consciousness. However, within a minute or so the patient was back to her baseline and refused medical evaluation. Today when she showed up at work she didn't "seem right" at times, whereas at other times, she seemed herself. For instance, her coworkers report that she is having difficulty performing simple tasks at work, and she responds slowly and at times inappropriately when answering questions. On interview, the patient answers most questions angrily and inappropriately, although at times, she answers lucidly. She denies experiencing headache, neck pain, visual symptoms, or loss of balance. She is not known to have any medical illnesses. On examination, she is afebrile, her blood pressure is 110/68 mmHg, and her pulse is 100 beats/min. She is awake but inattentive easily losing her focus. Her general examination is notable for the absence of nuchal rigidity and no obvious head trauma. Her Mini Mental State Examination (MMSE) is 24/30 having difficulty with orientation, concentration, and recall. She fluctuates throughout the examination at times being more appropriate than others. Her Glasgow Coma Scale is 14 broken down as E4 V4 M6 the only deficiency being verbal as she is disoriented. She does not have aphasia or dysarthria but does ramble and is tangential. Her neurologic examination shows intact cranial nerves and intact pinprick. The sensory, motor, and cerebellar examination cannot be adequately assessed because she is uncooperative, although her movements appear symmetric. The deep tendon reflexes are hyperreflexic throughout with bilateral Babinski signs present.

◆ **What is the most likely diagnosis?**

◆ **What is the next diagnostic step?**

ANSWERS TO CASE 9: Delirium from Head Trauma

Summary: A 23-year-old woman without medical illnesses presents with acute alteration in mental status 24 hours after sustaining head trauma with brief loss of consciousness. Her examination shows attentional deficits, disorganized thinking, altered psychomotor activity, difficulty focusing, memory deficits, and disorientation. Additionally, it seems that there has been some fluctuation to her symptoms. The examination is notable for absent nuchal rigidity and generalized hyperreflexia with bilateral Babinski signs.

◆ **Most likely diagnosis:** Delirium from subarachnoid hemorrhage.

◆ **Next Diagnostic Step:** CT scan of the head, complete blood count (CBC), comprehensive metabolic panel, and urine toxicology screen.

Analysis

Objectives

1. Be familiar with the clinical presentation of delirium.
2. Learn the differential diagnosis of delirium including medical and trauma related causes.
3. Describe how to evaluate a patient with delirium.

Considerations

This 23-year-old woman presents with acute fluctuating levels of attention, confusion, and altered psychomotor activity following head trauma associated with loss of consciousness (concussion). Her examination shows an altered MMSE and Glasgow Coma Scale with generalized hyperreflexia and bilateral Babinski sign. The findings of attentional deficits, disorganized thinking, altered psychomotor activity, difficulty focusing, memory deficits, and disorientation are characteristic for delirium. Importantly, not all patients with altered mental status have delirium. **The hallmarks of delirium are cognitive impairment, impaired attention, and fluctuating course.** Altered mental status can be from coma, stupor, and so forth. Given the history of trauma and signs of central nervous system dysfunction (inattention, confusion, and generalized hyperreflexia) the diagnosis of delirium from trauma related head injuries needs to be entertained. This can include epidural hematoma, subdural hematoma, or intracerebral hemorrhage besides subarachnoid hemorrhage. The lack of symptoms such as vomiting, headache, seizures, and the fact that she was lucid for at least the day of the trauma makes it highly unlikely to be an epidural hematoma or intracerebral hemorrhage. The lack of focal neurological findings argues against an acute subdural hematoma or intracerebral hemorrhage. The most likely diagnosis is thus subarachnoid hemorrhage, however, this needs to be evaluated by imaging studies such as a CT head with contrast.

In this particular case the focus should be on the history of trauma the patient sustained prior to the onset of her delirium. A CT head without contrast will evaluate for epidural or subdural hematomas, intraparenchymal hemorrhage, or subarachnoid hemorrhage. Her CT shows a subarachnoid hemorrhage, which should prompt immediate neurosurgical consultation and management in the intensive care unit (ICU). A history of illicit drug abuse should cause concern for other drug use warranting a toxicology screen. Lastly, metabolic disorders such as hypoglycemia or hyponatremia should be considered. These can be evaluated by the comprehensive metabolic panel. One key point is that head trauma can lead to the syndrome of inappropriate antidiuretic hormone secretion (SIADH), which can cause hyponatremia and delirium or altered mental status.

APPROACH TO DELIRIUM

Definitions

Delirium: A neurobehavioral disorder with a **fluctuating** course entailing inattention and acute alteration in mental status.

Glasgow Coma Scale: The Glasgow Coma Scale (Table 9–1) was developed to delineate categories of head injury and levels of consciousness in patients with traumatic brain injury. The scale is divided into three categories consisting of eye-opening (E), verbal response (V), and motor response (M). The maximum score is 15, and the minimum score is 3: GCS = E + M + V.

Subarachnoid hemorrhage: Hemorrhage within the subarachnoid space that is caused by rupture of an aneurysm, arteriovenous malformation, neoplasm, angioma, cortical thrombosis, mycotic aneurysm tear, spread of blood or dissection from an intraparenchymal hemorrhage or trauma.

Babinski sign: Extension of the big toe followed by abduction of the other toes when the lateral sole of the foot is stimulated. It is performed by stroking the foot at the heel and moving the stimulus toward the toes. It is a sensitive and reliable sign of cortical spinal tract disease. It is also known as the plantar reflex.

Attention: The ability to focus on specific stimuli while excluding others.

Table 9–1
GLASGOW COMA SCORE

EYE OPENING (E)	VERBAL RESPONSE (V)	MOTOR RESPONSE (M)
4 = Spontaneous	5 = Normal conversation	6 = Normal
3 = To voice	4 = Disoriented conversation	5 = Localizes to pain
2 = To pain	3 = Words, but not coherent	4 = Withdraws to pain
1 = None	2 = No words—only sounds	3 = Decorticate posture
	1 = None	2 = Decerebrate
		1 = None
		Total = E + V + M

Clinical Approach

The presentation of **acute mental status change, abnormal attention, and a fluctuating course** should alert the clinician to **delirium**. Delirium is a disorder caused by many different etiologies and is the most common neurobehavioral disorder in hospitals. It has been reported that up to 40% of hospitalized patients in ICUs have delirium. There are various recognized risk factors for delirium, the most common being age (particularly older than the age of 80), preexisting cognitive impairment, dehydration and electrolyte disturbances and gender (men more so than women).

Patients admitted with delirium to hospitals account for 10–24% of all admissions with up to 26% of these resulting in death. Almost 80% of patients near the time of death will experience delirium.

The pathophysiology of delirium is not well established, but there is evidence to suggest that there are multiple neurotransmitter abnormalities affecting acetylcholine, dopamine, and serotonin levels that leads to reversible impairment of cerebral oxidative metabolism.

There is also an inflammatory component to the mechanism of delirium with some studies showing that cytokines such as interleukin-1 and interleukin-6 are upregulated. The central nervous system pathways involved in delirium are not well established, but the ascending reticular formation in the upper brainstem, prefrontal cortex, posterior parietal cortex, and the thalamus seem to be involved.

Clinical characteristics of delirium include an acute change in mental status with a fluctuating course, disorganized thinking, and attentional deficits. Other characteristics are listed in the Table 9–2. Delirium should be differentiated from dementia, which is usually marked by a slow onset chronic cognitive disorder.

Table 9–2
DELIRIUM RISK FACTORS

Elderly, i.e., >80 years old; gender: men > women

Preexisting cognitive impairment; number and severity of medical illnesses

Dehydration/electrolyte disturbances; infections: urinary/pulmonary

Hypoxemia/cardiorespiratory failure; malnutrition

Drug abuse: EtOH or hypnotic dependency; sleep disturbance

Fever/hypothermia; polypharmacy/analgesic use

Depression; fractures

Physical trauma; burns

Sleep disturbance; visual/auditory impairment

EtOH, alcohol consumption and/or dependency

The diagnosis of delirium is clinical, with an emphasis on evaluating level of attention. Attention can be evaluated by serial reversal test (such as asking the patient to spell a word backwards). The history should include a review of medications patients take and information obtained from friends or family. The neurological examination may not show focal signs or may show myoclonus, dysarthria, tremor, motor abnormalities, or asterixis. Laboratory evaluation should include a comprehensive metabolic panel, glucose, blood urea nitrogen (BUN), liver function studies, electrolyte levels, a complete blood count (CBC) to evaluate for infection, thyroid function studies to evaluate for endocrinopathy, and ammonia to evaluate for hepatic encephalopathy. Arterial blood gas (ABG) or pulse oximetry should be obtained if the patient has a history of lung disease or smoking. Urine toxicology studies in those individuals with a history of drug abuse or at risk for drug abuse should be requested as well. A CT scan of the head or MRI brain scan needs to be performed with the choice of study depending on ease of obtaining and clinical scenario. Other studies to consider depending on the clinical picture include chest radiograph (evaluates for pneumonia), electrocardiograph (ECG) (exclude myocardial infarction or arrhythmia), electroencephalograph (EEG), and lumbar puncture if there is concern for central nervous system (CNS) infection.

The differential diagnosis for delirium is extensive (see Table 9–3) and includes metabolic causes, infections, drug-related causes, primary neurologic abnormalities, trauma, and perioperative causes. Importantly **delirium must be differentiated from dementia.** Typically demented patients have a history of chronic (>6 months) progression with normal attention (except advanced cases) and level of consciousness. Perceptual disturbances and fluctuating course are less common with dementia.

Table 9–3
SELECTED LISTING OF ETIOLOGIES OF DELIRIUM

Etiologies

Metabolic disorders: hypoglycemia, hyponatremia, uremia, hypoxia, hypo/hypercalcemia, endocrinopathies (thyroid, pituitary), vitamin deficiencies, hepatic encephalopathy, toxic exposures (lead, carbon monoxide, mercury, organic solvents)

Neurological: head trauma, cerebrovascular accidents, brain tumors, epilepsy, hypertensive encephalopathy

Infections: encephalitis, meningitis, neurosyphilis, HIV, brain abscesses

Drug related: narcotics, sedatives, hypnotics, anticholinergics, antihistamine agents, beta-blockers, antiparkinson medications, illicit drug (cocaine, amphetamines, hallucinogens)

Perioperative: anesthetics, hypoxia, hypotension, fluid and electrolyte abnormalities, sepsis, embolism, cardiac or orthopedic surgery

Other: cardiovascular, CNS vasculitis, dehydration, sensory deprivation

Treatment is dependent on the etiology of delirium with the use of drug-related treatments being directed toward symptoms such as agitation, hallucinations, paranoia, and so on. The most common medications used include **lorazepam**, haloperidol (**Haldol**), or **risperidone**. Elderly patients who are hospitalized, particularly in the ICU setting, often become disoriented and are prone to delirium; introducing familiar faces and objects and a routine is important in this setting.

Comprehension Questions

[9.1]   An 82-year-old man presents to the emergency room with acute disorientation, hallucinations, and agitation. He had been healthy until last year when he developed diabetes mellitus and suffered a myocardial infarction. His examination is normal except for the symptoms mentioned above. Which of the following is the best next step?

   A. Obtain a stat CT scan of the head followed by a lumbar puncture
   B. Review his medication list and talk to family or caregivers about his cognitive state earlier that week
   C. Obtain a CBC with dialysis/plasma urea ratio (D-P), comprehensive metabolic panel, and urinalysis
   D. Begin treatment with risperidone

[9.2]   A 21-year-old man is brought in by emergency medical services (EMS) to the emergency room with agitation, disorientation, hyperalertness, and recent personality changes. He is not known to have any medical problems and had been doing well until yesterday after attending a fraternity party. No one else is known to be ill, and he has not had fever or complained of headache or other symptoms. His examination is unremarkable except for mildly elevated blood pressure of 146/90 mmHg. What is the diagnosis?

   A. Bacterial meningitis
   B. Brain tumor
   C. Cerebrovascular accident
   D. Hallucinogen use

[9.3]   Which of the following statements is true regarding delirium?

   A. Up to 60% of delirium cases result in death
   B. Less than 10% of all cases presenting to the hospital involve delirium
   C. Delirium is distinguished from dementia based on a fluctuating level of attention
   D. Neuroimaging is indicated only with a history of trauma

Answers

[9.1]   **B.** History is key in trying to determine etiology of delirium so obtaining further information from caregivers or family including reviewing his medication list is critical. It is possible that his symptoms are caused by medications he is taking or that he has suffered another myocardial infarction and complained of chest pain before having an alteration in mental status. Obtaining a CBC with D-P, comprehensive metabolic panel, and urinalysis are important and will need to be performed but are not the next step in this patient's evaluation.

[9.2]   **D.** The most likely culprit of his delirium is hallucinogen use as he is in an age group at risk for this. He does not have fever or meningismus to suggest bacterial meningitis, and the lack of focal findings on examination argues against a brain tumor or stroke.

[9.3]   **C.** Typically demented patients have a history of chronic (>6 months) progression with normal attention (except advanced cases) and level of consciousness. Perceptual disturbances and fluctuating course are less common with dementia.

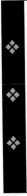

CLINICAL PEARLS

❖ Delirium is differentiated from dementia by having acute changes in mentation with fluctuating altered levels of consciousness and attention.

❖ Delirium has a myriad of etiologies including toxins, fluid/electrolyte or acid/base disturbances, infections such as urinary tract infections or pneumonia.

❖ Delirium often lasts only approximately 1 week, although it can take several weeks for cognitive function to return to normal levels. Full recovery is common.

REFERENCES

Chan D, Brennan NJ. Delirium: making the diagnosis, improving the prognosis. Geriatrics 1999 Mar;54(3):28–30, 36, 39–42.

Mendez Ashala, M. Delirium. In: Bradley WG, Daroff, RB, Fenichel G, Jankovic J. Neurology in clinical practice, 4th ed. Philadelphia, PA: Butterworth-Heinemann; 2003.

Sipahimalani A, Masand PS. Use of risperidone in delirium: case reports. Ann Clin Psychiatry 1997 Jun;9(2):105–107.

A 15-year-old right-hand dominant male became briefly unconscious after being tackled in a high school football game. He was unresponsive for approximately 30 seconds then slowly regained awareness over the following 2 minutes. He reported no neck pain but did complain of a moderate generalized headache as well as nausea and tinnitus. When tested on the sideline 5 minutes after his injury he was oriented only to place and the name of his coach, did not know the month, day, or year, could not recall who was President, and had no memory of the series of plays immediately prior to becoming unconscious. His speech was quite slow and deliberate. His pupils were equal, round, and reactive to light, and he had no facial asymmetry. Finger-to-nose testing was somewhat slow and deliberate with mild past-pointing. His gait was mildly wide-based and unsteady. When tested again 15 minutes after his injury he was oriented to person, place, and time, but still had no memory of the events preceding his injury, and his gait remained unsteady. He was taken to a local emergency room for further evaluation. Regarding the remainder of his history, he was a neurodevelopmentally normal young man who had never previously experienced loss of consciousness. He had no other medical problems and was not taking any medications. He had not recently been ill. There was no history of neurologic problems in the family.

◆ **What is the most likely diagnosis?**

◆ **What is the next diagnostic step?**

◆ **What is the next step in therapy?**

ANSWERS TO CASE 10: Cerebral Contusion

Summary: This previously healthy and neurodevelopmentally normal 15-year-old male experienced brief loss of consciousness during a football game with mild but persistent neurologic symptoms more than 15 minutes after the initial injury. He is now in the emergency room for evaluation.

◆ **Most likely diagnosis:** Grade 3 concussion

◆ **Next diagnostic step:** CT scan without contrast

◆ **Next step in therapy:** Observation, reassurance, and education

Analysis

Objectives

1. Be aware of the basic epidemiology of concussion.
2. Understand clinical criteria for obtaining head imaging following a concussion.
3. Know current "return-to-play" guidelines for sports-related concussions.
4. Be aware of the clinical features and usual course of the post-concussion syndrome.

Considerations

The neurologic status of this 15-year-old male is now steadily improving following his sports-related concussion. There are no focal or lateralizing findings on his neurologic examination to suggest a significant central nervous system injury. Nevertheless, given his persistent retrograde amnesia (his inability to remember the events preceding his injury), it would be prudent to obtain a noncontrast head CT looking for hemorrhage or other significant abnormality. He can then be observed in the emergency room until he returns entirely to his neurologic baseline, or he could be admitted to the hospital for overnight observation. It will be important to discuss with the family what postconcussive symptoms they should expect as well as any symptoms that should prompt seeking medical attention.

APPROACH TO CEREBRAL CONTUSION

Epidemiology

Although there is no universally accepted definition of concussion, the term is generally taken to refer to a traumatic alteration in cognitive function with or without loss of consciousness. As such, concussion is best thought of as a mild traumatic brain injury (TBI). It is a very common occurrence, with an incidence of approximately 50 people per 100,000 in the United States. More than 300,000 sports-related traumatic brain injuries occur every year, and football is the most common venue in which they take place. It has been estimated that at least one player experiences a concussion in every game of football. Rates of concussion are also high in soccer, ice hockey, and basketball. While sports and bicycle accidents are the most common causes of concussion in patients 5 to 14 years of age, falls and motor vehicle accidents are the more common precipitants in adults.

Pathophysiology

Because the ascending reticular-activating system (ARAS) is a key structure mediating wakefulness, transient interruption of its function can be partly responsible for temporary loss of consciousness following head injury. The junction between the thalamus and the midbrain, which contains reticular neurons of the ARAS, seems to be particularly susceptible to the forces produced by rapid deceleration of the head as it strikes a fixed object. The pathophysiology of other symptoms, such as anterograde and retrograde memory difficulties, is less clear. Certainly more severe traumatic brain injuries can be associated with diffuse axonal injury as well as cortical contusions leading to dysfunction.

Classification of Concussion

There are several different schemes available to classify concussions, but the one most commonly used is that developed by the American Academy of Neurology. According to this system:

- A grade 1 concussion involves no loss of consciousness and all symptoms resolve within 15 minutes.
- A grade 2 concussion involves no loss of consciousness but symptoms last longer than 15 minutes.
- A grade 3 concussion involves loss of consciousness for any period of time.

Such a grading system is useful in thinking about management as well as in considering possible return to play for sports-related concussions. It should be noted that this scheme is currently undergoing revision.

Initial Management of Concussion

In any patient with a head injury immediate thought must be given to whether or not there is a concomitant **cervical spine injury**. If any suspicion exists then the spine must be immobilized, and the patient transported to an emergency room for evaluation. If a spinal injury is suspected, taking off the football helmet should only be performed by a health care provider experienced in its removal. Apart from the spine, the possibility of intracranial hemorrhage is the principal concern in the setting of a concussive injury. This is relatively uncommon, complicating only 10% of such injuries, but must be considered as its presence will change subsequent management. A noncontrast head CT is more than sufficiently sensitive to detect clinically significant bleeding. An MRI scan is not necessary.

An important clinical question is to determine which patients require imaging and which do not. Clearly any patient with focal neurologic findings, persistent mental status changes, or worsening neurologic status requires imaging. Conversely, patients who experience only very brief transient confusion without any subsequent symptoms (a grade 1 concussion) are very unlikely to have any significant intracranial pathology. The *New Orleans Criteria* recommends a head CT if any of the following are true: (1) persistent headache, (2) emesis, (3) age: older than 60 years, (4) drug or alcohol intoxication, (5) persistent anterograde amnesia, (6) evidence of soft-tissue or bony injury above the clavicles, or (7) a seizure. Imaging is often recommended for children younger than 16 years of age because clear validated clinical criteria do not yet exist.

The next issue will be for how long and in what context to observe the patient. Clearly individuals with hemorrhage or other acute abnormalities on imaging will require hospitalization and careful monitoring. Relatively small surface contusions are not uncommon and are very unlikely to portend any significant neurologic problem other than headache. Such patients should be observed overnight in the hospital but can be discharged the next day if their neurologic examination is normal. Patients with normal head CTs and normal neurologic examinations who sustained a **grade 1 or grade 2 concussion can safely be discharged home** from the emergency room after 2 hours of observation. The practice of discharging patients with the instruction to wake them up at intervals to make sure that they can be aroused is not recommended. If such monitoring is necessary, it would be better performed in a hospital setting.

Prior to discharge it is important to clarify with the patient and the family what symptoms are to be expected and what symptoms should prompt a phone call or return visit. The postconcussive syndrome, discussed below, is quite common and symptoms such as headache, dizziness, irritability, and difficulty concentrating are to be expected. However, worsening cognitive function, new sensory or motor symptoms, increasing drowsiness, or significant emesis should prompt a return for further evaluation.

Postconcussion Syndrome

Following a concussion, up to 90% of patients will continue to experience headaches and dizziness for at least 1 month. Between 30% and 80% of patients develop a more extensive constellation of symptoms within 4 weeks of their head injury referred to as the postconcussion syndrome (PCS). These individuals report other symptoms such as irritability, depression, insomnia, and subjective intellectual dysfunction. Fatigue, anxiety, and excessive noise sensitivity can also be seen. Some patients report becoming unusually sensitive to the effects of alcohol. Many patients who develop PCS also become preoccupied with fears of brain damage. PCS appears to be more likely to develop in non–sports-related concussions such as those following motor vehicle accidents or falls. The peak of symptom intensity is generally 1 week after injury, and most patients are symptom free by 3 months. However, approximately 25% of patients will still be symptomatic after 6 months, and 10% report symptoms 1 year following injury. Particularly in patients with such unrelenting symptoms, it remains unclear and somewhat controversial how much is caused by psychogenic factors and how much is caused by residual pathophysiologic effects of the initial TBI. Psychiatric consultation would most certainly be warranted in patients with persistent PCS. More detailed neuroimaging using an MRI should also be considered in these patients to fully exclude significant parenchymal injury. Educating patients at the time of their initial injury regarding common symptoms and the benign self-limited nature of PCS is likely to be helpful.

Return to Play Guidelines

For sports-related concussions, an important consideration is when the athlete will be able to return to playing. Guidelines to assist in this decision have been developed by the American Academy of Neurology (AAN), although they are currently being revised.

Grade 1 concussion should be removed from the game for at least 15 minutes and assessed at 5 minute intervals. If there was no loss of consciousness and the symptoms have resolved completely by 15 minutes (the definition of a grade 1 concussion) then the athlete can return to play.

Grade 2 concussion (symptoms persisting longer than 15 minutes without initial loss of consciousness) merits removal from the game for the remainder of the day. If the athlete's neurologic examination is normal, he or she may return to play in 1 week.

Grade 3 concussion (any concussion associated with loss of consciousness) merits transport to an emergency room for evaluation and possible neuroimaging. Following this evaluation the patient's neurologic examination should be repeated both at rest and after exertion. If the examination is normal and the initial loss of consciousness was brief then the player can return after 1 week. If the loss of consciousness was more prolonged then 2 weeks are recommended.

These recommendations apply to athletes experiencing their first concussion of the season. For a second concussion, the guidelines would be to return to play (if asymptomatic): after 1 week for a grade 1 concussion, after 2 weeks for a grade 2 concussion, and after 1 month of being symptom free for a grade 3 concussion. Neurologic testing on the sideline should include orientation, digit string repetition, 5-minute word recall, recall of recent events and game events, pupillary symmetry, finger-to-nose testing, tandem gait, and Romberg testing. These tests should be performed at rest and, if normal, also after exertion (40 yard sprint, 5 push-ups, 5 sit-ups, and 5 knee bends).

Comprehension Questions

[10.1] Which of the following patients should have a head CT performed?

    A. A 27-year-old who was momentarily dazed after striking his head on a tree branch but is back to baseline within 5 minutes

    B. An 18-year-old ice hockey player who did not lose consciousness after being hit by a flying puck but did have significant dizziness and ataxia that resolved after 30 minutes

    C. A 68-year-old who slipped and hit his head on the pavement, was unconscious for less than 30 seconds, and was back to baseline within 5 minutes

    D. A 22-year-old who suffered a grade 2 concussion 1 week ago and who continues to have a mild to moderate headache

[10.2] Which of the following is true regarding return to play guidelines for sports-related concussions?

    A. The number of concussions experienced during a season do not matter as long as they do not involve loss of consciousness

    B. As long as an athlete is symptom-free at rest they can return to play after a grade 2 concussion

    C. Only players with a grade 1 concussion should be allowed to return to the game that same day

    D. Any loss of consciousness necessitates removing the athlete from play for the remainder of the season

[10.3] Which of the following is true regarding postconcussion syndrome?

    A. It is an uncommon sequelae of traumatic brain injury

    B. A characteristic symptom would be progressively increasing lethargy

    C. It is only found in patients who are involved in litigation

    D. It is usually self-limited and resolves over weeks to months

Answers

[10.1] **C.** Any patient who has experienced loss of consciousness should have a head CT obtained. Also, patients older than 60 years of age should be imaged given the higher incidence of hemorrhage with increasing age.

[10.2] **C.** Only players with a grade 1 concussion can be allowed to return to the game that same day. Athletes should be tested both at rest as well as after exertion.

[10.3] **D.** The postconcussion syndrome is a common sequelae of head injury and usually resolves over weeks to months. It is not a form of malingering. Progressively increasing lethargy would be concerning for an evolving hemorrhage or other serious process.

CLINICAL PEARLS

❖ Concussion is a brief, transient loss of consciousness associated with a short period of amnesia caused by blunt head trauma or sudden deceleration.

❖ The subjective memory impairments that patients with postconcussion syndrome (PCS) report are not associated with significant memory problems on formal neuropsychologic testing. Much of the problem with memory in PCS can actually represent difficulty with concentration.

❖ Patients with a prolonged course of postconcussion syndrome have a high rate of premorbid depression and anxiety. This is another reason why these patients are likely to benefit from psychiatric consultation.

❖ Whether or not repeated minor concussions can produce chronic cognitive problems remains controversial. It is clear that recurrent grade 3 concussions, such as what occurs in boxing, can result in long-term consequences.

❖ A brief convulsion occurring at the time of the initial head injury does not require treatment with anticonvulsant medication and is not associated with a significantly increased risk of epilepsy.

❖ The period of postconcussive amnesia is usually roughly proportional to the duration of unconsciousness.

❖ A concussion is a traumatic injury to the brain as a result of a violent blow, shaking, deceleration, or spinning.

REFERENCES

Buzzini SR, Guskiewicz KM. Sport-related concussion in the young athlete. Curr Opin Pediatr 2006;18:376.

Chachad S, Khan A. Concussion in the athlete: a review. Clin Pediatr (Phila) 2006;45:285.

Kelly JP, Rosenberg JH. The diagnosis and management of concussion in sports. Neurology 1997;48:575.

Ropper A, Gorson K. Concussion. N Engl J Med 2007;356:166.

A 68-year-old woman was brought to the emergency room after suddenly developing speech difficulty and weakness of the right arm and leg. She was in her usual state of health when she was observed by family members to become mute and slump in her chair. Her past medical history is significant for hypertension and angina for which she takes a beta-blocker, atenolol, and a calcium channel blocker, amlodipine. The patient's temperature is 36.6°C (98°F); heart rate, 84 beats/min; and blood pressure, 172/86 mmHg. Her physical examination reveals no carotid bruit and an irregularly irregular cardiac rhythm. Neurologic examination shows an alert, attentive patient who is able to follow some simple commands but has severe impairment of word fluency, naming, and repetition. There is a left gaze deviation and right lower facial droop. There is severe weakness of the right upper extremity and, to a lesser degree, weakness of the right lower extremity. The left limbs display full antigravity power without drift for 5 seconds. An electrocardiogram reveals atrial fibrillation.

◆ **Most likely diagnosis and what part of the brain is affected?**

◆ **What is the best next diagnostic step?**

◆ **What is the best next step in therapy?**

ANSWERS TO CASE 11: Acute Cerebral Infarct

Summary: A 68-year-old woman presents with the sudden onset of right hemiparesis and aphasia, risk factors of hypertension and coronary artery disease, and physical findings of atrial fibrillation.

◆ **Most likely diagnosis:** Acute left hemispheric stroke in the anterior circulation

◆ **Next diagnostic step:** Head CT scan

◆ **Next step in therapy:** Thrombolytic therapy if ischemic stroke and eligible by criteria

Analysis

Objectives

1. Understand the clinical presentation of stroke.
2. Be familiar with the evaluation and treatment of stroke.
3. Describe the risk factors and pathophysiology of stroke.

Considerations

The most likely diagnosis in a patient with abrupt onset of focal neurologic deficits is an acute cerebrovascular event. This patient's neurologic deficits, right hemiparesis, aphasia, and gaze paresis, point to a perfusion defect in the left middle cerebral artery territory. Focal neurologic deficits can include hemiparesis, hemisensory loss, speech disturbance, homonymous hemianopia, or hemiataxia. Other diagnostic considerations include a seizure with postictal Todd paralysis or complicated migraine. If the acuity of onset is less certain, a brain tumor, subdural hematoma, multiple sclerosis, herpes encephalitis, or a brain abscess can mimic a stroke albeit with a subacute tempo. The distinction between a stroke and a transient ischemic attack rests on the duration of symptoms. The symptoms of a transient ischemic attack resolve within 24 hours, usually lasting from several minutes to 1 to 2 hours. **Distinguishing between an ischemic stroke and an intracerebral hemorrhage requires a brain imaging study**, either CT or MRI. The etiologies and treatment of ischemic stroke and intracerebral hemorrhage are quite different. **Because intervention can improve outcome, the patient should be rapidly assessed for possible thrombolytic therapy (hemorrhagic stroke is a contraindication).** The treatment of hemorrhagic stroke is primarily supportive and involves the control of hypertension. Careful monitoring of intracranial pressure, hyperventilation, and osmotic therapy, and occasionally surgical decompression are employed.

APPROACH TO ACUTE CEREBRAL INFARCT

Definitions

Ischemic stroke: Cerebral infarction associated with neurologic symptoms of greater than 24-hour duration.

Transient ischemic attack: A cerebral ischemic event associated with focal neurologic deficits lasting less than 24 hours and generally no evidence of cerebral infarction.

Intracerebral hemorrhage: A cerebrovascular event characterized by arterial rupture and parenchymal hemorrhage.

Homonymous hemianopia: The loss of one-half of the field of view on the same side in both eyes.

Todd's paralysis: A brief period of transient (temporary) paralysis following a seizure.

Clinical Approach

Stroke, or cerebrovascular accident, is a neurologic deficit of sudden onset attributable to the loss of perfusion of a portion of the brain from vascular occlusion or hemorrhage. **Ischemic stroke is caused by vascular insufficiency**, whereas **hemorrhagic stroke is associated with a mass effect from the blood clot impinging on brain tissue.** Understanding the vascular supply to the brain can help in correlating the neurologic finding to the likely artery occluded. The carotid arteries are the vascular supply for the frontal and parietal lobes and most of the temporal lobes and basal ganglia. The main branches of the carotid artery are the middle cerebral and the anterior cerebral arteries. The vertebrobasilar territory encompasses the brainstem, cerebellum, occipital lobes, and thalami. The posterior inferior cerebellar artery derives from the vertebral artery. The posterior cerebral, superior cerebellar, and anterior inferior cerebellar arteries are branches of the basilar artery.

When a patient presents with weakness, numbness, or speech difficulties, a brain imaging study such as a CT or MRI is extremely valuable to distinguish between an ischemic stroke and an intracerebral hemorrhage and to help rule out a stroke mimic. An electrocardiogram and laboratory studies including a complete blood count, glucose, prothrombin time (PT), and partial thromboplastin time (PTT) are also essential.

The patient should be admitted to a unit that provides neurologic and cardiac monitoring. Intravenous fluids to maintain euvolemia (normal volume status) should be provided, and measures implemented to avoid aspiration pneumonia, deep venous thrombosis, and fever. Acute blood pressure elevation is often encountered in the stroke patient; in general, **the blood pressure should not be lowered in the first few days of an ischemic stroke unless extremely elevated.** Iatrogenic hypotension can exacerbate focal cerebral ischemia and worsen neurologic outcome.

The diagnostic evaluation for an ischemic stroke can include a carotid ultrasound, echocardiogram, magnetic resonance angiogram of the head and neck, and/or a cerebral arteriogram. A fasting lipid panel is usually warranted, and other laboratory studies such as serum B_{12}, folate, homocysteine levels, hemoglobin A1C, erythrocyte sedimentation rate (ESR), rapid plasma reagin (RPR), HIV, and toxicology screens can be useful to identify stroke risk factors.

Etiologies

The most common etiologies of ischemic stroke include cardiac embolism, large vessel atherothrombosis, and small vessel intracranial occlusive disease, although the comprehensive list of potential stroke etiologies is quite extensive (see also Case 13). As many as 30% of ischemic strokes are cryptogenic (without discernible etiology) after a thorough diagnostic evaluation.

Acknowledged sources of cardiac embolism to the brain include **atrial fibrillation**, mechanical prosthetic heart valves, acute myocardial infarction, low left ventricular ejection fraction <30%, patent foramen ovale, and endocarditis. Large vessel atherosclerosis can affect the carotid bifurcation, the major intracranial vessels, or the extracranial vertebral artery. Small vessel strokes, also known as **lacunar strokes**, are characterized by classic clinical syndromes such as pure motor stroke or pure sensory stroke and related to occlusive disease of penetrating arteries in the brain usually associated with hypertension and/or diabetes. Risk factors for stroke are similar to those of coronary heart disease and include elderly age, hypertension, smoking, diabetes, hyperlipidemia, heart disease, hyperhomocysteinemia, and family history.

Clinical Presentation

Hemiparesis, aphasia, and gaze paresis, point to an anatomic localization in the left middle cerebral artery territory (Fig. 11–1). Cortical symptoms such as **aphasia** (impairment of the ability to use or comprehend words), neglect, **agnosia** (loss of ability to recognize objects, persons, sounds, shapes or smells), and **apraxia** (loss of the ability to execute or carry out learned purposeful movements) indicate a lesion in the anterior (or carotid) circulation. Symptoms such as diplopia, vertigo, crossed neurologic findings, and homonymous hemianopia, however, suggest a **posterior (or vertebrobasilar) circulation lesion.** The symptoms of an intracerebral hemorrhage cannot be reliably distinguished from those of an ischemic stroke on clinical grounds alone. The presence of headache, depressed level of consciousness, or extreme elevations of blood pressure, however, can raise the suspicion of a **hemorrhagic stroke.**

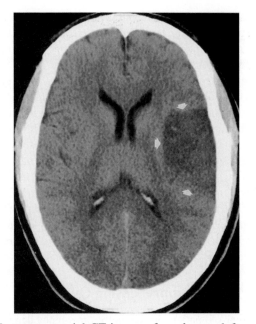

Figure 11–1. Noncontrast axial CT image of a subacute left major coronary artery infarction. *(With permission from Chen MY, Pope TL, Ott DJ. Basic radiology. McGraw-Hill Medical/Lange Clinical Science; 2004: Fig. 12–20.)*

Treatment

Treatment of ischemic stroke starts with assessment of eligibility for thrombolysis. Treatment must be initiated urgently. **Intravenous tissue plasminogen activator (t-PA)** can significantly improve the odds of neurologic recovery, but must be administered within 3 hours of onset of stroke symptoms. t-PA is associated with a risk of intracranial hemorrhage. Thus, urgent imaging of the brain such as CT scan is imperative to assess for hemorrhagic stroke. Contraindications to t-PA include active bleeding, recent stroke, or history of intracerebral hemorrhage. Other acute stroke treatments are currently under investigation and can in the near future include endovascular/intra-arterial and/or neuroprotective therapies. Patients who are not candidates for thrombolytic therapy should be treated with aspirin unless contraindicated.

    Secondary stroke prevention should be implemented right away. Antiplatelet drugs such as **aspirin**, clopidogrel, or the combination of aspirin and extended release dipyridamole are the mainstays of stroke prevention treatment for most patients with ischemic stroke and transient ischemic attack (TIA). Patients with high-risk cardioembolic conditions such as **atrial fibrillation,**

however, warrant long-term anticoagulation with warfarin, which has been demonstrated to be superior to antiplatelet treatment for this indication.

Risk factor management is crucial to preventing recurrent stroke. Long-term control of hypertension is especially important. Treatment should be initiated approximately 1 week after ischemic stroke. Statins for hyperlipidemia lower the odds of stroke recurrence, and current guidelines recommend a target low density lipoprotein (LDL) of under 100 mg/dL. Carotid stenosis in a patient with ischemic stroke or TIA is an indication for carotid endarterectomy or, in a patient who is a poor surgical candidate, carotid stenting. Rehabilitation is especially beneficial for patients who have gait difficulty or aphasia, or who require assistance in activities of daily living or help resuming gainful employment after a stroke.

The treatment of **hemorrhagic stroke** is primarily supportive and involves control of hypertension. Intracranial pressure should be monitored and addressed with hyperventilation and osmotic therapy, or surgical decompression when appropriate. Thrombolytic therapy is contraindicated.

Comprehension Questions

[11.1] An 81-year-old patient arrives in the emergency department with acute left hemiparesis and neglect. What finding is most important in determining noneligibility for thrombolytic treatment?

A. Time of symptom onset of 2 hours
B. History of any previous myocardial infarction
C. Patient taking any antihypertensive medication
D. Recent gastrointestinal (GI) bleeding

[11.2] For this patient in question 11.1, what study is most useful to rule out an intracerebral hemorrhage?

A. Electrocardiogram
B. Brain CT
C. Complete blood count
D. Cerebral arteriogram

[11.3] After receiving stroke therapy, the patient is being discharged home on physical therapy. The usual treatment would include long-term antiplatelet treatment; however, it is not used in this patient's case. Which of the following is most likely to be present such that antiplatelet therapy is not prescribed?

A. The patient has diabetes
B. The patient has ischemic heart disease
C. The patient has carotid stenosis
D. The patient has atrial fibrillation

Answers

[11.1] **D.** A history of bleeding issues can contraindicate the use of an anticoagulant.

[11.2] **B.** The head CT scan is reliable and rapid in assessing for cerebral hemorrhagic stroke.

[11.3] **D.** When atrial fibrillation is present, then warfarin therapy is used rather than antiplatelet therapy.

CLINICAL PEARLS

❖ Sudden onset of focal neurologic deficits equals stroke until proven otherwise.

❖ Time is brain viability; treat ischemic stroke with thrombolytics within 3 hours to preserve brain tissue.

❖ Stroke risk factors are similar to those of ischemic heart disease.

❖ Cortical symptoms suggest a carotid territory stroke; brainstem or cerebellar findings suggest a vertebrobasilar territory stroke.

REFERENCES

Mohr JP, Choi D, Grotta J, et al. pathophysiology, diagnosis, and management, 4th ed. Churchill Livingstone; 2004.

Ropper AH, Brown RH. Adams and Victor's principles of neurology, 8th ed. New York: McGraw-Hill; 2005.

A 50-year-old female is brought by her husband to the Emergency Center after experiencing sudden onset of severe headache associated with vomiting, neck stiffness, and left-sided weakness. She was noted to complain of the worst headache of her life shortly before she became progressively confused. Two weeks ago she returned from jogging noting a moderate headache with nausea and photophobia. She has a history of hypertension and tobacco use. On examination, her temperature is 37.6°C (99.8°F); heart rate, 120 beats/min; respiration rate, 32 breaths/min; and blood pressure, 180/90 mmHg. She is stuporous and moaning incoherently. Her right pupil is dilated with papilledema and ipsilateral ptosis, and she vomits when a light is shone in her eyes. She has a left lower face drooped and does not withdraw her left arm and leg to pain as briskly compared to the right. Her neck is rigid. Her chest examination reveals tachycardia and bibasilar crackles. During the examination, her head suddenly turns to the left, and she exhibits generalized tonic-clonic activity. STAT laboratory tests show a sodium level of 125 mEq/L. The electrocardiograph (ECG) shows prolonged QT interval and T-wave inversion.

◆ **What is the most likely diagnosis?**

◆ **What is the next diagnostic step?**

◆ **What is the next step in therapy?**

ANSWERS TO CASE 12: Subarachnoid Hemorrhage

Summary: A 50-year-old female with a history of hypertension and tobacco use presents with sudden onset of the worse headache of her life associated with confusion, vomiting, neck stiffness, and left-sided weakness. She was noted to complain of a headache 1 week ago. She is now hypertensive. Her neurologic examination is significant for stupor, right cranial nerve III paralysis, left-sided weakness, neck stiffness, and a seizure. Her workup is significant for hyponatremia and ECG changes.

◆ **Most likely diagnosis:** Subarachnoid hemorrhage

◆ **Next diagnostic step:** Noncontrast CT of the head

◆ **Next step in therapy:** Cerebral angiography

Analysis

Objectives

1. Identify the epidemiology and risk factors for subarachnoid hemorrhage.
2. Understand the prognosis and complications of subarachnoid hemorrhage.
3. Know a diagnostic and therapeutic approach to subarachnoid hemorrhage.

Considerations

This 50-year-old woman has multiple risk factors for subarachnoid hemorrhage caused by an underlying aneurysm, including her age (mean age for subarachnoid hemorrhage is 50 years of age), sex (slightly higher risk for females), hypertension, and tobacco use. The complaint of "the worst headache of my life" to describe its sudden severe onset is classic, and may or may not be associated with altered mentation and focal neurologic deficits. There is usually a history of a recent moderate headache as a result of *sentinel bleed*, as in her case after running, and 60% of subarachnoid hemorrhages occur during physical or emotional strain, head trauma, defecation, or coitus. The clinical severity of the subarachnoid hemorrhage is graded based on the degree of stupor, nuchal rigidity, focal neurologic deficits, and elevation of intracranial pressure. Our patient exhibits neurogenic pulmonary edema, a rare complication of subarachnoid hemorrhage. Her neurologic signs localize to a ruptured right posterior communicating artery aneurysm, with the bleed causing compression of the nearby ipsilateral cranial nerve III with mydriasis, ptosis, and impaired extraocular movements. Her contralateral hemiparesis and complex partial seizure with secondary generalization can result from either parenchymal extension of the hemorrhage with edema or middle cerebral artery vasospasm, all three of which are complications of subarachnoid hemorrhage. Hyponatremia is frequently seen on chemistries, correlating with an elevation of atrial natriuretic factor, cerebral salt wasting, and syndrome of inappropriate antidiuretic hormone. ECG changes, especially QT prolongation, T-wave inversion, and arrhythmias, are also systemic complications common to subarachnoid hemorrhage.

APPROACH TO SUBARACHNOID HEMORRHAGE

Definitions

Subarachnoid space: The spongy interval between the arachnoid mater and the pia mater. The headache and nuchal rigidity is caused by chemical inflammation of the pia arachnoid from blood degradation products in this space.

Sentinel bleed: Intermittent aneurysmal subarachnoid hemorrhage causing lesser headaches that precede the "worst headache" that occurs with rupture of the aneurysm.

Vasospasm: Most alarming complication of aneurysmal subarachnoid hemorrhage in which irritation causes constriction of major cerebral arteries, vasospasm lethargy, and cerebral infarction. Vasospasm occurs mostly with aneurysms rather than other causes of subarachnoid hemorrhage, and peaks after 4 to 14 days. Transcranial Doppler can be used to detect a change in flow velocity in an affected middle cerebral artery.

Acute communicating hydrocephalus: Complication that occurs because of obstruction of the subarachnoid granulations in the venous sinuses by the subarachnoid blood. CT shows enlarged lateral, third, and fourth ventricles, with clinical signs of headache, vomiting, blurry and double vision, somnolence, and syncope.

Clinical Approach

Etiologies

Subarachnoid hemorrhage is the underlying cause of approximately 10% of stroke presentations and results from a number of etiologies. **Ruptured saccular or berry aneurysms account for up to 80% of nontraumatic subarachnoid hemorrhage**, and portend the worst prognosis. More than three-fourths of intracerebral aneurysms arise in the anterior circulation. The most frequent sites of aneurysms are in the anterior communicating artery (up to one-third of aneurysmal subarachnoid hemorrhages), followed by the bifurcation of the internal carotid artery with the posterior communicating artery, and the bifurcation of the internal carotid artery with the middle cerebral artery. One-fourth of patients will have more than one aneurysm, with risk for rupture increasing with size of the aneurysm. Fibromuscular dysplasia is an associated etiology in one-fourth of aneurysm patients, whereas polycystic kidney disease is related to 3% of cases. Other risk factors for aneurysms include chronic severe hypertension with diastolic blood pressure greater than 110 mmHg, liver disease, tobacco and alcohol use, vasculitides, collagen vascular disorders such as Marfan syndrome, infections (mycotic aneurysms), and oral contraception. Nonaneurysmal causes of subarachnoid hemorrhage include trauma, arteriovenous malformations, and cocaine or amphetamine abuse.

Diagnosis and Prognosis

Head CT without contrast is the most sensitive neuroimaging study for detecting subarachnoid bleeding, appearing as hyperdensity within the cerebral convexities, cisterns, and parenchyma (Fig. 12–1). Intraventricular hemorrhage portends a worse prognosis and increased risk for hydrocephalus. Sensitivity of CT is greatest 24 hours after the event with 50% still detectable after 1 week. Negative head CT occurs in 10–15% of cases, and should be further evaluated with **lumbar puncture looking for xanthochromia** (yellowish discoloration of CSF) and increased red blood cells. Cerebrospinal fluid (CSF) studies are most sensitive 12 hours after onset, but can be negative in 10–15% of patients as well, in which case the prognosis is better. CT, MRI, or conventional angiography can be used to screen for an underlying aneurysm (Fig. 12–2).

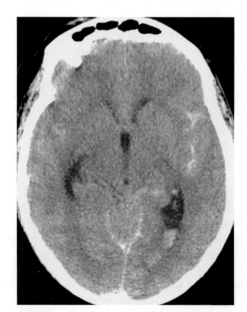

Figure 12–1. Noncontrast CT scan subarachnoid blood in the left sylvian fissure (bright) and within the left lateral ventricle. *(With permission from Kasper DL, Braunwal E, Fauci A, et al. Harrison's principles of internal medicine, 16th ed. New York: McGraw-Hill; 2004: Fig. 349–14b.)*

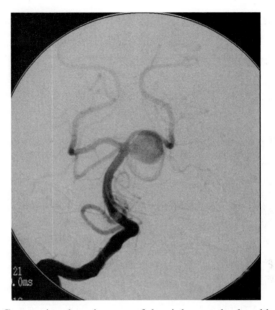

Figure 12–2. Conventional angiogram of the right vertebral and basilar artery showing the large aneurysm. *(With permission from Kasper DL, Braunwal E, Fauci A, et al. Harrison's principles of internal medicine, 16th ed. New York: McGraw-Hill; 2004: Fig. 349–14c.)*

Up to 60% of patients die in the first 30 days after a subarachnoid hemorrhage, 10% instantly without warning. First month mortality is 40% for hospitalized patients, with worsening of mortality to 50–80% with rebleeding. Severity of cases and their prognoses can be graded based upon alertness and presence of focal signs.

  Grade I subarachnoid hemorrhage (SAH) patients are alert with mild headache and nuchal rigidity and have a 5% chance of deteriorating with a 3–5% mortality risk.

  Grade II patients have moderate-to-severe headache and nuchal rigidity, and a 6–10% mortality.

  Grade III patients have added confusion.

  Grade IV patients have stupor and moderate hemiparesis.

  Grade V patients are comatose with signs of severe increased intracranial pressure, and they have the worst prognosis with 80% chance of deteriorating, 25–30% rebleeding rate, and 50–70% mortality. Delayed vasospasm is a calamitous complication that occurs in up to 20% of cases.

Treatment

Grade I and II subarachnoid hemorrhage may be observed after diagnostic measures. **Emergent conventional angiography is warranted if ruptured aneurysm is suspected and neurosurgical intervention is required.** Repeat angiography can be necessary if the underlying etiology is obscured by vasospasm. **Endovascular coiling** is indicated to reduce rebleeding in low-grade cases of subarachnoid hemorrhage and has been shown to be superior to clipping. **Clipping** should be performed in the first 48 hours after onset or be delayed for 2 weeks to avoid the window of greatest risk for vasospasm, especially with complicated high-grade cases. The mainstay of medical management is to reduce vasospasm through *Triple H* **therapy** (hypertensive hypervolemic hemodilution) to maintain cerebral perfusion, and nimodipine, a calcium channel blocker. It is also important to address other complications including metabolic derangements (hyponatremia, syndrome of inappropriate antidiuretic hormone secretion [SIADH], cerebral salt wasting), respiratory (neurogenic pulmonary edema) and cardiac (arrhythmias) complications, seizures, and hydrocephalus, which may require ventriculostomy.

Comprehension Questions

Match the following etiologies (A–C) to the clinical situation [12.1] to [12.3]:

    A. Anterior communicating artery aneurysm
    B. Posterior communicating artery aneurysm
    C. Vasospasm

[12.1] A 35-year-old woman was admitted last week for a subarachnoid hemorrhage caused by a left major coronary artery (MCA) aneurysm. Today during rounds she appears much less alert.

[12.2] A 45-year-old man with a history of alcohol consumption complains of a "thunderclap headache," nausea, and blurry vision with right anisocoria and diplopia on exam.

[12.3] A 20-year-old woman is found to have hypertension, kidney cysts, and intermittent headaches.

[12.4] An emergency room physician consults you for the best study to evaluate possible subarachnoid hemorrhage.

    A. Transcranial Doppler Study
    B. Electroencephalograph (EEG)
    C. PET scan of brain
    D. CT scan of head without contrast
    E. Brain MRI without contrast

[12.5] An internist consults you for the best study to evaluate hyperacute onset of left hemiparesis 1 week after admission for a subarachnoid hemorrhage. Which of the following would be most appropriate?

Answers

[12.1] **C.** Delayed vasospasm lethargy (and also acute hydrocephalus) can arise days after a ruptured aneurysm with subarachnoid hemorrhage. Emergent neuroimaging should be performed to assess the need for angiography or ventriculostomy.

[12.2] **B.** Ipsilateral ptosis, pupil dilation, and ophthalmoplegia result from compression of the third nerve by a posterior communicating artery aneurysm and bleed.

[12.3] **A.** The most common site for a cerebral aneurysm in polycystic kidney disease is in the anterior communicating artery, although multiple aneurysms may be observed.

[12.4] **D.** Head CT without contrast is a rapid and sensitive imaging modality to detect subarachnoid blood. If it is negative and a high suspicion remains, a lumbar puncture should be performed.

[12.5] **E.** Diffusion-weighted MRI is more sensitive than CT for detecting hyperacute ischemic injury caused by vasospasm, although conventional angiography is usually needed to confirm vasospasm. For acute changes in level of consciousness, CT head is preferred as a faster way to evaluate for hydrocephalus and need for ventriculostomy.

CLINICAL PEARLS

❖ Most cases of subarachnoid hemorrhage with no history of head trauma are caused by an underlying aneurysm.

❖ Subarachnoid hemorrhage severity and prognosis is assessed by the degree of change in consciousness, headache, nausea and vomiting, nuchal rigidity, focal deficits, and seizures.

❖ Mass effect from edema and parenchymal spread, vasospasm from subarachnoid involvement, and hydrocephalus from intraventricular spread are all serious delayed neurologic complications of subarachnoid hemorrhage that may not be apparent on the initial evaluation.

❖ *Triple H* therapy and nimodipine are important parts of medical management of subarachnoid hemorrhage. Endovascular coiling and clipping are surgical options with appropriate windows of intervention.

REFERENCES

Al-Shahi R, White PM, Davenport RJ, Lindsay KW. Subarachnoid haemorrhage. BMJ 2006 Jul 29;333(7561):235–240.

Feigin VL, Findlay M. Advances in subarachnoid hemorrhage. Stroke 2006 Feb;37(2):305–308.

A 22-year-old previously healthy college student presented to the emergency department with the complaint of gait instability and a droopy right eyelid. He began noticing these symptoms 2 days ago, the morning after his fraternity brother put him in a playful "choke hold." He managed to break free after a struggle and subsequently noticed a right temporal headache after the wrestling match. The patient's temperature is 36.4°C (97.6°F); heart rate, 64 beats/min; and blood pressure, 118/78 mmHg. General physical examination is unremarkable. The neurologic examination reveals ptosis of the right eye and anisocoria, with a pupillary diameter of 2 mm on the right and 4 mm on the left. Light reactivity is intact directly and consensually. Extraocular movements are normal. There is a mild left hemiparesis involving left face, arm, and leg. Gait is hemiparetic, and the patient tends to fall without assistance. The electrocardiogram is normal. Complete blood count, electrolytes, blood urea nitrogen (BUN), creatinine, glucose, urinalysis, prothrombin time (PT), and partial thromboplastin time (PTT) are normal. Noncontrast head CT shows an area of acute hypodensity in the right frontoparietal region.

◆ **What is the most likely diagnosis and mechanism?**

◆ **What is the next diagnostic step?**

ANSWERS TO CASE 13: Stroke in a Young Patient

Summary: A 22-year-old patient presenting with a right Horner syndrome and right hemispheric ischemic stroke after minor neck trauma.

◆ **Most likely diagnosis and mechanism:** Acute ischemic stroke caused by right carotid artery dissection as a result of trauma

◆ **Next diagnostic step:** Cerebral arteriogram

Analysis

Objectives

1. Understand that stroke occurs in patients of all ages.
2. Recognize the less typical stroke etiologies that often affect younger patients.
3. Be familiar with the diagnostic workup of stroke in the young patient.

Considerations

The clinical diagnosis of a stroke relies on the appropriate clinical history, neurologic findings, and supportive brain imaging studies. Although the majority of strokes occur in patients 65 years of age or older, tens of thousands of strokes per year nonetheless occur in patients 55 years of age or younger in the Unites States. Just as in older patients, the clinical suspicion of stroke should come to the forefront when focal neurologic deficits emerge acutely. This particular patient underwent a "choke hold," which occluded the right carotid artery, leading to ischemia to the right frontal aspect of the brain.

APPROACH TO STROKE IN A YOUNG PATIENT

Definitions

Carotid dissection: A tear in the carotid arterial wall that can result in luminal obstruction, thromboembolic complications, and/or pseudoaneurysm formation. Dissections can also occur in the vertebral arteries, or less commonly, the large intracranial arteries.

Patent foramen ovale: A persistent opening in the interatrial septum associated with paradoxical embolism in patients with cryptogenic stroke.

Arteriovenous malformations: Congenital high-pressure, high-flow cerebral vascular malformations characterized by direct arteriovenous shunting.

Clinical Approach

The diagnostic evaluation in a younger stroke patient may need to be more extensive because the likelihood is greater of a nonatherosclerotic etiology.

Some of these are discussed below. The workup can include a brain MRI, cerebral angiography or magnetic resonance angiography (MRA) of the intracranial and cervical vessels, transesophageal echocardiogram, and laboratory studies including lipid panel, homocysteine, protein C, protein S, antithrombin III, anticardiolipin antibody, lupus anticoagulant, factor V Leiden mutation, prothrombin gene mutation, and a toxicology screen. Other studies that can be indicated in the appropriate clinical setting might include lumbar puncture, HIV serology, blood cultures, vasculitis serologies, and screening for sickle cell disease.

Etiologies and Clinical Presentations

The main causes of stroke in older stroke patients remain important causes of stroke in younger adults, especially in younger patients who possess the traditional atherosclerotic risk factors of hypertension, heart disease, diabetes, and hyperlipidemia. The largest categories of stroke in the general population are cardioembolic, large-vessel atherothrombotic, and lacunar. A **patent foramen ovale (PFO)** is detectable in approximately 15% of the general population, but its prevalence is threefold higher in young patients with cryptogenic ischemic stroke. The mechanism is presumed to be paradoxical embolism. Transesophageal echocardiography (TEE) is the most reliable way to detect a PFO. Atrial septal aneurysms are also linked to cryptogenic stroke and best evaluated by TEE.

Craniocervical dissection is commonly but not always preceded by head or neck trauma such as a motor vehicle accident, chiropractic neck manipulation, or a bout of severe coughing (Fig. 13–1). Dissections can present with headache or thromboembolic cerebrovascular events. **Carotid dissection** is often associated with a **Horner syndrome**, that is, ipsilateral ptosis and miosis. Fibromuscular dysplasia, Ehlers-Danlos syndrome, and Marfan syndrome are predisposing factors to spontaneous craniocervical dissection.

Arteriovenous malformations and the lower-flow cavernous angiomas are associated with intracerebral hemorrhage as well as seizures and other neurologic presentations. Moyamoya disease is an idiopathic noninflammatory cerebral vasculopathy characterized by progressive occlusion of the large arteries at the circle of Willis. The characteristic *moyamoya* vessels refer to the small penetrating arteries that hypertrophy in response to chronic cerebral ischemia.

Drugs of abuse, especially cocaine and amphetamines, are associated with both ischemic and hemorrhagic stroke. Oral contraceptives are a risk factor for thromboembolic stroke, especially in women who smoke. A history of intravenous drug abuse should raise the suspicion of endocarditis and HIV disease. Other rarer infectious etiologies of stroke include tuberculous meningitis and varicella zoster.

Hypercoagulable conditions can predispose to stroke. These include malignancy, antiphospholipid antibodies, protein C deficiency, protein S deficiency, antithrombin III deficiency, factor V Leiden mutation, prothrombin gene mutation, and hyperhomocysteinemia. Some of these entities are most clearly linked to venous thromboembolism, which is particularly relevant to patients with cerebral venous thrombosis or a PFO.

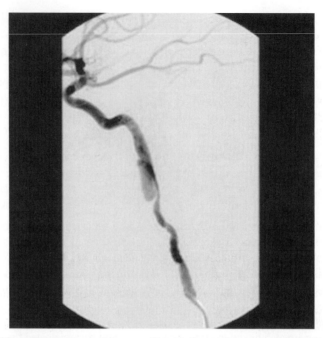

Figure 13–1. Cerebral arteriogram of internal carotid artery (ICA) dissection. *(With permission of Brunicardi FC, Andersen DK, Billiar TR, et al. Schwartz's principles of surgery, 8th ed. New York: McGraw-Hill; 2004: Fig. 22–92.)*

Treatment

Treatment, of course, is tailored to the specific stroke etiology. Antithrombotic drugs are a mainstay of therapy for most patients with ischemic stroke. Very few randomized clinical trials have been performed to help guide the choice of antiplatelet or anticoagulant treatment for the specific stroke subtypes discussed above. One such trial revealed no significant difference between aspirin and warfarin in patients with ischemic stroke associated with an antiphospholipid antibody.

Endovascular closure of PFO is currently under investigation. Because a substantial proportion of carotid or vertebral dissections spontaneously recanalize, stenting is usually reserved for patients who show no vessel recanalization after 3 to 6 months. The treatment of arteriovenous malformations can employ a combination of surgery, radiation, and endovascular therapies. Surgical revascularization procedures such as encephaloduroarteriosynangiosis or superficial temporal artery-middle cerebral artery (STA-MCA) bypass are frequently performed for moyamoya disease.

Comprehension Questions

[13.1] Which of the following risk factors is more common in an individual older than age 55 years?

A. Atrial fibrillation
B. Patent foramen ovale
C. Carotid dissection
D. Moyamoya disease

[13.2] A 45-year-old man is brought into the emergency room with symptoms of a stroke. After a search for an etiology, the neurosurgeon states that the patient is not a candidate for a surgical or endovascular intervention. Which of the following is most likely to be present in this patient's condition?

A. Arteriovenous malformation
B. Antiphospholipid antibodies
C. Moyamoya disease
D. Carotid dissection

[13.3] An 18-year-old male is seen by his pediatrician for right-sided arm weakness. The pediatrician is suspicious of a patent foramen ovale. Which of the following is the best examination to confirm this finding?

A. Electrocardiogram (ECG)
B. Auscultation of the heart
C. Echocardiogram
D. Arterial blood gas

Answers

[13.1] **A.** Atrial fibrillation is more common in older adults. The other etiologies should be considered in a young patient presenting with a stroke.

[13.2] **B.** Antiphospholipid syndrome is typically treated medically rather than surgically. The other choices present are often treated interventionally.

[13.3] **C.** Transesophageal echocardiography is the best test to detect a patent foramen ovale.

CLINICAL PEARLS

❖ Horner syndrome in a patient with headache and recent head or neck injury suggests carotid dissection.
❖ The etiology most often discovered in a young patient with cryptogenic stroke is a patent foramen ovale.
❖ The young patient is more likely to have an "unusual" cause of stroke, although up to 16% of no etiology is found.
❖ Three percent of cerebral infarcts occur in patients younger than 40 years of age.

REFERENCES

Mohr JP, Choi D, Grotta J, et al. Stroke: pathophysiology, diagnosis, and management, 4th ed. Philadelphia, PA: Churchill Livingstone; 2004.

Ropper AH, Brown RH. Adams and Victor's principles of neurology, 8th ed. New York: McGraw-Hill; 2005.

A 23-year-old graduate student was studying late at night for an examination. He recalls studying, but his next memory is being on the floor and aching throughout his body. He was incontinent of urine but not stool and felt slightly confused. No one was with him, and he did not know what to do. He called his mother, who recommended he go to the local emergency room.

The student was too busy and decided not to go to the hospital. He called the school infirmary the next day, and their physicians examined him. His vital signs were normal, and the neurologic examination, including motor and sensory evaluation, reflexes, and cranial nerve function were normal. His entire neurologic and physical examinations were normal. He asked for advice.

◆ **What is the most likely diagnosis?**

◆ **What is the next diagnostic step?**

◆ **What is the next step in therapy?**

ANSWERS TO CASE 14: New Onset Seizure: Adult

Summary: A 23-year-old man lost consciousness and when he awoke, he was confused, incontinent of urine, and had muscle soreness. His examination the following day was normal.

◆ **Most likely diagnosis:** Seizure disorder

◆ **Next diagnostic step:** MRI of the brain and electroencephalograph (EEG)

◆ **Next step in therapy:** Potential anticonvulsant medication, discuss driving

Analysis

Objectives

1. Know diagnostic approach to first seizure in an adult, including the importance of history, examination, and testing.
2. Understand the different types of therapy and arguments for and against treatment of first seizure.
3. Describe the workup and follow-up for the patient.

Considerations

This young man had an episode in which he lost consciousness. Case 16 discusses the difference between syncope versus seizure. Briefly, if someone has loss of consciousness and experiences subsequent confusion, he or she probably had a seizure unless he or she experienced head trauma. The diffuse muscle aches also suggest convulsion. Further, the urinary incontinence also suggests seizure, although if someone experienced syncope and had a full bladder, he or she might also have urinary incontinence. Stool incontinence, which this patient did not have, usually suggests seizure and is rare with syncope. It is important to know whether this patient had previous seizures or previous episodes of loss of consciousness (he did not). It is also important to know whether he has a family history of seizures, which he did not. Lastly, one needs to know whether he had any predisposing factors to seizures, such as increased alcohol consumption, drugs that can lower seizure threshold (e.g., cocaine, amphetamines), or sleep deprivation.

The fact that this man was up late can lower his seizure threshold. Patients with seizures have a greater likelihood of seizing as they enter or exit stage 2 sleep. Adult onset seizure is caused by tumor or stroke until proven otherwise, but in young patients such as ours, although these diagnoses should be screened, most have epilepsy without ascertainable cause. They need to be followed to be certain they do not have a tumor, and the most important part of the follow-up is the examination.

EEG is important, perhaps more as a baseline and to help decide whether the patient has seizures, but understand that the diagnosis of seizure rests with the history, not EEG testing. EEGs provide a window in time during which the electrical activity of the brain is evaluated. A normal EEG does not mean that the patient did not seize. It is also important to obtain brain imaging (e.g., MRI) to be certain there is no underlying tumor, although some might argue that this is unnecessary if you follow the patient.

It is important to sit down with the patient and decide on a plan. Patients need to be instructed to contact the Department of Public Safety regarding their driving, cautioned about being in situations in which they can harm themselves (i.e., being on a roof, swimming alone, etc.) if they have a seizure. The physician should also discuss the indication, dosing, and side effects of anticonvulsant medication and prescribe a medication based on the case.

APPROACH TO ADULT ONSET SEIZURE

Definitions

Loss of consciousness: Not being aware of one's surroundings. These patients usually have a window of time they cannot recall.

Seizure: Temporary, self-limited cerebral dysfunction as a result of abnormal, self-limited hypersynchronous electrical discharge of cortical neurons. There are many kinds of seizures, each with characteristic behavioral changes and each usually with particular EEG recordings.

Clinical Approach

Etiologies

The current classification of seizures relates to the 1981 Classification of Epileptic Seizures promulgated by the International League Against Epilepsy. Essentially, seizures are considered to relate to only one of the two cerebral hemispheres (these are referred to as partial or focal seizures) or both hemispheres of the brain (generalized seizures). Where the seizure pattern initiates and where it spreads determines the type of seizure, relates to prognosis, and frequently warrants different therapies.

Partial seizures are further subdivided depending on whether the patient has a change in level of (or loses) consciousness. In *simple partial seizures*, patients do not lose consciousness, but in *complex partial seizures* they do have an alteration or loss of consciousness.

In *generalized seizures*, the seizure usually has a focal onset (e.g., the right hand twitches, then the right arm twitches, and then the patient loses consciousness), although the focal onset may not always be clinically detected. Subcategorization of these generalized seizures primarily reflects the type of motor disturbances present during the convulsion (e.g., tonic-clonic, tonic, atonic, myoclonus).

Epilepsy is also classified as to the cause, whether idiopathic, symptomatic, or cryptogenic. There is considerable controversy about this issue. The *idiopathic epilepsy syndromes*, whether focal or generalized, include: benign neonatal convulsions, benign childhood epilepsy, childhood/juvenile absence epilepsy, juvenile myoclonic epilepsy, and idiopathic epilepsy (i.e., not otherwise specified).

Symptomatic epilepsy syndromes can be focal or generalized and include: infantile spasms (West syndrome), Lennox-Gastaut syndrome, early myoclonic encephalopathy, epilepsia partialis continua, Landau-Kleffner syndrome (acquired epileptic aphasia), temporal lobe epilepsy, frontal lobe epilepsy, posttraumatic epilepsy, and other forms not specified. There are other epilepsy syndromes of uncertain classification, including neonatal and febrile seizures, and reflex epilepsy.

Clinical Presentation

Seizure disorders can present as intermittent events. The initial event, whether reported by the patient or witnessed by an observer, is often clinically reliable as to whether a seizure begins with a focal onset or is immediately generalized. However, the physician must recognize that the patient may not remember initial focal symptoms because of postseizure (i.e., postictal) memory loss, consciousness can be rapidly impaired following a focal onset, or the area of the brain in which the seizure begins may not have focal symptoms.

In many cases, the classification of the kind of seizure the patient has is more important than the actual description of the seizure. This is because other relevant clinical information, of which the seizure may be only one variable, is also important. Within this context, the history (i.e., brain trauma, recent fever or headaches rendering suspicion for meningitis, family history of epilepsy, etc.) is important, as is the neurologic examination. Further, the results of EEG, neuroimaging, and blood tests are also important. These blood tests should include electrolytes, glucose, calcium, magnesium, renal and liver function, complete blood counts, and, if clinically suspected, lumbar puncture to rule out meningitis, and toxicology screens in the urine and blood.

Approximately 10–25% of patients who complain of a seizure without an obvious cause see a physician after having only one seizure. This is usually a tonic-clonic event and most have no risk factors for epilepsy. These patients usually have a normal neurologic examination, normal EEG, and normal radiographic testing. Of these patients, one-quarter will prove to have epilepsy.

There have been multiple studies and discourse on what to do for these patients because three-quarters will never seize again but one-quarter will. What is known is that treatment following the first seizure decreases the relapse rate, but there is no evidence that this treatment alters the prognosis of epilepsy.

Many neurologists wait until the second seizure before initiating treatment. The physician should discuss with the patient (or parents or both) the implications

Table 14–1

THERAPY FOR VARIOUS SEIZURE DISORDERS

Simple and complex partial seizures	carbamazepine, valproate, gabapentin, lamotrigine, topiramate, phenytoin
Secondary generalized	carbamazepine, valproate, gabapentin, lamotrigine, topiramate, phenytoin
Primary generalized	
Tonic-clonic	valproate, lamotrigine, topiramate, carbamazepine, phenytoin
Absence	valproate, lamotrigine, ethosuximide, zonisamide
Myoclonic	valproate, clonazepam, levetiracetam
Tonic	valproate, felbamate, clonazepam, zonisamide

of treating or not treating, discussing medicolegal issues, driving laws in the patient's state, and usually options for therapy.

Different seizures have different therapies. Table 14–1 provides a reasonable guideline for treatment of different seizures.

Comprehension Questions

[14.1] A 61-year-old woman with a long history of type 2 diabetes is admitted to the hospital because of poorly controlled disease. During her hospitalization she develops continuous tonic movements of her right arm and hand. A serum glucose is measured as >600 mg/dL. Which of the following is the most appropriate step in management?

A. Noncontrast CT brain scan
B. Intravenous (IV) administration of lorazepam
C. Insulin drip and frequent serum glucose monitoring
D. Securing the airway

[14.2] A 45-year-old man with history of embolic stroke 1 year ago presents with a generalized seizure. Which of the following is the most likely best choice?

A. Seizures are likely to continue to occur in this individual
B. Embolic strokes require a patent foramen ovale
C. This patient likely has a partial seizure disorder
D. This patient likely has diabetes

[14.3] A 7-year-old girl with history of muscle jerks in the early morning, or
with sleep deprivation, presents with a generalized tonic clonic seizure
after a late night playing video games. Which of the following is the
most likely diagnosis?

A. Juvenile myoclonic epilepsy
B. Myasthenia gravis
C. Systemic lupus erythematosus
D. Rheumatoid arthritis

Answers

[14.1] **D.** The ABC's are always the first step. Securing the airway is the first priority. Simple focal seizures are often caused by focal lesions in the brain,
however, physiologic or metabolic insults such as electrolyte imbalances,
significant elevated blood glucose, or drugs/toxins can also induce simple
or complex seizures and should be evaluated and managed.

[14.2] **A.** Epilepsy is likely to continue in this patient. Similar to sleep deprivation, acute alcohol ingestion or intoxication can be associated with a
seizure in the absence of preexisting lesions or risk factors.

[14.3] **A.** Juvenile myoclonic epilepsy is one of the most common epilepsy
syndromes. It accounts for 7% of all cases of epilepsy and is associated
with myoclonic seizures (quick little jerks of the arms, shoulder, or
occasionally the legs), usually in the early morning, soon after awakening. The myoclonic jerks sometimes are followed by a tonic-clonic
seizure in the context of sleep deprivation or alcohol ingestion.

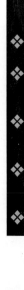

CLINICAL PEARLS

❖ Seizures can be associated with just about any type of intermittent
symptom.

❖ In patients who complain of a singular seizure, without a known
antecedent event, 10–25% will develop epilepsy (i.e., have more
seizures).

❖ The classification of epilepsy is based on whether the seizures are
partial or generalized and also the cause (i.e., idiopathic, symptomatic, cryptogenic) of the seizure.

❖ Sudden unexplained death in epilepsy is now emerging more frequently in research literature, adding weight and validity to this
once questionable entity.

❖ In 7 out of 10 people with epilepsy, no cause can be found.

REFERENCES

Bazil CW, Morrell MJ, Pedley TA. Epilepsy. In: Rowland LP, ed. Merritt's neurology, 11th ed. Philadelphia, PA: Lippincott Williams & Wilkins; 2005:990–1014.
Schacter SC. Epilepsy. In: Evans RW, ed. Saunders manual of neurologic practice. Philadelphia, PA: Saunders/Elsevier; 2003:244–265.

A 23-year-old graduate student was studying late at night for an examination, talking to his friends. All of a sudden, he began smacking his lips, stared into space, seemed confused, and kept mumbling the same word repeatedly. This episode lasted approximately 20 seconds. During the episode, his friends tried to constrain him, but he became combative. Within a few more seconds, he suddenly became asymptomatic although he seemed slightly confused for 5 to 10 more seconds. His friends wanted to take him to the emergency room, but he refused.

◆ **What is the most likely diagnosis?**

◆ **What is the next diagnostic step?**

◆ **What is the next step in therapy?**

ANSWERS TO CASE 15: Absence Versus Complex Partial Seizure

Summary: A 23-year-old man appeared suddenly confused and engaged in repetitive motor (including speech) behaviors. He then suddenly became asymptomatic.

◆ **Most likely diagnosis:** Complex partial seizure

◆ **Next diagnostic step:** Obtain an MRI and electroencephalograph (EEG)

◆ **Next step in therapy:** Initiate anticonvulsant medication or, if he is taking medication, alter dosage or prescribe new medicines; discuss driving

Analysis

Objectives

1. Know diagnostic approach to differential diagnosis of absence seizures and complex partial seizure, including their evaluation.
2. Understand the different types of therapy for these seizures.

Considerations

In this case of a 23-year-old college student, **complex partial seizures** is the most likely diagnosis given his age and presentation, although absence seizures are also a possibility. **Simple partial seizures** reflect epileptic discharge(s) occurring in a limited and often focal area of the cerebral cortex. Just about any symptom or sign can relate to this *epileptogenic focus*, depending on location. Thus, the patient can have any type of aura adumbrating the seizure, or any type of observable manifestation during a simple partial seizure, whether this is a simple motor movement (e.g., Jacksonian seizure, adversive seizure), unilateral sensory aberration, complex emotional episode, or a visual, auditory, or olfactory hallucination. The most common aura for any focal-onset seizure, including simple partial seizure, is sensation of abdominal discomfort. However, other auras for seizures (especially simple partial seizure) can include a feeling of unreality, detachment from the environment, *déjà vu*, or *jamais vu*. During a simple partial seizure, the patient is usually able to interact appropriately with their environment, except for possible limitations imposed by the seizure itself. In this case, the patient was unable to interact with his environment and therefore did not have a simple partial seizure.

Complex partial seizures differ from the above. These seizures, defined by impaired consciousness and associated with bilateral spread of seizure discharge, involve at a minimum the basal forebrain and limbic areas. In addition to impaired consciousness, these patients can exhibit automatisms, such as lip smacking, chewing, gesturing, repeated swallowing, repeating words or phrases, walking, running, undressing, snapping fingers, clumsy perseveration of an ongoing motor task, or some other type of complex motor activity that is not specifically directed and is not appropriate. If these patients are physically restrained during the seizure, they may become hostile or aggressive. Following the seizure, these patients are often transiently confused and disoriented; this can last several minutes. In patients with complex partial seizures, approximately three-quarters of the seizure foci arise in the temporal lobe. The remainder of the seizure foci arise in the frontal or occipital lobes. The patient's symptoms and signs will reflect where that seizure foci arises and where it spreads. These seizures can occur several times a day and last several minutes.

Absence seizures (petit mal) are another type of seizure and are sometimes confused with complex partial seizures. Absence seizures present with momentary lapses in awareness, however, they are not accompanied by automatisms seen with complex partial seizures, but are characterized by motionless staring and stoppage of any ongoing activity. Absence spells begin and end abruptly, occur without aura, and are not associated with postictal confusion. Sometimes, mild myoclonic contractions of the eyelid or facial muscles, loss of muscle tone, or automatisms (see above) can accompany longer attacks. Unlike complex partial seizures, absence seizures occur many times during a day and rarely last more than 10–15 seconds.

If the beginning and end of the absence spell is not distinct, or if tonic and autonomic components also occur, these spells are referred to as *atypical absence seizures*. Absence spells seldom begin *de novo* in adults, usually having their onset in childhood, usually beginning between ages 4 and 14, with 70% stopping by age 18. The children who get them usually have normal development and intelligence. **Atypical absence seizures** usually occur in cognitively challenged children with epilepsy or in patients having epileptic encephalopathy, such as the Lennox-Gastaut syndrome.

APPROACH TO ABSENCE AND PARTIAL COMPLEX SEIZURES

Definitions

Absence seizures: Absence seizures are brief episodes of staring that usually occur in childhood and last 5 to 10 seconds. If the seizure lasts beyond 10 seconds, there can also be eye blinking and lip smacking. They usually occur in clusters and can occur dozens or hundreds of times a day.

Complex partial seizure: previously called *temporal lobe seizures* or *psychomotor seizures*. *Complex* refers to loss of consciousness and lack of awareness of the patient's surroundings. Patients often engage in repetitive behavior, known as automatisms. This is the most common type of seizure in adults with epilepsy. Patients appear to be awake but do not respond normally to their environment. The "spell" usually lasts less than 3 minutes and can be immediately preceded by simple partial seizure.

Clinical Approach

Clinical Features and Epidemiology

Complex partial seizures cause impaired consciousness and arise from a single brain region. Impaired consciousness implies decreased responsiveness and awareness of self and surroundings. During a complex partial seizure, the patient may not communicate, respond to commands, or remember events that occurred. Consciousness might not be impaired completely. During a complex partial seizure, some patients may make simple verbal responses, follow simple commands, or continue to perform simple or, less commonly, complex motor behaviors such as operating a car. Complex partial seizures typically arise from the temporal lobe but can arise from any cortical region.

Automatisms are motor or verbal behaviors that commonly accompany complex partial seizures. The behavior is often repeated inappropriately or is inappropriate for the situation. Verbal automatisms range from simple vocalizations, such as moaning, to more complex, comprehensible, stereotyped speech. Motor automatisms are classified as simple or complex. Simple motor automatisms include oral automatisms (e.g., lip smacking, chewing, swallowing) and manual automatisms (e.g., picking, fumbling, patting). Unilateral manual automatisms accompanied by contralateral arm dystonia usually indicates seizure onset from the cerebral hemisphere ipsilateral to the manual automatisms.

Complex motor automatisms are more elaborate, coordinated movements involving bilateral extremities. Examples of complex motor automatisms are cycling movements of the legs and stereotyped swimming movements. De novo automatisms often begin after seizure onset. In other cases, perseverative automatisms occur as repetitions of motor activity that began before the seizure. Bizarre automatisms such as alternating limb movements, right-to-left head rolling, or sexual automatisms can occur with frontal-lobe seizures.

Automatisms also can occur during nonepileptic states of confusion (e.g., metabolic encephalopathy), after ictus, and during absence seizures and thus can be confused with complex partial epilepsy. However, there are clinical features that often help distinguish absence from complex partial seizures (Table 15–1).

Partial seizures often begin with a brief aura (simple partial seizure) lasting seconds and then become complex partial seizures. The type of aura is related to the site of cortical onset. Temporal-lobe seizures often begin with a rising abdominal sensation, fear, unreality, or déjà vu. Parietal-lobe seizures can begin with an electrical sensation, tingling, or numbness. Occipital-lobe seizures can begin with visual changes, such as the perception of colored lines, spots, or shapes or even a loss of vision.

Table 15–1

COMPLEX PARTIAL VERSUS ABSENCE SEIZURES

FEATURE	COMPLEX PARTIAL	ABSENCE
Onset	Can have simple partial onset	Abrupt
Duration	Usually >30 s	Usually <30 s
Automatisms	Present	Duration dependent
Awareness	No	No
Ending	Gradual postictal	Abrupt

Complex partial seizures of the temporal lobe often begin with a motionless stare followed by simple oral or motor automatisms. In contrast, frontal-lobe seizures often begin with vigorous motor automatisms or stereotyped clonic or tonic activity. Extratemporal-lobe seizures can spread quickly to the frontal lobe and produce motor behaviors similar to those associated with complex partial seizures of the frontal lobe. Tonic and dystonic arm posturing can occur in the arm contralateral to the seizure focus. Sustained head or eye turning contralateral to the seizure focus can occur immediately before or simultaneously with clonic or tonic activity elsewhere.

Complex partial seizures often last 30 seconds to 2 minutes. Longer seizures can occur, particularly when the seizures become generalized convulsions. Complex partial status epilepticus can also occur with prolonged episodes of waxing and waning of consciousness.

In the United States, for people younger than 60 years of age, the incidence of partial seizures is 20 cases per 100,000 person-years. For people aged 60–80 years, incidence increases to 80 cases per 100,000 person-years. The prevalence of epilepsy is 0.5–1 case per 100 persons. Complex partial seizures occur in approximately 35% of persons with epilepsy. Internationally, partial seizures are more common in countries where **cysticercosis** is prevalent.

The mortality rate among individuals with epilepsy is two to three times that of the general population. Most deaths are as a result of the underlying cause of epilepsy. Sudden unexpected death in epilepsy (SUDEP) occurs with no apparent cause. The incidence of SUDEP is 1 case per 370–1110 patient-years among people with epilepsy. SUDEP is most common among those with frequent, medically intractable seizures. Individuals with epilepsy are at increased risk for trauma, burns, and aspiration.

Etiology and Pathogenesis

Unlike absence seizures that have a genetic basis or are associated with abnormal neurodevelopment, the etiopathogenesis of complex partial seizures can include brain trauma, encephalitis, meningitis, stroke, perinatal brain injuries, vascular malformations, cortical dysplasia, and neoplasms. Febrile seizures of childhood that are unusually prolonged, frequent, or associated with focal neurologic features can increase risk for later development of complex partial seizures. In most patients, **complex partial seizures represent a symptom of underlying temporal-lobe epilepsy,** the cause of which is unknown. Characteristic pathologic changes, called *mesial temporal sclerosis*, are most often visible on brain MRI. In addition, single-photon emission CT (SPECT) ictal studies show hypoperfusion of bilateral frontal and parietal association cortex, and hyperfusion of the mediodorsal thalamus and rostral brainstem. Ictal effects on these structures by means of the spread of epileptic discharges or a transsynaptic mechanism can mediate impaired consciousness during complex partial seizures.

Evaluation and Treatment

A thorough history and neurologic examination, as well as appropriate diagnostic studies for these disturbances (usually including blood tests, brain imaging, EEG, and sometimes ongoing EEG monitoring) are often necessary. First aid care is found in Table 15–2. Laboratory studies to determine the serum anticonvulsant drug concentrations are indicated for known or suspected patients with epilepsy. Otherwise, laboratory studies should be directed at ruling out metabolic or toxic triggers of seizures, including electrolyte and glucose levels and a drug screen.

For **complex partial seizures, cranial MRI** can be indicated to detect focal brain lesions and often shows reduced hippocampal volume or increased signal on fluid attenuation inversion recovery (FLAIR). T2-weighted MRI identifies sclerosis of mesial temporal lobe in 80–90% of cases. Gadolinium enhancement is indicated if a neoplasm or vascular malformation is suspected. In addition, special imaging protocols can be required for subtle cortical changes from cortical dysplasia, which are often overlooked with standard imaging protocols. In idiopathic absence seizures, neuroimaging is often normal.

EEG should be performed in every patient who has experienced a "spell" that may be a possible seizure. Epileptiform discharges can indicate the type of seizure and site of the seizure focus. In **absence seizures, the EEG is often**

Table 15–2
FIRST AID FOR SEIZURES

- Do not restrain the person.
- Remove dangerous objects from the person's path.
- Calmly direct the person to sit down and guide him or her from dangerous situations. Use force only in an emergency to protect the person from immediate harm, such as walking in front of an oncoming car.
- Observe, but do not approach, a person who appears angry or combative.
- Remain with the person until he or she is fully alert.

diagnostic showing regular and symmetrical 3 Hz, possible 2- to 4-Hz spike-and-slow-wave complexes, and possible **multiple spike-and-slow-wave complexes.** However, a negative interictal EEG does not exclude a diagnosis of epilepsy, especially complex partial seizures. If the waking EEG is negative, a sleep-deprived EEG can demonstrate epileptiform abnormalities. When the EEG and history are nondiagnostic, prolonged EEG-video monitoring is useful for differential diagnosis. Ambulatory EEG can be used in some instances, although it provides less information about seizure behavior than EEG-video monitoring. Lumbar puncture should be performed when an inflammatory or infectious brain disorder (e.g., encephalitis) is suspected, however, it is unnecessary in every seizure evaluation.

Treatment and Management

Anticonvulsant therapy is generally indicated when patients have more than one seizure. The goal is to make the patient seizure free. Even one seizure per year can prevent the patient from working and/or driving. Therapy with one agent is generally preferred to therapy with two or more anticonvulsants, especially because cognitive adverse effects are common with anticonvulsants, especially traditional drugs, including phenytoin, phenobarbital, carbamazepine, and valproic acid. The newer anticonvulsants are increasingly being used because of fewer side effects and drug-drug interaction, a higher therapeutic index, higher dose tolerance, and they do not require drug-concentration monitoring. These drugs include gabapentin, lamotrigine, levetiracetam, oxcarbazepine, pregabalin, tiagabine, topiramate, and zonisamide.

If a diagnosis of absence seizures is made, often in association with a syndrome, the likelihood of other coexistent seizure types, such as myoclonic or tonic-clonic, should be considered. Ethosuximide is one anticonvulsant that is only indicated for absence seizures and would not be indicated for this case presentation. **Valproic acid is also effective against absence, myoclonic, and tonic-clonic (as well as partial) seizures** and for this case, is a consideration.

Although many anticonvulsants are listed as category D (unsafe in pregnancy), the use of anticonvulsants during pregnancy is warranted if necessary to control seizures. Nevertheless, all women of childbearing age should be instructed about effective birth control while taking anticonvulsants and be prescribed up to 4 mg of folic acid daily to lower the risks of congenital defects, including neural tube defects. Of the anticonvulsants, **valproate is more likely than other anticonvulsants to cause congenital birth defects in a dose-related fashion.**

Initiation of anticonvulsant therapy requires laboratory screening and monitoring and regular patient evaluation for efficacy and/or side effect. Once therapy is initiated and maintained at therapeutic doses, subsequent, periodic blood and urine monitoring in otherwise asymptomatic patients receiving anticonvulsants does not help in identifying patients at risk for life-threatening adverse drug reactions. However, mild elevations in transaminase levels and mild depressions in blood cell counts often occur with anticonvulsant therapy and are generally observed. Patients should be educated about how to recognize the signs of a severe adverse drug reaction, which can vary depending on the drug but include dizziness, vertigo, double vision, gait disturbances or ataxia, rash, and mental confusion.

For patients in which diagnostic studies are unyielding or seizures remain refractory to adequate treatment, a referral to an epilepsy specialist is indicated. An epilepsy specialist can evaluate the patient with EEG-video monitoring, evaluate current and past therapies, optimize treatment, and evaluate the patient for possible epilepsy surgery. Surgical intervention is indicated for patients who have frequent, disabling seizures despite adequate trials of two or more anticonvulsants. Such procedures include temporal lobectomy, extratemporal resections, corpus callosotomy, placement of a vagus-nerve stimulator, hemispherectomy, and multiple subpial transections.

Lifestyle and Activity

All persons with uncontrolled seizures must be advised to refrain from high-risk activities that put themselves and/or others in danger in the event of a seizure. These activities include, but are not limited to the following: operating a motor vehicle, operating a stove or other dangerous machinery, and working at heights. These patients should be advised to contact the appropriate state agency regarding driving regulations. Some states require physician reporting of drivers who experience seizures. These activity restrictions should be reviewed in detail (and documented in the medical record) with the patient, family, and/or caregivers.

Comprehension Questions

[15.1] A 24-year-old female is diagnosed with a complex partial seizure disorder. Which of the following would be typical automatisms that can occur in complex partial seizures?

A. Lip smacking, chewing, gesturing
B. Singing and coughing
C. Choreiform dance-like movements
D. Rigid arm motions directed laterally

[15.2] A 9-year-old boy is diagnosed with absence seizures. Which of the following would most likely best describes his seizure episodes?

A. Tremulousness of the right arm in the absence of other movement disorder
B. Momentary lapses in awareness, accompanied by motionless staring and cessation of any ongoing activity
C. Alternate flexion and extension and rigidity of the arms and legs
D. Sudden loss of posture and falling unconscious to the floor

[15.3] A 35-year-old man is diagnosed with a seizure disorder. There is no history of trauma or medical condition. What is the most common type of seizure in adults with epilepsy?

    A. Absence seizures
    B. Complex partial seizures
    C. Grand mal seizures
    D. Todd paralysis

Answers

[15.1] **A.** Lip smacking, chewing, and swallowing are common findings in complex partial seizures.

[15.2] **B.** Absence seizures are typified by staring off episodes without conscious awareness.

[15.3] **B.** The most common type of seizure with epilepsy in adults is complex partial seizures.

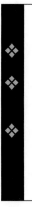

CLINICAL PEARLS

❖ Complex partial seizures are the most common form of seizure in adults.

❖ The differential of complex partial seizure includes absence seizures and also multiple medical disturbances, including transient ischemic attacks.

❖ In approximately one-third of women with seizures, there is a relationship between seizures and the menstrual cycle, and the seizure frequency can double. This is often called catamenial seizure exacerbation or catamenial epilepsy.

REFERENCES

Bazil CW, Morrell MJ, Pedley TA. Epilepsy. In: Rowland LP, ed. Merritt's neurology, 11th ed. Philadelphia, PA: Lippincott Williams & Wilkins; 2005:990–1014.

Murro AM. Complex partial seizures. Available at: http://www.emedicine.com/NEURO/topic74.htm. Accessed March 20, 2007.

Schacter SC. Epilepsy. In: Evans RW, ed. Saunders manual of neurologic practice. Philadelphia, PA: Saunders/Elsevier; 2003:244–265.

A 52-year-old healthy white male is brought to the emergency room (ER) after he has had a car accident in which he hit the dividing rail. He apparently did not suffer any significant injuries and at the time of the examination was fully awake. On further questioning, he reported driving on the highway and then without any warning hit the rail. He immediately stopped the car. His wife, who was in the car with him, stated that he suddenly stopped responding in the middle of the sentence, and the car started to go to the left. When they hit the rail, he woke up and braked the car. He denies feeling lightheaded, nausea, or warning prior to the loss of consciousness. He also denied feeling ill or disoriented on awakening, and he was immediately aware of his surroundings. There was no evidence of tongue biting or urinary incontinence, or convulsive jerking. In the ER, the patient had an unremarkable examination, laboratory work, and CT scan of his head. He was admitted for 24-hour observation, and a neurologist was consulted. The patient admitted to two previous syncopal episodes, both in his office, and both without provocation. On one occasion he was seated, on the second occasion he was standing and suffered a fall. In neither case did he have any warning or postevent confusion. After the second episode he scheduled an appointment with his family doctor but did not have the chance to see him prior to the accident. On review of systems, the patient complained of frequent fatigue and lack of energy over the last year but attributed it to work schedule and lack of adequate exercise. His detailed neurologic examination showed no abnormal findings.

◆ **What is the most likely diagnosis?**

◆ **What is the next diagnostic step?**

◆ **What is the next step in therapy?**

ANSWERS TO CASE 16: Cardiogenic Syncope Related to Bradycardia

Summary: This 64-year-old man presents with an acute and temporary loss of consciousness and history of two similar episodes in the past. These episodes were not associated with warning signs or symptoms nor followed by persistent confusion, weakness, or findings on examination.

◆ **Most likely diagnosis:** Cardiogenic syncope related to bradycardia

◆ **Next diagnostic step:** Cardiac evaluation and invasive electrophysiology

◆ **Next step in therapy:** Pacemaker placement

Analysis

Objectives

1. Know common causes of acute loss of consciousness or syncope.
2. Describe the workup for syncope.
3. Be familiar with the management of syncope.

Clinical Considerations

In this case, the patient suffered an acute loss of consciousness that was without any provocation or premonitory symptoms including nausea, sweating, or abdominal discomfort. He did not become pale or ashen according to his wife. The event occurred while he was sitting in his car, and he regained consciousness quickly. These findings are less consistent with a vasovagal or orthostatic syncope because it was not associated with a change in position from sitting or lying down to standing or upright and was not associated with signs and symptoms suggestive of low blood pressure.

His wife denied any convulsions or postictal confusion, and the patient denied any premonitory symptoms. On examination there was no evidence of tongue biting or urinary incontinence, making a good case against an epileptic seizure. Therefore the most likely diagnosis in this patient is cardiogenic syncope. An evaluation should be performed including a tilt-table testing. The patient should also have an MRI of the brain with and without contrast and electroencephalograph (EEG). Routine laboratory tests should be undertaken to assess for metabolic or endocrine problems; complete blood count (CBC) for evidence of anemia or infection. An electrocardiograph (ECG) and 24-hour Holter monitoring are usually obtained. After an evaluation and follow-up, the patient may have repeated bouts of syncope, which requires more extensive evaluation and therapy. This particular patient experienced repeated syncopal episodes. There was a negative workup, an invasive electrophysiological study was ordered, and the patient was diagnosed with "sick sinus syndrome." The treatment was an implanted dual chamber pacemaker, and the patient was discharged home with resolution of syncope and fatigue.

APPROACH TO CARDIOGENIC SYNCOPE

Definitions

Syncope: A sudden brief loss of consciousness (LOC).

Orthostatic syncope: Syncope associated with a sudden change in position from supine to sitting up or sitting to standing up.

Electroencephalography: The neurophysiologic measurement of the electrical activity of the brain by recording from electrodes placed on the scalp or, in special cases, subdurally or in the cerebral cortex.

Epilepsy: Neurologic condition that makes people susceptible to seizures. A seizure is a change in sensation, awareness, or behavior brought about by a brief electrical disturbance in the brain.

Tilt-table testing: Test to evaluate how the body regulates blood pressure in response to some very simple stresses while lying on a special table. It involves cardiac monitoring (ECG), blood pressure monitoring, and intravenous (IV) infusion of drugs to stress the system.

Sick sinus syndrome: A type of bradycardia in which the sinoatrial (**SA**) or **sinus node** is not working as it should.

Clinical Approach

Syncope can result from a variety of cardiovascular and noncardiovascular causes. The most common pathophysiologic mechanism for cardiovascular syncope is decreased cerebral blood flow with resultant cerebral hypoxia, which prompts immediate and forceful rearrangement of posture to ensure an adequate flow of the blood to the central nervous system (CNS). Decreased cerebral blood flow is most commonly caused by decreased cardiac output (CO) and arrhythmias. Heart rate below 35 and above 150 beats/min can cause syncope even without the presence of cardiovascular disease. Although bradycardia can occur at any age, it occurs most frequently in the elderly and is usually caused by ischemia or fibrosis of the conduction system. Digitalis, beta-blockers, and calcium channel blockers can also cause bradycardia. However, supraventricular or ventricular tachyarrhythmias that cause syncope can be related to cardiac ischemia or electrolyte abnormalities.

Among the most common non–cardiac-related mechanisms of syncope are peripheral vasodilation, decreased venous return to the heart, and hypovolemia.

History is critical in making the correct diagnosis in the case of syncope. It should guide the evaluation and not the other way around. Syncope of cardiac etiology occurs suddenly and ends abruptly without warning or post-event confusion. The postural changes are often not necessary for the termination of the event. This presentation is the most common sequela of the arrhythmia and requires careful electrophysiological study as well as cardiac catheterization to rule out ischemia as the cause of the conduction defect.

Exertional syncope suggests cardiac outflow obstruction, mainly caused by aortic stenosis, and therefore warrants echocardiogram as the first step in evaluation. Cough or micturition syncope as well as syncope occurring during any natural or iatrogenic Valsalva maneuver, implicates decrease in venous return and can be present even in healthy individuals.

Vasovagal syncope is not a serious or life-threatening condition but is an abnormal reflex. This results in a drop in blood pressure leading to decreased blood flow to the brain resulting in dizziness or fainting. The mechanism of vasovagal syncope is the subject of a great deal of research. It is typically precipitated by unpleasant physical or emotional syncope most commonly pain, sight of blood or gastrointestinal discomfort. It usually occurs in the upright position, and the patient describes a sensation of lightheadedness, dimmed vision and hearing, depersonalization, sweating, nausea, and increased heart rate. The patient usually wakes up immediately after the event but if prevented from obtaining a supine position, usually by well-wishing observers, syncope can be prolonged and accompanied by brief convulsions (so-called *convulsive syncope*). This almost always precipitates neurologic consult for the new onset seizures.

The picture is often complicated by the **spontaneous micturition**, which is widely believed to be a sign of **epileptic activity**. Contrary to popular belief, incontinence can be the result of any syncopal episode if the patient happens to have a full bladder prior to the event. Most often, if clearly elucidated, a pure vasovagal episode in the patient without any risk factors for cardiovascular disease and a normal post-event physical examination does not require any further evaluation.

Syncope caused by epileptic seizure is abrupt in onset and most of the time associated with focal or generalized tonic or clonic muscular activity, clearly described by the witnesses. **Tongue biting and urinary incontinence are common** but by no means required for the diagnosis. Most of the time the patient experiences at least brief postictal confusion, making it the single most important sign for the differentiation from other causes of syncope.

In patients with known epilepsy, defined as recurrent seizures, between which there is complete recovery, evaluation should be centered over the **antiepileptic medications**. Blood levels should be checked for the current medications and if low, the cause or causes need to be elucidated. The most common causes are noncompliance or introduction of the new medication that interferes with the absorption or metabolism of the current antiepileptic drug or drugs. Frequently, however, recurrent seizures happen despite adequate blood level of antiepileptic medication. It can be a result of concurrent acute illness, behavioral changes (staying up all night, skipping meals, or drinking alcohol) or simply inadequate seizure control.

Orthostatic syncope has different etiology in elderly (e.g., over 50 years) and young patients. When occurring in the young it is most often confused with epilepsy because of age and absence of cardiovascular risk factors. Orthostatic syncope almost always happens with the sudden change of posture from lying or sitting to standing or after prolonged standing without moving. The classic example is a young soldier fainting during the military parade on a hot summer afternoon. When this happens in young and otherwise healthy individuals, it always requires a table-tilt test, because sequential measurements of orthostatic blood pressure changes in the clinic may not be enough.

In the elderly, however, orthostatic syncope is often caused by hypovolemia, or increased venous pooling as seen after prolonged bed rest. The other contributing factor in this population is polypharmacy that often includes combination of beta-blocker, loop diuretic, and nitrate; combining dehydration, vasodilatation and delayed cardiac response to cause sudden orthostatic changes in blood pressure without adequate compensatory response.

The other possibility for the orthostatic hypotension leading to the syncope is autonomic nervous system abnormality. By far the most common cause of dysautonomia is diabetic neuropathy, where interruption of the sympathetic reflex arc inhibits adequate adrenergic response to standing. The other less frequent causes of autonomic failure are amyloidosis, syphilis, spinal cord injury or syringomyelia, alcoholic neuropathy, or acute inflammatory demyelinating polyradiculoneuropathy (AIDP) also known as Guillain-Barré syndrome, which can all affect the peripheral or central autonomic pathways. Orthostatic hypotension is also one of the cardinal features of multiple system atrophy, an atypical Parkinsonian syndrome, which consists of a variable combination of parkinsonism, cerebellar dysfunction, dysautonomia, and pyramidal symptoms. However, orthostatic hypotension can be present later and often to a milder degree in idiopathic Parkinson disease, and often aggravated by the use of dopaminergic agents.

Evaluation

Patients suspected of cardiogenic syncope or any nonepileptic syncope should undergo an extensive evaluation including 12-lead ECG, two-dimensional-echocardiography, 24-hour Holter monitoring for arrhythmias, and possibly cardiac catheterization. Patients should have serial orthostatic blood pressure measurements to document a decrease in blood pressure or increase in heart rate with postural changes, which is associated with orthostatic syncope.

Discussion

Bradycardias are caused by two problems: disease of the sinus node or disease of the conduction system. *The sinus node* is the pacemaker of the heart. The electrical impulse that generates the heart beat arises in the sinus node. Disease of the sinus node, therefore, can result in the lack of sufficient electrical impulses (and thus a lack of sufficient heart beats) to maintain the body's needs. Sinus node disease that leads to symptoms caused by a slow heart rate is called *sick sinus syndrome*. Most sinus node disease is related to simple deterioration in sinus node function caused by aging. Likewise, tachyarrhythmias caused by Wolff-Parkinson-White syndrome or prolonged-QT syndrome can also lead to insufficient cardiac output and syncope.

Treatment

In the case of syncope, diagnosis is the most difficult part. The treatment is only as effective as the diagnosis is correct. In the case of vasovagal syncope, treatment often is not required.

Orthostatic hypotension can be treated by avoiding hypovolemia, electrolyte imbalance, and excess alcohol intake. If this is not enough increased salt intake and fludrocortisone can be recommended. If orthostasis is related to venous pooling in the legs, fitted elastic hose can enhance the venous return and cardiac output. Obviously, if seizures were found to be the cause of the syncope, they have to be treated with appropriate antiepileptic medications, and the patient needs to be referred to as epileptologist for further evaluation. Tachyarrhythmias are treated with variety of antiarrhythmic drugs, the discussion of which is beyond this case. Sick sinus syndrome, if symptomatic, is often treated with permanent pacing, to avoid an onset of fatal arrhythmia or sinus arrest.

Comprehension Questions

[16.1] A 22-year-old nursing student passes out when observing a woman giving birth.

    A. Seizure
    B. Vasovagal syncope
    C. Orthostatic hypotension
    D. Cardiogenic syncope

[16.2] A 17-year-high school football player passes out on the field while running practice sprints.

    A. Vasovagal syncope
    B. Exertional syncope
    C. Seizure
    D. Orthostatic hypotension

[16.3] A 43-year-old woman with history of previous brain trauma is found unconsciousness in her home by a visiting neighbor. She has urinated on herself, and there is a small amount of blood and saliva coming from the side of her mouth.

    A. Cardiogenic syncope
    B. Vasovagal syncope
    C. Seizure
    D. Orthostatic hypotension

Answers

[16.1] **B.** This is most likely caused by a vasovagal reflex (drop in blood pressure) in response to painful or emotionally charged stimulus and is usually non–life threatening.

[16.2] **B.** Exertional syncope is caused by insufficient cardiac output necessary to meet exertional demands. This is usually caused by cardiac outflow obstruction often associated with aortic or subaortic stenosis and requires an echocardiogram.

[16.3] **C.** Seizure is the most likely diagnosis given a prior history of brain trauma, which can predispose to a seizure focus. Although clinical signs such as incontinence and tongue laceration are not specific for seizure, in the context of a possible cerebral focus, seizure is the most appropriate answer.

CLINICAL PEARLS

❖ It is prudent to ask for clarification when the patient complains of "dizziness."

❖ Vertigo and lightheadedness should be differentiated because their evaluations are very different.

❖ Lightheadedness often includes dimmed vision, nausea, palpitations, and diaphoresis before syncope.

❖ Tongue biting and urinary incontinence is not pathognomonic for seizure activity, nor does the absence of those signs exclude epileptic seizures.

REFERENCES

Armour A, Ardell J. Basic and clinical neurocardiology. Oxford: Oxford University Press; 2004.

Kosinski DJ, Wolfe DA, Grubb BP. Neurocardiogenic syncope: a review of pathophysiology, diagnosis and treatment. Cardiovasc Rev Rep 1993;14:22–29.

Linzer M, Yang EH, Estes NA 3rd, et al. Diagnosing syncope. Part 1: value of history, physical examination, and electrocardiography. Clinical Efficacy Assessment Project of the American College of Physicians. Ann Intern Med 1997 Jun 15; 126(12):989–996.

Linzer M, Yang EH, Estes NA 3rd, et al. Diagnosing syncope. Part 2: unexplained syncope. Clinical Efficacy Assessment Project of the American College of Physicians. Ann Intern Med 1997 Jul 1;127(1):76–86.

A 23-year-old graduate student was studying late at night for an examination, telling his friends that he was not at all worried about his forthcoming examinations. Suddenly, he stood from his chair, stared at the wall, and fell to the floor, his arms and legs uncontrollably shaking. He complained during this episode that he was hurting. He then began mumbling incoherently. He was never incontinent of urine or stool and did not bite his tongue. His friends were able to escort him to the bed, following which he stared vacuously, continually asking where he was and who they were. His friends took him to the emergency room.

◆ **What is the most likely diagnosis?**

◆ **What is the next diagnostic step?**

◆ **What is the most likely useful consultation?**

ANSWERS TO CASE 17: Pseudoseizure

Summary: A 23-year-old man suddenly "seized" in all four extremities, remained conscious, complaining about pain and querying his surroundings.

◆ **Most likely diagnosis:** Pseudoseizure.

◆ **Next diagnostic step:** See a physician. Have a careful neurologic assessment and psychiatric assessment as well. Blood studies, brain imaging, electroencephalograph (EEG), and EEG monitoring may need to be obtained.

◆ **Consultation:** Initiate interaction with psychiatrist and recognize that patients with pseudoseizures may also have associated bona fide seizures.

Analysis

Objectives

1. Know diagnostic approach to pseudoseizures.
2. Understand that pseudoseizures reflect psychodynamic issues and can be associated with bona fide organic seizures.

Considerations

Pseudoseizures are one of the most misunderstood areas in neurology. A good example that helps clarify this situation is asthma. Patients with asthma can become upset and develop an asthmatic attack. Or, they can make themselves agitated and bring on an asthmatic attack. And, they can feign asthmatic symptoms. Similarly, patients, with epilepsy can have emotional angst that prompts a seizure, they can feign a seizure, and they can also have psychiatric disturbance in which they are not "pretending" to seize but have characteristics of seizure that are nonphysiologic. The patient in this case is having four-extremity motor activity yet is wide awake and aware of his surroundings. This level of consciousness is inconsistent with bilateral cerebral hemisphere epileptic activity.

APPROACH TO PSEUDOSEIZURES

Definitions

Pseudoseizures: An attack resembling an epileptic seizure but having purely psychological causes; it lacks the electroencephalographic characteristics of epilepsy and the patient may be able to stop it by an act of will.
Malingering: Intentional production of false or exaggerated symptoms motivated by external incentives, such as obtaining compensation or drugs, avoiding work or military duty, or evading criminal prosecution. Malingering is not considered a mental illness.

Clinical Approach

Etiologies and Clinical Presentation

Hysterical attacks have been described by Briquet (1887), Charcot (1887–1889), and Breuer and Freud (1895). There are multiple theories, spawning the advent of psychiatry, and recently intertwined with numerous overlapping neurologic theories. Originally termed hysterical seizures, these attacks are associated with loss of impulse, especially in stressful situations, and were formerly (and erroneously) defined as only involving women. Current knowledge reveals that these "spells" are more common in young adults and in female adolescents.

The attacks often consist of storms of movements that are difficult to define precisely. Patients may arch their backs, engage in bizarre movements, and can have pelvic movements as well. **Rotatory head movements**, kicking, and bicycling movements can also occur. Patients can experience episodes of loss of consciousness, twitching or jerking, and unusual emotional states, such as intense feelings of fear or déjà vu. The episodes can last 20 minutes, but are **not associated** with **electrical abnormalities** in the brain as is the case with epileptic seizures. Most investigators agree that falls during these psychogenic attacks never physically traumatize the patient. Tongue biting and urinary incontinence can occur but are not common.

Pseudoseizure has been equated with psychogenic seizures. In some series, approximately 1–2% of patients with pseudoseizures also had bona fide organic seizures. Pseudoseizures should not be confused with malingering, which can be very difficult to separate. The boundaries between conscious and subconscious behavior in psychogenic seizures can be difficult to detect. True malingerers can prove quite resourceful in pretending to have focal abnormalities on examination, even producing voluntary Babinski signs. Even for trained medical professionals, the differences between epileptic seizures and pseudoseizures are difficult to recognize. Physicians believe pseudoseizures are psychologic defense mechanisms induced by stress or episodes of severe emotional trauma. The seizures happen when patients try to avoid or forget the trauma. It is not at all uncommon that patients referred to an epilepsy center, after monitoring, turn out to have pseudoseizures. The diagnosis of nonepileptic seizures has become more prevalent with a better understanding of the psychologic issues related to these events and correlation of these changes with normal brain activity. It is important for the physician to recognize that these patients are often calling for help, and it is inappropriate to view them as "crocks" or feel anger toward them, thinking that they might be trying to "fake out" the doctor.

Certainly, a thorough history and neurologic examination are important, as are EEG recordings and brain imaging. In difficult cases, ongoing EEG monitoring might be necessary, to assess brain physiological function and processing during the episode. Psychiatric assessment is also very important. **A good rule is that bilateral seizure activity without confusion or unconscious** (i.e., able to talk coherently to the examiner while their arms and legs are shaking),

is rarely organic. This is because bilateral seizure activity in the brain is usually associated with altered consciousness because both hemispheres in the brain are compromised.

Pseudoseizures should be queried when a patient with seizures has a normal neurologic evaluation/assessment (often including normal EEG monitoring during the seizure), and the seizures are not only refractory to treatment but are also influencing family members and impacting the patient's life (this can also occur in organic seizures) in areas with psychodynamic meaning/ importance.

Treatment

The earlier in the syndrome the patient is diagnosed, the better the chances for complete recovery, however, diagnosing and treating this disorder is not easy. The diagnosis requires an inpatient admission where the patient is continuously monitored by both an EEG and video camera. Both the EEG readings and tapes are scanned by medical professionals. On diagnosis, patients receive an outline for treatment. This plan includes a discussion of the illness with the patient, termination of anticonvulsant medicines, which are sedating and worsen the problem, and counseling services. Many patients are also treated for depression or anxiety. A multidisciplinary approach is the best management for patients to help resolve both the old and new stresses in their lives, and a significant portion of the patient's symptoms can be eliminated.

Comprehension Questions

[17.1] A 35-year-old man is suspected to have pseudoseizure. Which of the following is the best method to confirm the diagnosis?

    A. Resting EEG monitoring
    B. Initiation of anti-epileptic therapy and observation
    C. Psychiatric evaluation
    D. Video EEG monitoring

[17.2] A 23-year-old man is noted to have tonic-clonic activity while yelling and screaming for a fire extinguisher. Which of the following is the most likely etiology?

    A. Malingering
    B. Psychological defense mechanism to a significant traumatic event
    C. Hypertensive encephalopathy
    D. Complex partial seizure

[17.3] Which of the following is the best evidence of pseudoseizure?

    A. Cocaine found on urine drug screen
    B. Oxygen saturation level of 80%
    C. Alert with generalized (bilateral) convulsions
    D. History of diabetes mellitus

Answers

[17.1] **D.** Up to 1–3% of patients with pseudoseizures have true, organic epilepsy. This is why patients often require invasive and/or noninvasive video EEG monitoring to determine whether true epileptic events are present. For the vast majority of patients with pseudoseizures, termination of anti-epileptic therapy is recommended.

[17.2] **B.** Pseudoseizure, like many psychoneurological syndromes, has psychological origin and is often associated with a past history of a significant emotional or physical traumatic life event(s).

[17.3] **C.** Generalized convulsions or bilateral convulsions are typically associated with loss of consciousness or significantly impaired alteration of consciousness, which can last several minutes after the ictal event.

CLINICAL PEARLS

❖ Pseudoseizures should be considered when patients bilaterally "seize" but maintain normal consciousness.

❖ Sexual abuse and head injury are important risk factors of pseudoseizures, reported in approximately one-third of patients.

❖ Asthma has been reported in 26.5% of pseudoseizure patients.

❖ Pseudoseizures can coexist with organic seizures in up to 3% of patients.

❖ Pseudoneurologic syndromes mimic almost any neurologic disease. Presenting syndromes can include pseudoparalysis, pseudosensory syndromes, pseudoseizures, pseudocoma, psychogenic movement disorders, and pseudoneuro-ophthalmologic syndromes.

REFERENCES

Bazil CW, Morrell MJ, Pedley TA. Epilepsy. In: Rowland LP, ed. Merritt's neurology, 11th ed. Philadelphia, PA: Lippincott Williams & Wilkins; 2005:990–1014.

Neidermeyer E. Nonepileptic attacks. In: Niedermeyer E, Lopes da Silva F, eds. Electroencephalography: basic principles, clinical applications, and related fields, 5th ed. Philadelphia: Lippincott Williams & Wilkins; 2005:621–630.

de Wet CJ, Mellers JD, Gardner WN, Toone BK. Pseudoseizures and asthma. J Neurol Neurosurg Psychiatry 2003 May;74(5):639–641.

University of Michigan. Adult health advisor: seizures. Available at: http://www.med.umich.edu/11ibr/aha/aha_seizure_crs.htm. Updated 2005.

A 24-year-old white female has a 12-year history of headaches. These headaches started in grade school, and the patient remembers missing school with her headaches. Typically, she gets one of these headaches one to two times per month. The headache starts over the right eye, and the headache is usually preceded by flashing lights and zigzag lines. Once the headache occurs, there is extreme nausea and vomiting, and the patient goes into a dark room to minimize her head pain. Generally, the headache lasts 4 to 6 hours, but the patient feels tired and listless for the next 24 hours. The patient feels that the headache worsens with her menstrual cycle, and certain foods especially red wine can exacerbate her headache. Her general and neurologic examinations are normal.

◆ **What is the most likely diagnosis?**

◆ **What is the next diagnostic step?**

◆ **What is the next step in therapy?**

ANSWERS TO CASE 18: Migraine Headache

Summary: A 24-year-old white female has a 12-year history of monthly headaches that started in grade school. The headache starts over the right eye and is preceded by flashing lights and zigzag lines. Once the headache occurs, there is extreme nausea and vomiting, and the patient goes into a dark room to help with her head pain. Generally, the headache lasts 4 to 6 hours, and worsens with menses and certain foods.

◆ **Most Likely Diagnosis:** Migraine headaches

◆ **Next Diagnostic Step:** MRI of the head

◆ **Next Step in Therapy:** Consider use of medications such as one of the triptans to help treat the headaches

Analysis

Objectives

1. Know how to recognize a migraine headache and be able to distinguish it from headaches of other etiologies.
2. Understand what medications are available to treat migraine headaches.
3. Be familiar with a workup for headaches and also be aware of other clinical disorders, which have headache as a prominent feature.

Considerations

When evaluating a patient for headache, the clinical history is of critical importance. The nature (type of pain and associated symptoms or triggers), severity, and duration of the headache is important in determining what type of headache it is and how to manage it. In this case, the patient has a prior history of headaches characterized as episodic and associated with nausea and vomiting, sensitivity to light (photophobia) and sound (phonophobia). Her examinations have been normal, and therefore, her clinical history is highly suggestive of a vascular or migrainous headache.

APPROACH TO MIGRAINE HEADACHES

Definitions

Migraine with aura: Formally referred to as **classic migraine**, in which the migraine begins with visual, auditory, smell, or taste disturbances 5 to 30 minutes before pain onset.

Migraine without aura: Formally referred to as **common migraine**, which is not typically associated with an aura.

Clinical Approach

The prevalence of migraine varies from 0.5–2% in the adult population. The sex distribution of migraine in children is approximately 1:1 but in adults, women predominate in a ratio of 3:1. It is thought that 24 million Americans suffer from migraine, 18 million females and 6 million males. Of migraineurs, 25% report greater than four attacks per month; 35% experience two to three attacks per month; and 40% have a single attack per month. Older literature has divided migraine into two large subgroups, common and classic migraine. Common migraine is now called migraine without aura, and classic migraine is now referred as migraine with aura. Migraine with aura approximates 25% of the entire migraine group.

Clinical Characteristics

Prodrome   The prodrome of migraine consists of nonspecific phenomenon that can occur days but more often hours before the actual head pain. These symptoms can be more mental such as depression, euphoria, and irritability or more constitutional such as increased urination, defecation, anorexia, or fluid retention. Often photophobia, phonophobia, and hyperosmia accompany the prodrome.

Aura   An aura or a prodrome can precede the actual head pain, but an aura is differentiated from a prodrome in that an aura is often associated with frank neurologic dysfunction usually transient in nature. Migraine with aura occurs in approximately 25% of migraine attacks. The aura can be seen from 5 minutes to 1 hour prior to the head pain. It is uncommon to have the aura occur simultaneously with the headache. Visual auras are the most common and include scotomas, teichopsias, fortification spectra, photopsias, and distortion of images. Sensory auras such as numbness and tingling in a limb are second most common, and aphasia and hemiparesis occur less often.

Headache Pain   The headache pain in migraine occurs unilaterally in 65% of migraineurs. It is usually located in the periorbital region and can extend to the cheek and ear. The pain can switch from side to side with different headaches. Migraine pain can occur in any place of the head and neck, including the posterior strap muscles of the cervical area. Typically, the head pain lasts at least 4 to 8 hours but can last for several days although this is rare. The quality of the pain can be mild to severe and usually has a pulsating and throbbing quality. The patient often is troubled by associated symptoms, which can occur with the actual head pain. These include nausea and vomiting, photophobia, and phonophobia and can be more disabling to the patient than the actual head pain.

Evaluation of the Migraine Patient

The evaluation of a migraine headache begins with a complete history and physical examination. If the history is consistent with the typical characteristics of migraine and the neurologic examination is normal then appropriate medication can be prescribed before any testing is undertaken. Caution is exercised if either the history is atypical (i.e., migraines in a male beginning after age 50) or if the neurologic examination is abnormal. If the physician feels that a workup is necessary then diagnostic studies can include: (1) routine blood studies, (2) sedimentation rate, (3) spinal fluid examination, and (4) an imaging study.

Routine Blood Studies

There are several systemic illnesses, which are associated with headaches. These include vasculitis, toxic exposures, metabolic diseases, severe hypertension, and infectious diseases. Routine blood chemistries (chemistry panel and complete blood count [CBC]), HIV testing, vasculitis screen, thyroid function studies, and serum protein electrophoresis can be ordered as part of a routine blood study screening.

Sedimentation Rate

In **headache patients who are older than 60 years of age, temporal arteritis** should be considered. Temporal arteritis is a granulomatous arteritis affecting medium and large sized arteries of the upper part of the body especially the temporal vessels of the head. The headaches are often precipitous and can be accompanied by complaints of pain and stiffness in the neck, shoulders, back, and sometimes in the pelvic girdle. The head pain is usually one-sided and in the temporal region. The major complication of temporal arteritis is unilateral loss of vision. In addition to the clinical story, ancillary data which helps make a diagnosis of temporal arteritis includes an elevated sedimentation rate and a positive temporal artery biopsy. If a firm diagnosis is made, a course of oral steroids is the treatment of choice.

Lumbar Puncture

A lumbar puncture (LP) should be considered in patients in whom new onset headaches are associated with either fever, stiff neck, or altered mental status. If the diagnostic considerations include subarachnoid hemorrhage or pseudotumor cerebri, a spinal tap should also be considered. If the LP is being done in a workup of headache, then the patient should have a scan performed before the LP is completed except in those conditions where bacterial meningitis is a strong consideration. In those cases the LP should be done immediately unless there is evidence of papilledema.

Imaging Study

If the history and neurologic examination do not suggest any focal findings then it would be unusual to find an abnormality on an imaging study. If the physician feels that an imaging study is indicated, MRI of the brain is usually ordered although, a CT scan is often adequate to identify any space occupying lesion, shift in midline structures, brain herniation, or presence of subarachnoid blood. If a lumbar puncture (LP) is indicated in the workup of headache, then head imaging should be done prior to the lumbar puncture.

Headaches in Special Clinical Settings

There are several clinical settings where headaches play a prominent feature:

Postspinal Headaches

Approximately 25% of patients will have a headache after lumbar puncture. These headaches are often better when lying down and worsen with sitting or standing up and can be associated with nausea and vomiting. These can occur with either a traumatic or an atraumatic tap. They generally improve over time with bedrest and fluids but for those post LP headaches that do not improve, an epidural blood patch (small injection of the patient's blood injected into the epidural space) at the site of the original spinal tap can be helpful.

Postcoital Cephalgia

Postcoital cephalgia occurs both before and after orgasm. It is seen equally in men and women. The head pain is usually sudden, often pulsatile, and can involve the entire head. Fewer than 2% of patients who are seen with subarachnoid hemorrhage have the hemorrhage occur during intercourse. Therefore, a benign etiology of postcoital cephalgia is usually the case, and patients should be pretreated prior to sexual relations with medication, usually a simple analgesic.

Pseudotumor Cerebri

Pseudotumor cerebri (benign intracranial hypertension) is manifested by increased intercranial pressure without evidence of a CNS malignancy. Patients with benign intracranial hypertension complain primarily of headaches often associated with visual disturbances. Pseudotumor cerebri is usually seen in female patients who are obese and often have menstrual irregularities.

Acute Glaucoma

Acute glaucoma is often characterized by sudden orbital or eye pain in the face of nausea and vomiting. The pain can begin after the use of anticholinergic drugs. An elevated intraocular pressure is the hallmark of acute angle-closure glaucoma.

Carotid Dissection

Patients with carotid dissection, often present with orbital or neck pain associated with neurologic findings suggestive of carotid disease. A Horner syndrome (a constellation of signs produced when sympathetic innervation to the eye is interrupted) on the ipsilateral dissected carotid side, can accompany these symptoms. Trauma to the neck or vigorous movements to the neck will often trigger the dissection.

Brain Tumor

Headaches associated with brain tumors often present as typical tension or migraine headache. The headaches can be quite frequent and can occur on a daily basis, often awakening the patient from sleep. Neurologic examination can be normal but can reveal focal abnormalities as well as papilledema on funduscopic examination. Headaches are the presenting feature in approximately 40% of brain tumor patients.

Sinusitis

The issue of whether chronic sinusitis can contribute to headaches is often unclear. Patients incorrectly assume that head pain in and above the eye is from sinus disease, and in truth of fact the majority of these patients actually have migraine headaches.

Subarachnoid Hemorrhage

Subarachnoid hemorrhage occurs from the following: (1) leakage of an arteriovenous malformation, (2) leakage of a ruptured aneurysm, or (3) trauma. Patients with subarachnoid hemorrhage often present with a debilitating headache described as the worst headache of their lives. It is of sudden onset and can be associated with nausea, vomiting, and stiff neck. A subarachnoid hemorrhage can look like a migraine attack especially if there is extreme nausea and vomiting. Subarachnoid hemorrhage is associated with blood in the subarachnoid space, which is usually documented on MRI or CT scanning. A lumbar puncture will confirm subarachnoid hemorrhage, where frank blood or xanthochromic staining of the cerebrospinal fluid (CSF) is noted. Patients with subarachnoid hemorrhage can decompensate quickly, and 50% of patients do not survive their subarachnoid bleed.

Abortive Treatment of Migraine

The treatment of an individual migraine attack once it has occurred is referred to as abortive therapy. Currently there are four medications used in abortive therapy: (1) the triptans; (2) ergotamine; (3) dihydroergotamine; and (4) isometheptene mucate, dichloralphenazone, acetaminophen (Midrin) (Table 18–1).

Triptans

There are now seven medications referred to as **triptans that are currently state of the art in the abortive treatment of migraine.** These include suma-triptan (Imitrex), almotriptan (Axert), rizatriptan (Maxalt), zolmitriptan (Zomig), eletriptan (Relpax), naratriptan (Amerge), and frovatriptan (Frova).

Table 18–1
MIGRAINE CHARACTERISTICS

CHARACTERISTIC	MIGRAINE
Onset	Teenage to age 40 occurs anytime during day
Location of pain	Half of face; frontal, usually in or about eye or cheek
Precipitating factor	Fatigue, stress; hypoglycemia; diet (tyramine, alcohol); sunlight; hormonal change (menstruation)
Frequency of attack	2–4 per month or sporadically; can be cyclic with menstruation
Sex distribution	70% female 30% male
Duration of attack	Head pain 4 hours, aura to postdrome 24–36 hours
Pain type and severity	Begins as dull ache, progress to stabbing pain; intense
Associated symptoms	Nausea and vomiting; photophobia, visual obscuration

Each individual drug has different formulations; thus, these drugs are available in oral, nasal spray, and intramuscular formulations. The drugs work as 5HT-1D serotonin receptor agonists. These drugs are 80% effective in the treatment of an individual migraine attack. They should be used early in the headache often during the prodrome but can also be used once the headache has started. The drugs can be repeated as early as 4 hours in headache reoccurrence, but no more than three doses per 24 hours should be used. The side effect profile of the group of seven triptans is similar and include occasional **nausea, vomiting, and numbness and tingling of the fingers and toes.** Clearcut **contraindications to the use of triptans include a history of coronary artery disease or hypertension.** If the patient has hemiplegia or blindness as an aura in a migraine attack, then triptans should not be used.

Ergotamine Derivatives

Ergotamines are no longer the cornerstone of the abortive treatment of migraine. When patients fail triptans then ergotamines should be considered. Usually a 2 mg sublingual tablet is prescribed and repeated for two doses each separated by 30 minutes if necessary. This dose can be repeated three times per day. Ergotamines should not be prescribed on an ongoing daily basis for chronic usage.

Dihydroergotamine

An episodic migraine, which can become more chronic and intractable, can respond to intramuscular or intravenous dihydroergotamine (DHE). The initial dose of DHE is 0.5 mg intravenously with 10 mg of metoclopramide or 5 mg prochlorperazine if nausea is present. If the headache improves, the dosage of DHE plus metoclopramide is repeated for two more doses separated by 8 hours and then one more dose of DHE alone. Nasal DHE is now available and can be used in the abortive treatment of migraine. In some patients, the nasal spray can replace intramuscular or intravenous use.

Midrin

Midrin is a medication that spans the gap between abortive and prophylactic therapy. The drug consists of **three components; acetaminophen (a simple analgesic), dichloralphenazone (a muscle relaxant), and isometheptene mucate (a vasoconstrictor).** If Midrin is used in an abortive fashion, patients are instructed to take two tablets at the onset of a headache or aura, then one tablet hourly for three additional doses (five tablets total). The drug can also be used as a prophylactic agent for muscle tension headaches taking one tablet twice a day scheduled, and then a third or even a fourth pill for a breakthrough headache during that day.

Table 18–2

COMMON TRIGGERS OF MIGRAINE HEADACHES

Chocolate, cheese, red wine, citrus fruits, coffee, tea, tomatoes, potatoes, irregular meals

Excessive or insufficient sleep

Changes in hormone balance in women (such as menses, the pill, or the menopause)

Stress or relaxation after a period of stress

Caffeine withdrawal

Physical activity

Smoking

Flashing lights or noise

Weather—high pressure conditions, changes in pressure, hot dry winds, change of season, exposure to sun and glare

Sexual arousal

Smells—paint, fumes from car heaters or perfume

Prophylactic Treatment of Migraine

Prophylactic therapy is used when there are at least three attacks per month, or if acute therapy is not effective. There are currently several classes of medication, used in the prophylactic treatment of migraine. These include anticonvulsants (topiramate [Topamax], divalproex [Depakote], and gabapentin [Neurontin]) beta-blockers (propranolol [Inderal]), calcium channel blockers (verapamil) and antidepressants (duloxetine [Cymbalta], amitriptyline [Elavil], and nortriptyline [Pamelor]). Other medications used in migraine prevention, but clearly now second-line agents include methysergide maleate (Sansert), lithium carbonate, clonidine, captopril, and monoamine oxidase inhibitors. Currently anticonvulsants are prescribed most frequently in the prophylactic treatment of migraine. The most common drug now prescribed is topiramate (Topamax). Side effects include sleepiness, numbness and tingling in the fingers and toes, and rarely blindness in one eye secondary to increased intraocular pressure. Divalproex (Depakote) has also been used successfully to treat migraine, starting out at a dose of 250 mg extended release (ER) at night for 1 week, followed by sequential increase in dosage each week if headaches do not come under control. Side effects include alopecia and tremor.

Beta-Blockers

Beta-blockers have been used in the prophylactic treatment of migraine since 1972. The most commonly prescribed beta-blocker is propranolol (Inderal).

The long-acting (LA) form is often prescribed, and the dose is usually increased until the blood pressure drops to 100/60 mmHg, and the pulse drops to 60 beats/min. Once a beta-blocker has been instituted, there can be a slight decrease in blood pressure and pulse. The major side effects seen with beta-blockers are depression, fatigue, alopecia, bradycardia, cold extremities, and postural dizziness. From a practical standpoint, in a population of migraineurs that is generally young and female, beta-blockers are often difficult to tolerate and are used when other groups of medications have failed.

Comprehension Questions

For each clinical presentation [18.1] to [18.4], choose the most appropriate diagnosis from the following list:

A. Subarachnoid headache
B. Sinusitis
C. Post-LP headache
D. Carotid dissection
E. Pseudotumor cerebri
F. Migraine with aura
G. Migraine without aura

[18.1] A 38-year-old man presents with right-sided neck pain and left-sided numbness of face, arm, and leg after a chiropractic manipulation of his neck.

[18.2] A 37-year-old woman presents with nasal congestion and post-nasal drip, complaining of bilateral pain above and around her eyes.

[18.3] A 21-year-old college student studying for final examinations complains of recurrent right temple pain, preceded by flashing lights, and followed by nausea lasting 3–5 hours.

[18.4] A 54-year-old man underwent a spinal tap 2 days prior for evaluation of foot numbness. He now complains a significant headache and nausea when he rises from a supine (lying flat) to an upright position.

Answers

[18.1] **D.** Carotid dissection is the most likely explanation in this case.

[18.2] **B.** Sinusitis is likely caused by the nasal congestion and can cause a frontal or maxillary headache.

[18.3] **F.** This is the typical presentation of migraine with aura.

[18.4] **C.** Post-LP headache is likely caused by the proximal relationship to the lumbar puncture.

CLINICAL PEARLS

❖ Rarer types of migraines include **hemiplegic** migraine (temporary stroke-like symptoms), **ophthalmoplegic** migraine (eye pain and oculomotor weakness), **basilar artery** migraine (dizziness, confusion, or lack of balance), **retinal** migraine (eye pain and vision loss), and **abdominal** migraine (abdominal pain, nausea, vomiting, and diarrhea).

❖ For women whose headaches have been closely linked with their menstrual periods, menopause can result in improvement in headaches, although it is rare for them to disappear entirely.

❖ In women experiencing spontaneous menopause, migraine headache improves in 67%, is unchanged in 24%, and worsens in 9%.

❖ Approximately 80% of people who get migraine headaches have a family history of migraine, which implicates genetics in susceptibility.

REFERENCES

Derman H. In: Current neurology, vol. 14. St. Louis: Mosby; 1994:179.

Saper, JR, Silberstein SD, Gordon CD, et al. Handbook of headache management, a practical guide to diagnosis and treatment of head, neck, and facial pain. Baltimore: Williams & Wilkins; 1993.

Silberstein, SD, Lipton RB, Goadsby PJ. Headache in clinical practice. London: Martin Dunitz; 2002.

A 38-year-old white female has a history of headaches for at least 10 years. The headaches now occur on a daily basis. They are of mild to moderate pain. Usually, the pain is located in the temples and often radiates to the neck. The patient also reports a different headache approximately three times per month that is located over one eye and is often associated with nausea, vomiting, photophobia, and phonophobia. These headaches are often worse during her menstrual cycle. The patient has a prior history of episodic migraine beginning in her 20s. They initially occurred one to three times per year, but then progressed to as much as one to three times per week. The patient has tried many over-the-counter (OTC) medications for her headaches and has used acetaminophen (Tylenol), aspirin, caffeine (Excedrin Migraine), ibuprofen, and naproxen sodium (Aleve) with regularity. She is currently taking three acetaminophen (Tylenol) every 4 hours and still gets a headache. She notes that when these headaches began, 2 acetaminophen (Tylenol) usually relieved the headache, but now even the 18 acetaminophen (Tylenol) per day do not impact her headache. Her general examination is within normal limits. Her neurological examination does not reveal neck stiffness or muscle rigidity, abnormal reflexes, weakness, or sensory changes.

◆ **What is the most likely diagnosis?**

◆ **What is the most likely next diagnostic step?**

◆ **What is the likely next step in therapy?**

ANSWERS TO CASE 19: Chronic Headache

Summary: A 38-year-old white female has a 10-year history of daily headaches, located in the temples and often radiating to the neck. The patient also reports a different headache approximately three times per month, which occurs over one eye and is often associated with nausea, vomiting, photophobia, and phonophobia, exacerbated by menses. The patient has a prior history of episodic migraine beginning in her 20s. Numerous OTC medications including large acetaminophen doses are unhelpful. Her general examination and neurologic examination are within normal limits.

◆ **Most Likely Diagnosis:** Chronic daily headache with analgesic rebound

◆ **Next Diagnostic Step:** Neurologic examination

◆ **Next Step in Therapy:** Taper acetaminophen (Tylenol) usage and consider treatment with valproic acid or topiramate

Analysis

Objectives

1. Recognize chronic daily headache and be able to distinguish it from migraine and other causes of headache.
2. Know what treatments are available for chronic daily headache including both medications and nonmedication intervention.
3. Know what workup is necessary for patients with chronic daily headache.

Considerations

When evaluating a patient for headache, the clinical history is of critical importance. The nature (type of pain and associated symptoms or triggers), severity, and duration of the headache is important in determining what type of headache it is and how to manage it. In this case, the patient has a prior history of headaches. Her headaches are described as two types. She reports pain around her temples and neck which occurs daily; these symptoms seem to be consistent with a tension type of headache. She also has a frequently recurring headache that occurs on one side and is associated with nausea and vomiting, and sensitivity to light and sound, which is suggestive of a migraine headache. The duration of these headaches is over many years. Although she has increased frequency, the character of her headaches has not changed. Her examination is normal. Therefore, her headaches are unlikely due to other etiologies, such as tumor, infection, or trauma. Nevertheless, if the patient has not had imaging of the head recently, an MRI or CT scan would be prudent. The history gives a record of episodic migraines in the past, which have become chronic daily headaches, transiently responsive to OTC analgesics. Once chronic daily headache is confirmed and other etiologies such as infection and brain tumor are ruled out, tapering of the acetaminophen and initiation of another medication such as the seizure medication valproic acid seems to be helpful in these conditions.

APPROACH TO CHRONIC HEADACHE

Definitions

Vascular headache: A type of headache, including migraine, thought to involve abnormal function of the brain's blood vessels or vascular system.

Migraine headache: The most common type of vascular headache is migraine—headaches that are usually characterized by severe pain on one or both sides of the head, upset stomach, or disturbed vision.

Photophobia: Light sensitivity or an intolerance to light.

Phonophobia: Heightened sensitivity to sound.

Clinical Approach

The clinical entity chronic daily headache encompasses several headache syndromes. These include chronic migraine headache, chronic tension type headache, and new daily persistent headache. All of these entities can be complicated by analgesic abuse.

Chronic Migraine Headache

Chronic migraine most often is seen in women who have had a history of intermittent migraine, which usually began in their teens or twenties. The headaches become much more frequent over the years, and these chronic migraine headaches are usually not associated with the photophobia, phonophobia, or nausea. Even as these headaches become more chronic, many patients still have intermittent episodic migraine, and these breakthrough, random migraine headaches can be associated with nausea, vomiting, photophobia, and phonophobia. A significant number of chronic migraine patients suffer from underlying depression and anxiety. The entity of transformed migraine speaks to this change from episodic migraine to a picture of chronic daily headache. Thus, chronic migraine has the following characteristics: daily or almost daily headache greater than 15 days a month. The patient suffers from headaches at least 4 hours a day, and there is usually a history of episodic migraine during this chronic phase. This transformation to a more chronic picture usually takes place over a 3- to 6-month period of time.

Chronic Tension Type Headache

Patients with a history of episodic tension headaches can progress to a more chronic tension type headache. There is usually the absence of the typical features of migraine except for **nausea**, which is usually not associated with vomiting. The patient usually is affected more than 15 days a month, with an average headache duration of greater than 4 hours per day. The pain is usually in the **temporal region, described as a pressing or tightening, which is of mild to moderate severity.** It is often in a **hatband** distribution. There can be associated pain and tenderness in the occipital area as well as in the posterior strap muscles of the neck. These patients can also have an occasional breakthrough migraine headache, but the dominant headache is clearly the more frequent bitemporal headache.

New Daily Persistent Headache

New daily persistent headache is the **acute development of a daily headache** over a short period of time, usually **less than 3 days**. There can be a precipitating event, often an antecedent viral illness. Typically patients with new daily persistent headaches are younger than those with chronic migraine. Once the headache has begun, the average frequency is greater than 15 days per month of headache, and the headache duration is usually greater than 4 hours a day if untreated. There is no prior history of tension type or migraine headaches. The acute onset of headache which is present less than 3 days is critical in making the diagnosis. It is important to consider that all of the chronic daily headache types may be exacerbated by analgesic rebound, and a vigorous attempt should be made to get patients off all OTC analgesics.

Evaluation

Most patients with chronic daily headache have been seen by multiple physicians because of the chronicity of the headache. Imaging studies have typically been performed in the past and are normal; if unavailable, then an MRI/magnetic resonance angiography (MRA) should be done to evaluate for ischemia, intracranial pressure, or a space occupying lesion. Serum chemistries, complete blood count (CBC) with differential, thyroid panel, and a sedimentation rate should be drawn. A lumbar puncture after MRI clearance should be considered in those patients with headache of acute origin over a short period of time to rule out an infectious or inflammatory cause(s).

Treatment

Success rates in the treatment of chronic daily headache is approximately 30%; but most patients can get some improvement in their head pain. There are both medical and nonmedical treatments available, and both should be pursued especially if there is a significant neck component to these headaches.

Nonmedical Treatment

The nonmedical treatment of chronic daily headache includes **biofeedback, stress management, psychological interventions, and lifestyle changes.** Many patients can benefit from physical therapy by a head and neck rehabilitation specialist. Massage therapy has also been shown to be helpful in certain patients.

Medical Therapy

As noted previously, the first intervention in a plan of medical therapy for chronic daily headache is **removal of any OTC medications,** which can include either **acetaminophen or aspirin**. Simple analgesics as tramadol and propoxyphene without acetaminophen can be used judiciously as a bridge to new prophylactic therapy. **Preventative** medicines that have been successful in the treatment of chronic daily headache include anticonvulsants, antidepressants, and other drugs, which can be successful in migraine. The initial medication is **sodium valproate (Depakote ER)** starting at 250 mg at night increasing to 750 mg as indicated. Topiramate (Topamax) can also be helpful, starting at a dose of 50 mg at night increasing to 50 mg twice a day over a 4 week period of time increasing the dose by 25 mg per week. Amitriptyline (Elavil) and nortriptyline (Pamelor) have also been helpful in chronic daily headache with dosing usually beginning at 25 mg or 50 mg at night and then increased to 100 mg as indicated. Beta-blockers such as propranolol (Inderal LA 80 mg) and calcium channel blockers such as verapamil (Isoptin SR 100 mg) have been used in chronic daily headache. Of all these medication groups, the anticonvulsants seem to be the most successful in the treatment of chronic daily headache. Recently, botulinum toxin injections have been used in chronic daily headache, especially in those patients with trigger points of head pain, or in those patients with significant cervical pain and spasm. The success rate of botulinum in some patients may approach 60%.

Comprehension Questions

[19.1] A 33-year-old woman is noted to have chronic daily headaches. The workup has been negative. Which of the following is an important principle in the management of this disorder?

    A. Maintain analgesic dose while using antiepileptic therapy
    B. Increase the analgesic dose while initiating biofeedback therapy
    C. Lower the analgesic dose while beginning other therapy
    D. Reassure the patient, and refer to psychiatrist

[19.2] A 33-year-old woman is noted to have daily severe headaches. Her physician prescribed botulinum toxin injections, which have been highly effective. Which of the following types of headaches is most likely to be present?

    A. Migraine vascular headache
    B. Cluster vascular headache
    C. Cervical muscle spasm
    D. Tension headache

[19.3] A 40-year-old woman comes into the physician's office with a 20-year history of headache nearly every day. She states that it is associated with some nausea. Acetaminophen (Tylenol) is helpful at times, although over the past 3 months, not as effective. The patient states that her doctors in the past have performed history and physical examinations and have found no problems. The neurologic examination is normal. Which of the following the best next step?

    A. Initiate beta-blocker
    B. Substitute aspirin for acetaminophen (Tylenol)
    C. CT imaging of the head
    D. Psychiatric evaluation

Answers

[19.1] **C.** Analgesic overuse often contributes to headache or migraines becoming chronic headaches. Therefore, the first intervention in a plan of medical therapy for chronic daily headache is removal of any OTC medications, which can include either acetaminophen or aspirin.

[19.2] **C.** At present, the anticonvulsants seem to be most effective in the treatment of chronic daily headache. Botulinum toxin injections have been used in chronic daily headache, especially in those patients with trigger points of head pain, or in those patients with significant cervical pain and spasm. Although, botulinum toxin injections is reported to be effective in the majority of patients, it is not considered first-line therapy.

[19.3] **C.** Although the majority of patients with chronic daily headache have relatively normal neuroimaging, any patient with recurrent or persistent headaches who has never been imaged, requires an MRI and/or MRA of the brain to evaluate for potential causes or exacerbating factors.

CLINICAL PEARLS

❖ Tension-type headaches, associated with a band-like constant bilateral pressure and pain from the forehead to the temples and to the neck, are the most common form of headache.

❖ Pseudotumor cerebri is a condition of increased cerebrospinal fluid pressure (overproduction or decreased absorption) associated with chronic headaches, often relieved with lumbar puncture.

❖ Disrupted sleep (hypersomnia or insomnia) is a very common trigger of headache and migraine.

❖ Transformed migraine is migraine disease that transforms into daily less severe headaches punctuated by severe and debilitating migraine attacks. Overuse of pain relievers is a major factor of transformed migraines.

REFERENCES

Derman H. In current neurology, vol. 14. St. Louis: Mosby; 1994:179.

Saper JR, Silberstein SD, Gordon CD, et al. Handbook of headache management, a practical guide to diagnosis and treatment of head, neck, and facial pain. Baltimore: Williams & Wilkins; 1993.

Silberstein SD, Lipton RB, Goadsby PJ. Headache in clinical practice. London: Martin Dunitz; 2002.

A 67-year-old woman was admitted to the hospital for extreme confusion and agitation. She had been doing reasonably well until 3–4 weeks prior to admission; however, her family says that her memory has been getting worse over the last 3 years. Initially she had problems remembering recent events and people's names and had a tendency to dwell in the past. She got lost several times driving, most recently in a familiar neighborhood. She has stopped cooking because she can no longer work her electric oven. Sometimes her words didn't make sense. Her social graces have remained preserved; however, and she is still quite pleasant to be around, although she tends to interact socially less and less. She still walks around the block every day, and her basic gait and coordination seems quite normal. Because she was crying intermittently recently, her family doctor began her on a progressively increasing dose of amitriptyline 1 month ago. Initially, she began sleeping well at night, but the last few days she was having visual hallucinations and shouting incoherently. On physical examination she was mildly tachycardic. She was inattentive and difficult to keep on task. She had numerous paraphasic errors but was otherwise fluent. Her neurologic examination was otherwise unremarkable.

◆ **What is the most likely diagnosis?**

◆ **What is the next diagnostic step?**

◆ **What is the next step in therapy?**

ANSWERS TO CASE 20: Alzheimer Dementia

Summary: A 67-year-old woman was admitted to the hospital for extreme confusion and agitation, but she has had short-term memory deficits over the last 3 years. She got lost several times driving, most recently in a familiar neighborhood. She has stopped cooking because she can no longer work her electric oven. Sometimes her words do not make sense. Her social graces have remained preserved; however, and she is still quite pleasant to be around, although she tends to interact socially less and less. Her gait seems normal. Because of depressive symptoms, she has been prescribed amitriptyline for 1 month. Initially, she began sleeping well at night, but the last few days she was having visual hallucinations and shouting incoherently. On physical examination she was mildly tachycardic. She was inattentive and difficult to keep on task. She had numerous paraphasic errors but was otherwise fluent. Her neurologic examination was otherwise unremarkable.

◆ **Most likely diagnosis:** Underlying dementia, probably Alzheimer disease, with superimposed delirium from amitriptyline

◆ **Next diagnostic step:** Discontinuation of amitriptyline, medical evaluation, and observation

◆ **Next step in therapy:** After observation and stabilization, consider treatment of underlying dementia

Analysis

Objectives

1. Understand the differentiation and differential diagnosis of different types of dementia.
2. Know the underlying pathophysiology of Alzheimer disease.
3. Understand the special susceptibilities of patients with dementia.

Considerations

This is case that has two main aspects to it: a several year history of apparent cognitive decline, and there is also a rather precipitous decline and agitation. The insidious onset and gradual progression is characteristic of degenerative disease, although other classes of diseases can sometimes mimic this time course. In this patient there has been decline of cognition but no change in fundamental neurologic function, that is, cranial nerves, motor, sensation, coordination, gait, and station. Preservation of long-term memory and profound deficits of short-term memory is typical. Thus, this is a disease that presents primarily as dementia. There is no presence of tremor or gait disturbance that can indicate Parkinson disease, or associated neurologic deficits of stroke. The differential diagnosis of dementia is extensive, and a thorough history and physical, brain imaging, and laboratory testing is in order.

The acute onset of agitation and delirium is likely caused by the antidepressant. This patient was administered amitriptyline for apparent depression. This is a tricyclic antidepressant but also has significant anticholinergic effects. It appears highly likely that she had a delirium superimposed on her dementia that was precipitated by amitriptyline. By virtue of her underlying condition, she was particularly susceptible to this event. With many conditions, and this is especially true of Alzheimer disease (AD), the effects of therapeutic agents are relatively modest, but can be of most help to patients by avoiding doing harm by administering medications that can make them worse. As AD progresses, a variety of behavioral problems ensue. Among these are disruptive behaviors, wandering, disinhibition, and agitation. In the differential diagnosis of dementia is the syndrome of pseudodementia caused by depressive syndromes. Some of the characteristics of depressive pseudodementia include manifestations of depressive syndromes such as withdrawal from social behaviors, disruption of the sleep wake cycle, and altered eating behavior. These are items that are common in depression rating scales, but are nonspecific and can be seen in demented patients without depression. A good behavioral clue to pseudodementia versus true dementia is the type of answers given on mental status testing. Whereas patients with mild dementias make "near misses" such as being a little off on the year or the month, patients with pseudodementia tend to respond with "I don't know." It is important to get patients to answer your questions. Patients with AD often know they are failing and so may not answer to avoid embarrassment. It is important to make the patient feel comfortable so one can get a handle on the qualitative aspects of the dementia. Depression is common, and the threshold to treat is currently very low. Antidepressants, however, do not improve patients with AD who do not have depression. In addition, these patients are susceptible to the side effects, especially of the older drugs with less pharmacologic specificity.

In this patient, the first order of business is to make sure she is medically stable. In addition, she should be checked for other causes of delirium including metabolic and pharmacologic agents as well as vitamin and hormonal deficiencies. Her amitriptyline should be discontinued, and she should be observed. She should improve and reach a stable baseline. At this point she can be examined more closely as to the nature of her dementia with imaging and cerebrospinal fluid (CSF) studies as indicated by the clinical picture. If she is felt to be depressed, she can be treated with a relatively specific selective serotonin reuptake inhibitor (SSRI). Treatment with an anticholinesterase such as Donepezil, which has been shown to delay disease progression, would be appropriate at this point. Memantine, an NMDA receptor antagonist, can also be considered since it has benefit in moderate stages of AD. Dementia is a prolonged disorder; it does not change overnight, and there is no need to treat it with the timing and urgency of a cardiac arrest. These patients can be very sensitive to the deleterious effect of medications. Medication should be titrated carefully, and two drugs should never be started at once.

APPROACH TO ALZHEIMER DEMENTIA

Definitions

Delirium: A transient, usually reversible, cause of cerebral dysfunction that manifests clinically with a wide range of neuropsychiatric abnormalities. The clinical hallmarks are decreased attention span and a waxing and waning type of confusion.

Paraphasic errors: The production of unintended syllables, words, or phrases during the effort to speak.

Nucleus basalis of Meynert: A group of nerve cells that has wide projections to the neocortex and is rich in acetylcholine and choline acetyltransferase.

Pseudodementia: A severe form of depression resulting from a progressive brain disorder in which cognitive changes mimic those of dementia.

Dementia: Impairment of memory and at least one other cognitive function (e.g., language, visual-spatial orientation, judgement) without alteration in consciousness; representing a decline from previous level of ability, and interfering with daily functioning and independent living.

Alzheimer disease: The leading cause of dementia, accounting for half of the cases involving elderly individuals, correlating to diffuse cortical atrophy and hippocampal atrophy with ventricular enlargement. The pathologic changes in the brains of AD patients include neurofibrillary tangles with a deposition of abnormal amyloid in the brain.

Multi-infarct dementia: Dementia in the setting of cerebrovascular disease, occurring after multiple cerebral infarctions, whether large or small (lacunar).

Approach to Dementia

Dementias can be characterized and categorized in a number of ways. One way is cortical versus subcortical. The features of both types of dementia are listed in **Table 20–1** and a differential diagnosis in **Table 20–2**. **Cortical dementias** tend to have involvement of cognitive functions while basic neurologic function is preserved. Language is affected although speech articulation is generally not. These differences diminish in later stages of the dementia, however. Cortical dementias can also be subdivided into **anterior and posterior** varieties. Anterior cortical dementia is typified by frontotemporal dementia. When the anterior half of the cortex is affected, it tends to produce problems with behavior, executive dysfunction. Patients can lose their social graces early while having memory and intellectual functions relatively preserved. Posterior cortical dementias tend to lose intellectual function while preserving social graces. **The prototype for posterior cortical dementias is Alzheimer disease.** This disorder almost invariably shows early involvement of recent memory, with language dysfunction (aphasia),

Table 20–1

CLINICAL CHARACTERISTICS OF CORTICAL AND SUBCORTICAL
DEMENTIAS

CHARACTERISTIC	CORTICAL	SUBCORTICAL
Verbal output		
Language	Aphasic	Normal
Speech	Normal	Abnormal (hypophonic, dysarthric, mute)
Mental Status		
Memory	Amnesia (learning deficit)	Forgetful (retrieval deficit)
Cognition	Abnormal (acalculia, poor judgement, impaired abstraction)	Abnormal (slowed, dilapidated)
Visuospatial	Abnormal	Abnormal
Affect	Abnormal (unconcerned or disinhibited)	Abnormal (apathetic or depressed)
Motor system		
Posture	Normal	Abnormal
Tone	Normal	Usually increased
Movements	Normal	Abnormal (tremor, chorea, asterixis, dystonia)
Gait	Normal	Abnormal

and apraxia and agnosia. When the Mini Mental State Examination (MMSE) is performed, delayed recall is generally affected first and even in mild dementia patients get 0/3 on the delayed recall task. **Olfaction** is the only "lower neurological function" that is shown to be reliably impaired even in early Alzheimer disease.

Of tremendous practical importance is the fact that virtually all dementias that are treatable for cure or at least may be amenable to slowed progression are **subcortical dementias.**

Alzheimer Disease is a degenerative disorder first described by Alois Alzheimer, who described the clinical presentation and the characteristic histologic changes consisting of **amyloid plaques and neurofibrillary tangles** (Fig. 20–1). The amyloid plaques stain positively with antibodies to amyloid precursor protein. AD can be caused by a variety of factors. There are known mutations in the amyloid precursor protein as well as two homologous proteins, presenilin-1 and presenilin-2 that tend to present with early-onset disease. In the past, AD was considered presenile dementia with onset younger than 65 years of age, however all age presentations are now considered as dementia of the Alzheimer type. Interference with metabolism of amyloid precursor protein is considered a critical step in the pathophysiology of AD. There are several

Table 20–2
CLASSIFICATION OF DEMENTIA BASED ON CORTICAL OR
SUBCORTICAL DYSFUNCTION

Cortical Dementias	Dementias with Combined Cortical and Subcortical Dysfunction
Alzheimer disease	Multi-infarct dementias
Frontal temporal dementias	Prion diseases
Pick disease (frontotemporal variant)	
Semantic dementia (temporal variant)	
Progressive nonfluent aphasia	
Subcortical Dementias	
Dementia with parkinsonism	Syphilis (general paresis)
Parkinson disease	Toxic/Metabolic encephalopathies
Huntington disease	Systemic illnesses
Progressive supranuclear palsy	Endocrinopathies
Multiple system atrophies	Deficiency states (B_{12})
Neurodegeneration with brain iron accumulation	Drug intoxications
Hydrocephalus	Heavy metal exposure
Dementia syndrome of depression	Industrial dementias
White matter diseases	Misc. dementia syndromes
Multiple sclerosis	Posttraumatic
HIV encephalopathy	Postanoxic
Vascular dementias	Neoplastic
Subcortical ischemic vascular disease	Mass lesions
Lacunar state	Paraneoplastic
Binswanger disease	
CADASIL	
Radiation-induced leukoencephalopathy	Corticobasal degeneration
	Dementia with Lewy bodies

CADASIL, cerebral autosomal dominant arteriopathy with subcortical infarcts and leukoencephalopathy.

studies now demonstrating that CSF Aβ1–42 is decreased whereas τ protein is increased in AD. This finding is diagnostically fairly specific but not very sensitive. Apolipoprotein protein E (APO-E) is involved in cholesterol metabolism and can play a role in amyloid metabolism. There are three main haplotypes for this protein and type ϵ4 is a risk factor for AD. It is possible to order an APO-E genotype from commercial laboratories. It is important to note however that the presence APO-E ϵ4 is only a risk factor and does not prove AD.

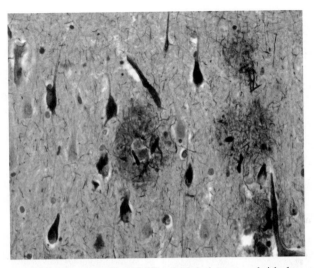

Figure 20–1. Photomicrograph (B&W) of Alzheimer amyloid plaque and neurofibrillary tangle. *(With permission from Ropper AH, Brown RH. Adams and Victor's principles of neurology, 8th ed. New York: McGraw-Hill; 2005: Fig. 39–1; 2006.)*

Imaging studies typically show cortical atrophy, especially the parietal and temporal cortices, with hippocampal atrophy. As a correlate, functional imaging studies show hypometabolism in the temporal and parietal cortices (Fig. 20–2A). There seems to be particular **degeneration of the cholinergic cells that project to the cortex from the basal forebrain**, particularly the nucleus basalis of Meynert. The main approach to enhancing cognition in patients with AD is by trying to **enhance cholinergic function by the administration of inhibitors of acetylcholinesterase** that penetrate the CNS. One of the consequences of cholinergic loss is also extreme sensitivity to the deleterious effects of anticholinergic medications.

Differential Diagnosis

If cognitive decline occurs with prominent mood disturbance, then one consideration is **depression** or pseudodementia. It is often difficult to distinguish which occurred first, because many elderly patients with cognitive decline and declining level of independent functioning suffer from a reactive depression. History from involved family members of the onset of symptoms, or history of prior depression or other psychiatric illness can help establish the diagnosis, and an empiric trial of antidepressants can be considered.

If the patient has a history of irregular stepwise decline in functioning, especially if the patient has had apparent stroke symptoms or transient ischemic events, or has known cardiovascular disease or atrial fibrillation, then **multi-infarct dementia** is the most likely diagnosis. This type of vascular dementia is the second most common cause of dementia in the United States,

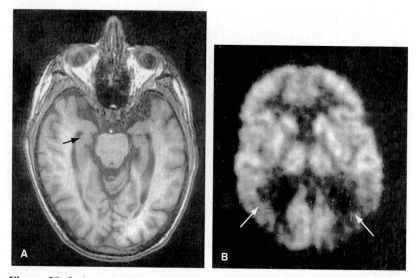

Figure 20–2. A. Axial T1-weighted magnetic resonance images of Alzheimer disease patient showing bilateral hippocampal atrophy and generalized atrophy. **B.** Positron emission tomographic scan with decreased activity in the parietal lobes bilaterally. *(With permission from Bird TD, Miller BL. Alzheimer's Disease and other Dementias. In: Kasper DL, Braunwal E, Fauci A, et al. Harrison's principles of internal medicine, 16th ed. New York: McGraw-Hill; 2005: Fig. 350–2b, 2d. p 2399.)*

comprising 10–20% of dementia. Other patients with cerebrovascular disease, especially as a result of long-standing hypertension, can develop diffuse sub-cortical white matter changes seen on imaging, and an insidious rather than sudden stepwise decline in cognitive function. This condition is often referred to as Binswanger disease.

Other common causes of dementia include cognitive decline caused by long-standing **alcoholism**, or dementia associated with **parkinsonism**. Both of these underlying conditions are readily discovered by the appropriate asso-ciated medical history.

Less common causes of dementia include medical conditions such as Wernicke encephalopathy as a result of thiamine (vitamin B_1) deficiency, **Vitamin B_{12}** deficiency caused by pernicious anemia, untreated **hypothy-roidism,** or chronic infections such as **HIV** dementia or **neurosyphilis.** A vari-ety of primary CNS diseases can lead to dementia including Huntington disease, multiple sclerosis, or neoplastic diseases such as primary or metastatic brain tumors (although they are much more likely to produce seizures or focal deficits rather than dementia), or leptomeningeal spread of various cancers. **Normal pressure hydrocephalus** is a potentially reversible form of dementia where the cerebral ventricles slowly enlarge as a result of disturbances to cerebral spinal fluid resorption. The classic triad is dementia, gait disturbance, and urinary or bowel incontinence. Relief of hydrocephalus through placement of a ventriculoperitoneal shunt can reverse the cognitive decline.

Treatment of Alzheimer Disease

For patients with Alzheimer disease, the average life expectancy after diagnosis is 7–10 years. The clinical course is characterized by the progressive decline of cognitive functions (memory, orientation, attention, and concentration) and the development of psychological and behavioral symptoms (wandering, aggression, anxiety, depression, and psychosis). The goals of treatment in AD are to (1) improve cognitive function, (2) reduce behavioral and psychological symptoms, and (3) improve the quality of life. Three agents are currently available: donepezil, rivastigmine, and galantamine. In addition, memantine, which is an inhibitor of excitatory amino acids, has been shown to be helpful especially in later dementia. Donepezil (Aricept) and rivastigmine (Exelon) are cholinesterase inhibitors that are effective in improving cognitive function and global clinical state. Antagonists to N-methyl-D-aspartate (NMDA) receptors, such as memantine, also seem to reduce the rate of decline in patients with Alzheimer dementia. Risperidone reduces psychotic symptoms and aggression in patients with dementia. Other issues include wakefulness, nightwalking and wandering, aggression, incontinence, and depression. A structured environment, with predictability, and judicious use of pharmacotherapy, such as SSRI for depression or a short-acting benzodiazepine for insomnia, are helpful. The primary caregiver is often overwhelmed and needs support. The Alzheimer Association is a national organization developed to give support to family members and can be contacted through www.alz.org.

Comprehension Questions

[20.1] The drugs donepezil, rivastigmine, and galanthamine are used in AD to try to raise the availability of what transmitter in the brain?

A. Dopamine
B. Norepinephrine
C. Glutamate
D. Acetylcholine

[20.2] Abnormal processing of which of these proteins is felt to be particularly important in the pathophysiology of Alzheimer's disease?

A. Acetylcholinesterase
B. Alpha-synuclein
C. Huntingtin
D. Amyloid precursor protein
E. A right spinal cord hemisection syndrome

[20.3] Which one of these abnormalities on the neurologic exam would be unusual in a patient with mild AD?

    A. Problems drawing a clock
    B. Impaired sense of smell
    C. Hyperreflexia with positive Babinski signs
    D. Impaired short-term memory

Answers

[20.1] **D.** These agents all inhibit acetylcholinesterase and hopefully result in elevated availability of acetylcholine in the cerebral cortex.

[20.2] **D.** There are abnormalities of amyloid precursor protein deposition, CSF levels demonstrated in AD and mutations in the protein have been shown to cause the clinical disorder.

[20.3] **C.** Impaired olfaction is the only abnormality except those on MMSE testing reliably demonstrated in patients with AD.

CLINICAL PEARLS

❖ Alzheimer disease is an anterior cortical dementia with insidious onset and gradual progression. In its early stages, affected patients have a normal neurologic exam except for the mental status examination and olfactory testing.

❖ Alzheimer disease is associated with neurofibrillary tangles with deposition of abnormal amyloid plaques in the brain.

❖ Patients with Alzheimer disease are unusually sensitive to deleterious effects of anticholinergic medications.

❖ Anticholinesterase medications have been shown to improve cognition and behavior in patients with Alzheimer disease.

❖ Although clear depressive syndromes should be treated in patients with Alzheimer disease, medications should not be routinely employed without appropriate symptomatology.

❖ Alzheimer disease is the most common type of dementia, followed by multi-infarct (vascular) dementia.

❖ Depression and reversible causes of dementia should be considered in the evaluation of a patient with memory loss and functional decline.

❖ A cholinesterase inhibitor such as donepezil is effective in improving cognitive function and global clinical state in patients with Alzheimer disease.

REFERENCES

Blennow K, de Leon MJ, Zetterberg H. Alzheimer's disease. Lancet 2006; 368:387–403.

Borson S, Raskind MA. Clinical features and pharmacologic treatment of behavioral symptoms of Alzheimer's disease. Neurology 1997;48(5 suppl 6):S17–24.

Jackson JC, Gordon SM, Hart RP, et al. The association between delirium and cognitive decline: a review of the empirical literature. Neuropsychol Rev 2004 Jun;14:87–98.

Lyketsos CG, Lee HB. Diagnosis and treatment of depression in Alzheimer's disease. A practical update for the clinician. Dement Geriatr Cogn Disord 2004; 17:55–64.

Muller-Thomsen T, Arlt S, Mann U, et al. Detecting depression in Alzheimer's disease: evaluation of four different scales. Arch Clin Neuropsychol 2005;20:271–6.

van der Flier WM, Scheltens P. Epidemiology and risk factors of dementia. J Neurol Neurosurg Psychiatry 2005;76(suppl 5):v2–7.

A 64-year-old woman was admitted for a possible seizure. The patient states that she has been having vivid nightmares and dreams for months and will often awake screaming or falling out of bed. She was brought to the hospital because of "thrashing around" and screaming "Stop" as witnessed by her niece. Her niece also stated that her aunt had shown a decline for the past year. She was previously an outgoing active person who lived independently. In the past 6 months, she has become more reclusive, and her son has had to take over her finances as a result of an accumulation of unpaid bills. She was recently placed on a psychotropic medicine by her primary care physician a few months earlier with marked worsening. It was discontinued. The patient also admits to seeing "things" at night and will occasionally hear "things." Neurologic examination is significant for mild bradykinesia, decreased right arm swing, and small stepped ambulation. There is also mild right arm rigidity without tremor. A neuropsychologic examination revealed changes in executive functioning (verbal fluency, attention, judgment) and difficulties performing previously learned tasks (dyspraxia).

◆ **What is the most likely diagnosis?**

◆ **What is the next diagnostic step?**

◆ **What is the next step in therapy?**

ANSWERS TO CASE 21: Dementia (Lewy Body)

Summary: The patient is a 64-year-old woman with progressive decline in personality, daily function, and depression. The patient's history is also significant for sleep disorders, including dream stage disturbance and auditory and visual hallucinations. Her examination reveals impairment in the extrapyramidal system and subcortical and cortical cognitive dysfunction consistent with a parkinsonian syndrome with a dementia.

◆ **Most likely diagnosis:** Diffuse Lewy body dementia

◆ **Next diagnostic step:** MRI of brain; neuropsychologic evaluation

◆ **Next step in therapy:** Anticholinesterase medications

Analysis

Objectives

1. Describe the typical presentation of Lewy body dementia.
2. Know the differential diagnosis of conditions with parkinsonism and dementia.
3. Understand the evaluation and management of Parkinson dementia syndromes.

Considerations

This is a woman who developed cognitive, behavioral, and motor dysfunction that is most likely caused by Lewy body dementia (LBD). Her history is significant for onset of cognitive and behavioral decline characterized by social isolation, inability to handle personal affairs, rapid eye movement (REM) sleep-related behavior disorders, and hallucinations. Dementia with LBD involves a predominant executive dysfunction and motor parkinsonism, in addition to a number of core and suggestive features that include fluctuating cognition, hallucinations, sensitivity to neuroleptics, and sleep-related disorders. Based on the temporal progression of dementia and behavioral decline, then sleep-related disorders and parkinsonism, diffuse Lewy body disease is the likely diagnosis. Her examination is highly suggestive of parkinsonism characterized by a festinating (short, small steps), ipsilateral decreased arm swing, and rigidity. Formal testing confirmed dysfunction including impaired verbal fluency, concentration, judgment, and apraxia. Her history is also significant for clinical worsening with an empiric trial of a psychotropic, not otherwise specified.

For this case, the differential diagnosis is Parkinson disease or its related disorders, Alzheimer disease (AD), CNS infections, or cerebrovascular disease.

Alzheimer patients present with a primary cortical dementia with memory impairment as a predominant feature. Parkinsonian features are not uncommon in AD, but often will show in advanced disease when cognitive impairment is severe. In addition, AD patient can inadvertently be treated with antipsychotics for associated behavioral disturbances and develop drug-induced parkinsonism. With Parkinson disease, patients can also have a dementia, but it is predominantly subcortical (slowed thought processes, retrieval, attention, and concentration) and is usually not a predominant clinical feature of the disease.

CNS infections such as HIV encephalitis or chronic fungal meningitis can present with slowly progressive dementia and motor dysfunction. Often the dementia and motor dysfunction are more global and include multiple cortical and subcortical deficits, extrapyramidal and pyramidal dysfunction, and a more rapid clinical course. Normal pressure hydrocephalus and cerebrovascular disease (particularly ischemic disease of the deep white matter) typically presents as what is called "lower body parkinsonism" with early gait and balance problems, lower body akinesia/bradykinesia, little or no tremor. Urinary abnormalities and the executive frontal lobe dysfunction are common. For both these disorders, neuroimaging often shows characteristic abnormalities.

APPROACH TO DIFFUSE LEWY BODY DEMENTIA

Definitions

Constructional apraxia: Difficulty in performing tasks involved with construction, for example, drawing a five-pointed star.

Executive function: Mental capacity to control and plan mental skills, the ability to sustain or flexibly direct attention, the inhibition of inappropriate behavioral or emotional responses, the planning of strategies for future behavior, the initiation and execution of these strategies, and the ability to flexibly switch among problem-solving strategies. It is mediated by the prefrontal lobes of the cerebral cortex.

Ideomotor apraxia: Disturbance of voluntary movement in which a person cannot translate an idea into movement.

REM-related disorders: A parasomnia involving dissociation of the characteristic stages of sleep. The major feature is loss of motor inhibition leading to a wide spectrum of behavioral release during sleep, that is, "acting out dreams."

Clinical Approach

Diffuse Lewy body dementia (DLBD) is felt to represent the second most common cause of dementia in developed countries in the Western Hemisphere. It accounts for 10–20% of dementias; however, the sensitivity and specificity of DLBD and common dementias are poor because pathology and clinical features can overlap between DLBD and dementias, such as AD. In fact, 40% of AD patients have the pathologic alterations felt to be specific for DLBD, the Lewy body. Epidemiologic studies are limited but suggest that men are more affected than woman, and the usual onset is in late 50's and beyond.

Clinical History and Features

DLBD is a progressive degenerative dementia but can overlap with other parkinsonian dementias and primary Alzheimer dementia, clinically and pathologically (Table 21–1 for diagnostic features of DLBD). However, when dementia precedes motor signs, particularly with visual hallucinations and episodes of reduced responsiveness, the diagnosis of DLBD should be considered. The following clinical features help distinguish DLBD from Alzheimer dementia: (1) fluctuations in cognitive function with varying levels of alertness and attention, (2) visual hallucinations, (3) parkinsonian motor features that appear relatively early in DLBD. Cognitive impairment in DLBD is characterized by more executive dysfunction and visual-spatial impairment rather than the anterograde memory loss of AD. It is not unusual for someone with DLBD to have a relative severe dementia by history, but to have relatively preserved delayed recall with severe constructional dyspraxia. This combination is virtually never seen in AD. When parkinsonism precedes cognitive dysfunction by more than 2 years, the disorder is referred to as Parkinson disease dementia. Although this differentiation seems largely semantic, knowing this clinical presentation is useful practically (Table 21–2). Other suggestive features of DLBD are nonvisual hallucinations, delusions, unexplained syncope, REM-sleep disorders, neuroleptic sensitivity.

Pathology

Frederick Lewy first described Lewy bodies (LBs) in 1914, which are cytoplasmic inclusions of the substantia nigra neurons in patients with idiopathic Parkinson disease (PD). By the 1960s, pathologists had described patients with dementia who had LBs of the neocortex. It was not until the mid 1980s, when sensitive immunocytochemical methods to identify LBs were developed, that dementia with LBs (DLB) was then recognized as being far more common than previously thought. However, there is considerable controversy at this point over whether DLB in PD are two different conditions or just part of a spectrum disorder with common underlying pathology.

Diagnostic Studies

Laboratory studies should include the routine dementia evaluation, including a chemistry panel, complete blood count (CBC), thyroid studies, vitamin B_{12} levels, syphilis serology, Lyme disease serology, or HIV testing, when appropriate.

Table 21–1
DIAGNOSTIC FEATURES OF DEMENTIA WITH LEWY BODIES

1. Central feature (essential for a diagnosis of possible or probable DLB):
   - Dementia defined as progressive cognitive decline of sufficient magnitude to interfere with normal social or occupational function; prominent or persistent memory impairment may not necessarily occur in the early stages but is usually evident with progression; deficits on tests of attention, executive function, and visuospatial ability may be especially prominent

2. Core features (two core features are sufficient for a diagnosis of probable DLB, one for possible DLB)
   - Fluctuating cognition with pronounced variations in attention and alertness
   - Recurrent visual hallucinations that are typically well formed and detailed
   - Spontaneous features of parkinsonism

3. Suggestive features (one or more of these in the presence of one or more core features is sufficient for a diagnosis of probable DLB; in the absence of any core features, one or more suggestive features is sufficient for a diagnosis of possible DLB; probable DLB should not be diagnosed on the basis of suggestive features alone)
   - REM-sleep behavior disorder
   - Severe neuroleptic sensitivity
   - Low dopamine-transporter uptake in basal ganglia demonstrated by SPECT or PET imaging

4. Supportive features (commonly present but not proven to have diagnostic specificity)
   - Repeated falls and syncope
   - Transient, unexplained loss of consciousness
   - Severe autonomic dysfunction
   - Hallucinations in other modalities
   - Systematized delusions
   - Depression
   - Relative preservation of mesial temporal lobe structures on computed tomography/magnetic resonance imaging
   - Reduced occipital activity on SPECT/PET
   - Low uptake MIBG myocardial scintigraphy
   - Prominent slow wave activity on EEG with temporal lobe transient sharp waves

DLB, dementia with Lewy bodies; EEG, electroencephalograph; MIBG, metaiodobenzylguanidine; PET, positron emission tomography; REM, rapid eye movement; SPECT, single-photon emission computed tomography.

Source: McKeith IG, Dickson DW, Lowe J, et al. Diagnosis and management of dementia with Lewy bodies: third report of the DLB Consortium. Neurology 2005;65:1863–1872.

Table 21–2
CLINICAL PHENOMENOLOGY OF DEMENTIA WITH LEWY BODIES

- Comparison to PD
  - Less severe parkinsonism
  - Less tremor
  - More postural instability

- Comparison to AD
  - More visuospatial deficit
  - Less language, memory encoding deficit

- Comparison to AD & PD
  - More fluctuation and hallucinations

AD, Alzheimer disease; PD, Parkinson disease.

Imaging studies are important to evaluate for other conditions that can mimic this disorder (vascular dementia, tumor, normal pressure hydrocephalus, etc). Patients with DLBD usually have less hippocampal atrophy than patients with AD (but more than control subjects). Whether this difference is clinically useful is under investigation, as is the diagnostic utility of functional imaging. Single-photon emission CT scanning or positron emission tomography scanning can show decreased occipital lobe blood flow or metabolism in DLB but not in AD. Reduced dopamine transporter activity in the basal ganglia is seen with positron emission tomography scanning or single-photon emission CT scanning.

Other Tests

In certain circumstances, **neuropsychologic testing** is helpful to differentiate DLB from AD and to establish a baseline for future comparison. Patients with DLB can have changes on **electroencephalography** earlier than patients with AD, but whether this difference is diagnostically useful is not clear. Cerebrospinal fluid (CSF) examination is not required in routine cases, but patients with AD have higher levels of tau protein in their CSF than patients with DLB. Patients with both LB variant-AD have intermediate values. CSF levels of beta-amyloid are lower than normal in DLB, AD, and LBV-AD. However, CSF beta-amyloid levels in DLB, LBV-AD, and AD do not differ from each other.

Treatment

There are no medications that have been shown to delay the degeneration of this disorder. Symptomatically, the **anticholinesterase medications** (i.e., rivastigmine, donepezil, and galanthamine) have been demonstrated to have

cognitive/behavioral symptom improvement. The cortical cholinergic depletion in DLB is actually much more severe than AD and so appears to be more
responsive to treatment. Cognitive and behavioral symptoms have been shown
to improve with this class of medications, however, not depression.
Neuroleptic agents should be used with extreme caution in these patients.
Patients, often treated for behavioral issues with neuroleptics, have been
described to have disastrous responses to this class of medicines, even when
using "atypical antipsychotics." For severe depression, **electroconvulsive
therapy** has been shown to be effective and safe. In addition, parkinsonian
motor signs have also been shown to improve with ECT.

Comprehension Questions

[21.1] A 68-year-old woman is diagnosed with dementia with Lewy bodies.
Her medications are mixed up with her husband's medication bottles.
Which of the following is most likely to be her husband's medication?

    A. Rivastigmine
    B. Donepezil
    C. Haloperidol
    D. Galanthamine

[21.2]. A 61-year-old man is brought into the doctor's office for memory loss
and confusion. Which of the following symptoms are most suggestive
of Alzheimer disease as opposed to dementia with Lewy bodies?

    A. Visual hallucinations
    B. Dramatic fluctuations in clinical condition
    C. Early anterograde memory loss
    D. Early shuffling gait

[21.3] A 73-year-old man is noted to have a slow onset of cognitive deficits. The
physical examination reveals no obvious etiology. Which of the following imaging findings are most suggestive of dementia with Lewy bodies?

    A. Medial temporal lobe atrophy
    B. Parietal temporal hypometabolism
    C. Atrophy of the midbrain
    D. Occipital lobe hypometabolism

Answers

[21.1] **C.** Haloperidol is a dopamine-receptor blocking agent that can have
severely deleterious consequences in this disorder. The other three are anti-
cholinesterases and have evidence for the use presented in the literature.

[21.2] **C.** Cognitive impairment in DLB is characterized by more executive
dysfunction and visuospatial impairment more than the anterograde
memory loss of AD.

[21.3] **D.** Occipital lobe hypometabolism is most typical of DLB. Medial temporal lobe atrophy and parietal temporal hypometabolism are characteristic of AD. Atrophy of the midbrain is characteristic of progressive supranuclear palsy.

CLINICAL PEARLS

❖ Lewy bodies are associated with a number of clinical syndromes, including Alzheimer's dementia and Parkinson disease.

❖ The typical clinical syndrome of DLB is relatively specific for the Lewy body pathology, but the converse is not necessarily so and can constitute part of a spectrum of synucleinopathies.

❖ Compared to AD, DLB is associated with a greater loss of acetylcholine and a smaller loss of acetylcholine (ACh)-receptors

❖ Levodopa can be effective for the parkinsonism but is often not very rewarding for behavioral or cognitive dysfunction.

❖ REM-related behavior disorders can be one of the first symptoms of DLBD, prior to the onset of significant cognitive or motor disturbance.

REFERENCES

Ballard C, Grace J, McKeith I, et al. Neuroleptic sensitivity in dementia with Lewy bodies and Alzheimer's disease. Lancet 1998;351:1032–1033.

Bonner LT, Tsuang DW, Cherrier MM, et al. Familial dementia with Lewy bodies with an atypical clinical presentation. J Geriatr Psychiatry Neurol 2003;16:59–64.

Geser F, Wenning GK, Poewe W, et al. How to diagnose dementia with Lewy bodies: state of the art. Mov Disord 2005 Aug;20(suppl 12):S11–20.

Korczyn AD, Reichmann H. Dementia with Lewy bodies. J Neurol Sci 2006;248:3–8.

McKeith IG, Dickson DW, Lowe J, et al. Diagnosis and management of dementia with Lewy bodies: third report of the DLB Consortium. Neurology 2005;65: 1863–1872.

Miyasaki JM, Shannon K, Voon V, et al; Quality Standards Subcommittee of the American Academy of Neurology. Practice parameter: evaluation and treatment of depression, psychosis, and dementia in Parkinson disease (an evidence-based review): report of the Quality Standards Subcommittee of the American Academy of Neurology. Neurology 2006;66:996–1002.

A 48-year-old man complained of "numbness and stiffness" in his arms for the past 4 months. His gait has gradually deteriorated because of unsteadiness. On examination the patient appeared older than his stated age. His hair was nearly completely gray. There was slight limitation of head movement to either side, but no pain with neck extension. His tongue was red and depilated. His gait was broad based, and he was unable to walk a straight line. He was able to stand with his feet together with his eyes open, but he nearly fell when his eyes were closed. He had normal arm coordination but was ataxic on the heel-knee-shin maneuver. Deep tendon reflexes (DTRs) were 3+ in the arms, trace at the knees, and absent at the ankles. Both plantar responses were extensor. There was a 2+ jaw jerk and a positive snout reflex. There was a stocking decrease in sensation and a marked decrease in vibration and joint position sense in the toes and ankles. Cranial nerves were normal, and there were mild problems with memory and calculation. T2-weighted MRI of the brain demonstrated extensive areas of high-intensity signal in the periventricular white matter. MRI of the spine showed a hyperintense signal along the posterior column of the spinal cord.

◆ **What is the most likely diagnosis?**

◆ **What is the next diagnostic step?**

◆ **What is the next step in therapy?**

ANSWERS TO CASE 22: Subacute Combined Degeneration of Spinal Cord

Summary: This is a 48-year-old patient with a progressive gait disorder characterized by sensory ataxia caused by impaired position sense and spasticity. His examination is significant for both peripheral and central nervous system involvement, primarily affecting the white matter fibers of the posterior columns of the spinal columns and pyramidal tracts and large myelinated peripheral nerve affecting coordination and muscle tone.

◆ **Most likely diagnosis:** Vitamin B_{12} deficiency

◆ **Next diagnostic step:** Vitamin B_{12} level and if positive, subsequent testing to determine the source of B_{12} malabsorption

◆ **Next step in therapy:** Intramuscular vitamin B_{12}

Analysis

Objectives

1. Understand the range of pathologic and clinical manifestations of vitamin B_{12} deficiency.
2. Know the differential diagnosis of vitamin B_{12} deficiency.
3. Understand the types of tests to confirm the diagnosis and etiology of vitamin B_{12} deficiency.
4. Be aware of the proper mode of repletion of vitamin B_{12}.

Considerations

The pertinent features of this case include the presentation, unsteadiness of gait, and numbness and stiffness. The physical examination helps localize the pathology. There was a stocking decrease in sensation, specifically vibration and joint position sense, which strongly suggests a neuropathy involving myelinated fibers. Involvement of the dorsal columns of the spinal cord, at or above the lumbar level is also a possibility. The pathologically increased reflexes in the arms along with the presence of primitive reflexes are "upper motor neuron signs" and suggest involvement of the corticospinal tract above the level of the cervical spinal cord. In this case, one would expect increased reflexes in the legs also, unless there is also a coexistent neuropathy. The ataxic heel knee to shin maneuver, also points to aberrant input to the cerebellum, which comes through large fibers. The mild problems on mental status examination indicate a cortical disorder. All of these findings suggest involvement at multiple levels of the nervous system. The imaging study confirms involvement of myelinated regions in the spinal cord, specifically the dorsal columns and in the brain.

Assuming all these signs/symptoms are manifestations of a single entity, a systemic disease should be considered, such as HIV-1 associated vacuolar myelopathy, Lyme disease, multiple sclerosis, neurosyphilis, or vitamin B_{12} deficiency. Neuropathic conditions would not be expected to give upper motor neuron signs. Another clue on physical diagnosis is the abnormal tongue and prematurely graying hair.

APPROACH TO SUBACUTE COMBINED DEGENERATION OF THE SPINAL CORD

Spinal cord diseases are common, and many are treatable if discovered early. The spinal cord is a tubular structure originating from the medulla of the brain and extending through the bony spine to the coccyx. Ascending sensory and descending motor white matter tracts are located peripherally; posterior columns govern joint position, vibration and pressure, lateral spinothalamic tracts pain and temperature, and ventral corticospinal tracts carry motor signals.

Vitamin B_{12} Deficiency

Vitamin B_{12} deficiency usually presents as paresthesias in the hands and feet and loss of vibratory sense. There is a diffuse effect on the spinal cord, primarily the posterior lateral columns, explaining the early loss of vibratory sense. Late in the course, optic atrophy and mental changes as well ataxia can occur. The macrocytic anemia is common.

Cyanocobalamin is a compound that is metabolized to a vitamin in the B complex commonly known as vitamin B_{12}. Vitamin B_{12} is the most chemically complex of all the vitamins. The structure of B_{12} is based on a corrin ring, which is similar to the porphyrin ring found in heme, chlorophyll, and cytochrome. The central metal ion is cobalt (Co). Once metabolized, cobalamin is a coenzyme in many biochemical reactions, including DNA synthesis, methionine synthesis from homocysteine, and conversion of propionyl into succinyl coenzyme A from methylmalonate. Dietary cobalamin (Cbl), obtained through animal foods, enters the stomach bound to animal proteins. Absorption requires many factors including stomach acid, R-protein, and intrinsic factor from parietal cells, and the distal 80 cm of the ileum for transport. Interference in any of these points can lead to malabsorption of vitamin B_{12}. In addition there are a number of inborn errors of metabolism that can both interfere with the absorption and action of vitamin B_{12}. The most common cause of vitamin B_{12} deficiency is malabsorption because of pernicious anemia, a condition where antibodies are generated to the parietal cells of the stomach, and the necessary proteins are not available. There are many other causes, however, that should be considered.

Pathologically, in experimental subacute combined degeneration (SCD), there is edema and destruction of myelin. Thus, the clinical presentation of SCD is caused by dorsal column, lateral corticospinal tract, and sometimes lateral spinothalamic tract dysfunction. The initial symptoms are usually paresthesia in the hands and feet. This condition can progress to sensory loss, gait ataxia, and distal weakness, particularly in the legs. If the disease goes untreated, an ataxic paraplegia can evolve. Specific findings on examination are loss of vibratory and joint position sense, weakness, spasticity, hyperreflexia, and extensor plantar responses. The syndrome of sensory loss as well as spastic paresis associated with pathologic lesions in the dorsal columns and lateral corticospinal tracts is referred to as *subacute combined degeneration*. There are also effects on other body systems, most conspicuously hematologic with the macrocytic anemia.

Differential Diagnosis

The manifestations of vitamin B_{12} deficiency are noted in Table 22–1. The differential diagnosis for progressive spastic paraplegia includes degenerative, demyelinating, infectious, inflammatory, neoplastic, nutritional, and vascular disorders. HIV-1 associated vacuolar myelopathy, Lyme disease, multiple sclerosis neurosyphilis, toxic neuropathy, Friedreich ataxia, and vitamin E deficiency.

Table 22–1
CLINICAL MANIFESTATIONS OF VITAMIN B_{12} DEFICIENCY

Neurologic
- Paresthesia
- Peripheral neuropathy
- Combined systems disease (demyelination of dorsal columns and corticospinal tract)

Behavioral
- Irritability, personality change
- Mild memory impairment, dementia
- Depression
- Psychosis

General
- Lemon-yellow waxy pallor, premature whitening of hair
- Flabby bulky frame
- Mild icterus
- Blotchy skin pigmentation in dark-skinned patients

Cardiovascular
- Tachycardia, congestive heart failure

Gastrointestinal
- Beefy, red, smooth, and sore tongue with loss of papillae that is more pronounced along edges

Hematologic
- Megaloblastic anemia; pancytopenia (leukopenia, thrombocytopenia)

The differential diagnosis of SCD is broad, but B_{12} deficiency should be considered in any patient with progressive sensory symptoms or weakness.

Laboratory Confirmation

Testing for vitamin B_{12} deficiency includes a direct assay of the vitamin as well as looking at the indirect effect of abnormal reactions resulting in altered metabolite levels. The definitions of Cbl (vitamin B_{12}) deficiency are as follows: Serum Cbl level <150 pmol/L on two separate occasions OR serum Cbl level <150 pmol/L AND total serum homocysteine level >13 μmol/L OR methylmalonic acid >0.4 μmol/L (in the absence of renal failure and folate and vitamin B_6 deficiencies). The hematologic manifestations of vitamin B_{12} deficiency can be mimicked by folate deficiency, but this does not mimic the neurologic manifestations. In addition, the multiple organ systems and subsystems affected are highly variable from patient to patient.

Confirmatory effects of the anatomic and physiologic consequences of B_{12} deficiency involve nerve conduction studies and MRI. Few reported cases of MR imaging of SCD exist. Findings in these cases include modest expansion of the cervical and thoracic spinal cord and increased signal intensity on T2-weighted images, primarily in the dorsal columns and lateral pyramidal tracts (Fig. 22–1).

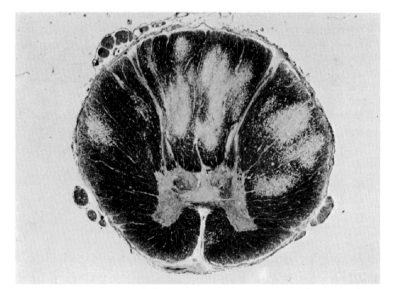

Figure 22–1. Degeneration of spinal cord in subacute combined degeneration on microscopy. (*With permission from Lichtam MA, Beutler E, Kaushansky K, et al. Williams hematology, 7th ed. New York: McGraw-Hill; 2005: Fig. 39–19.*)

Treatment

Treatment of vitamin B_{12} deficiency involves administering the vitamin in a fashion to bypass the pathologic steps in the transport process. This usually involves intramuscular administration of the vitamin, first to build up stores and then on a monthly basis. Specifically, 1000 µg/d for 1 week, then 1000 µg/wk for 1 month. Then 1000 µg/mo until the cause of deficiency is corrected, or for life in the case of pernicious anemia. This is effective for all forms of deficiency. There are also methods of oral administration that are sometimes effective. Treatment can reverse or stop most if not all of the sequelae of vitamin B_{12} deficiency.

Comprehension Questions

[22.1] Vitamin B_{12} repletion by which of the following routes will be effective in virtually all causes of B_{12} deficiency?

A. Concentrated oral vitamin B_{12}
B. Nasal vitamin B_{12} administration
C. A diet high in red meats
D. Intramuscular B_{12} administration

[22.2] Which feature of the clinical picture might make you most suspicious of vitamin B_{12} deficiency as a cause for a patient with spastic paresis and sensory loss?

A. Severe signs and symptoms developing over 1 day
B. Loss of pain and temperature sensation in excess of vibration and joint position sense
C. Severe weakness with spasticity and loss of all sensory modalities in the legs with a neurogenic bladder
D. Anemia with an increased mean corpuscular volume (MCV) and hypersegmented polymorphonuclear cells

[22.3] Which feature of vitamin B_{12} deficiency is not mimicked in at least some cases of typical multiple sclerosis?

A. Loss of vibration and joint position sensation in the feet
B. Positive Babinski signs
C. Slowed nerve conduction velocities
D. Increased signal on T2 imaging in the spinal cord

Answers

[22.1] **D.** The other forms require some aspect of the body's B_{12} absorption system.

[22.2] **D.** Megaloblastic anemia is the characteristic finding in vitamin B_{12} deficiency. The clinical picture usually develops over months, not days. Usually all limbs are involved to some extent, and severe involvement of the legs and not arms makes one consider an anatomic lesion in the spinal cord. In addition, vibration and joint position sense are usually involved much more than pain and temperature.

[22.3] **C.** Multiple sclerosis is by and large a disorder of the central nervous system and does not affect peripheral nerve conduction studies.

CLINICAL PEARLS

❖ Vitamin B_{12} deficiency typically affects peripheral nerves, as well as the dorsal columns and lateral corticospinal tracts giving a syndrome of spasticity with ataxia as a result of loss of joint position sense. There are many more neurologic signs, however, that can variably be seen.

❖ Nerve conduction studies can show both demyelinating and denervation features in vitamin B_{12} deficiency.

❖ The most common cause of vitamin B_{12} deficiency is pernicious anemia.

❖ Intramuscular administration of vitamin B_{12} is the most effective way of treating this condition and can reverse or stop the neurologic features.

❖ Vitamin B_{12} deficiency is associated with a macrocytic anemia.

REFERENCES

Andrès E, Loukili NH, Noel E, et al. Vitamin B_{12} (cobalamin) deficiency in elderly patients. CMAJ 2004;171(3):251–259.

Healton EB, Savage DG, Brust JC, et al. Neurological aspects of cobalamine deficiency. Medicine 1991;70:229–244.

Larner AJ, Zeman AZJ, Allen CMC, et al. MRI appearances in subacute combined degeneration of the spinal cord due to vitamin B_{12} deficiency. J Neurol Neurosurg Psychiatry 1997;62:99–100.

Ravina B, Loevner LA, Bank W. MR findings in subacute combined degeneration of the spinal cord: a case of reversible cervical myelopathy. AJR Am J Roentgenol 2000;174:863–865.

Reynolds E. Vitamin B_{12}, folic acid, and the nervous system. Lancet Neurol 2006 Nov;5(11):949–960.

Scalabrino G. Cobalamin (vitamin B[12]) in subacute combined degeneration and beyond: traditional interpretations and novel theories. Exp Neurol 2005;192:463–479.

A 23-year-old graduate student was studying late at night for an examination. As he looked at his textbook, he realized he was having difficulty reading through his left eye. When he covered his left eye, visual input through the right eye seemed normal. However, when he covered his right eye, his visual input was blurred. He also noted left ocular pain when he moved his eyes. He had no pain in his right eye and had no headache, dizziness, pain, or numbness. Aside from his left monocular visual compromise, he had no symptoms. Further, he had no history of any previous symptoms. He decided to go to sleep and went to the infirmary the following day.

◆ **What is the most likely diagnosis?**

◆ **What is the next diagnostic step?**

◆ **What is the next step in therapy?**

ANSWERS TO CASE 23: Optic Neuritis

Summary: A 23-year-old man suddenly developed left monocular visual complaints and left eye pain with ocular movement. Otherwise, he had no symptoms.

◆   **Most likely diagnosis:** Optic neuritis.

◆   **Next step in therapy:** Therapy may or may not be indicated. Depending on the evaluation, a short course of steroids might prove helpful.

Analysis

Objectives

1.   Understand the differential diagnosis of monocular visual compromise.
2.   Understand the evaluation for optic neuritis.
3.   Understand the relationship between optic neuritis and multiple sclerosis.
4.   Understand when and how to treat optic neuritis.

Considerations

Optic neuritis usually is associated with an acute, usually unilateral, loss of visual acuity or visual field or both. Ninety percent of patients with optic neuritis have ocular pain, usually with eye movement. This disturbance can occur at any age but usually occurs in young adults, younger than 40 years old. Within several weeks following onset of symptoms, approximately 90% of patients with optic neuritis experience visual improvement to normal vision, or only marginal compromise. Visual recovery can continue for months, sometimes for as long as 1 year. Some patients have residual deficits in contrast sensitivity, color vision, depth perception, light brightness, visual acuity, or visual field. The patient in this case should see a physician, have a careful neurologic assessment, and have blood studies. Brain imaging might be indicated. Lumbar puncture for assessment of possible demyelinating disease might also be necessary.

APPROACH TO OPTIC NEURITIS

Definitions

Optic neuropathy: Unilateral or bilateral impairment of optic nerve function. The diagnosis is usually made clinically. Differential diagnosis: congenital, hereditary, infectious, inflammatory, infiltrative, ischemic, demyelinating (optic neuritis), and compressive etiologies.

Optic neuritis: A general term for idiopathic, inflammatory, infectious, or demyelinating optic neuropathy.

Anterior optic neuritis: Also called *papillitis*. This condition refers to swelling of the optic nerve.

Retrobulbar neuritis: Also called *posterior optic neuritis*. Patients have symptoms because of compromise of the optic nerve, but the optic nerve appears normal.

Clinical Approach

Optic neuritis is defined as inflammation of the optic nerve. It is one of the causes of acute loss of vision associated with pain mainly because of demyelination and can be idiopathic and isolated. However, this disease has a very strong association with multiple sclerosis (MS).

Epidemiology

Whites of northern European descent are affected eight times more frequently than blacks and Asians. Whites of Mediterranean ancestry are at intermediate risk. African blacks and Asians are rarely affected. In the United States, the male-to-female ratio for optic neuritis is 1:1.8. The mean age of onset is approximately 30 years, with most patients presenting from 20–40 years of age.

The condition is rare in children and is usually related to a postinfectious or parainfectious demyelination. Optic neuritis in children is less likely to progress to MS, but, in some reports, it has a worse prognosis for full vision recovery. In patients older than 50 years of age, optic neuritis is less common and can be mistaken for ischemic optic neuropathy, which is more common in persons in this age group.

Etiologies and Clinical Presentation

Patients with optic neuritis experience an acute, usually unilateral loss of visual acuity or compromise of visual field; sometimes, they have both a loss of acuity and field compromise. These symptoms usually occur suddenly but can worsen over the next several days to weeks. Usually, eye movement causes pain in the involved eye.

Examination reveals decreased visual acuity or visual field compromise (or both), and an *afferent pupillary defect*. This deficit is associated with a dilated pupil in the involved eye. This dilated pupil does not constrict well to direct light and, when light is directed into that eye, the pupil of the other (normal) eye does not contract, signifying afferent compromise of light to the involved eye.

However, when light is directly shined into the normal eye, not only does the pupil of that normal eye constrict, but the (already dilated) pupil of the involved eye constricts, signifying that the efferent output to the pupil of the involved eye is normal (Fig. 23–1).

The etiology of optic neuritis is usually idiopathic or caused by demyelinating disease. Sometimes, optic neuritis is caused by other disorders, such as noted in Table 24–1 of case 24. Indications for laboratory testing depends on the

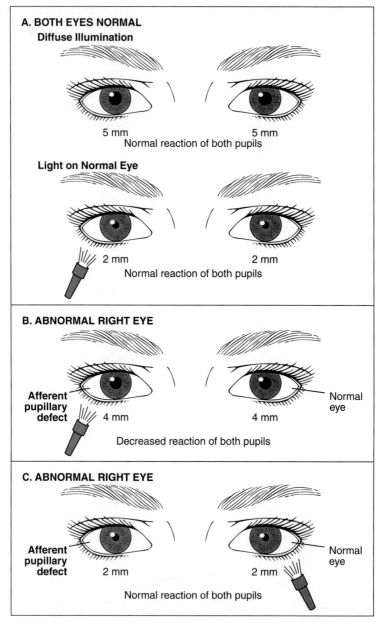

Figure 23–1. Afferent pupillary defect. (*With permission from Riordan-Eva P, Hoyt WF, Neuroophthalmology. In: Riordan-Eva P, Asbury T, Whitcher JP, General Ophthalmology, 16th ed. New York: McGraw-Hill; 2003: Fig. 14–32, p 268.*)

patient's other symptoms, or lack thereof. At issue is whether the patient has MS, which often requires a thorough evaluation to rule out other causes. Many neurologists do not obtain any tests but, instead, follow the patient. Others pursue chest radiograph, blood studies (e.g., syphilis, collagen vascular disease, serum chemistries, complete blood count, sedimentation rate, serum protein electrophoresis), and lumbar puncture for assessment of possible demyelinating disease. MRI of the brain (with and without contrast) in patients with optic neuritis is usually not necessary for the diagnosis but is a powerful predictor of the patient developing MS. Absence of pain or a normal MRI of the brain suggests decreased risk.

The 5-year cumulative probability of clinically definite MS in patients with optic neuritis is 30%. If, at the onset of symptoms, the MRI of the brain reveals no lesions, this risk decreases to 16%. If the patient has three or more lesions on their MRI, the risk increases to 51 percent. Aside from three or more lesions on the MRI suggesting increased risk of developing MS, other factors that also suggest increased risk include prior nonspecific neurologic symptoms; increased immunoglobulins or oligoclonal bands in the cerebrospinal fluid; previous optic neuritis; testing positive for human leukocyte antigens HLA-DR2 or HLA-B7.

Diagnosis

The diagnosis of optic neuritis is usually made on clinical grounds, supplemented by ophthalmologic examination findings. However, in atypical cases (e.g., prolonged or severe pain, lack of visual recovery, atypical visual-field loss, evidence of orbital inflammation), MRI is used to further characterize and to exclude other disease processes. The real contribution of imaging in the setting of optic neuritis is made by imaging the brain, not the optic nerves themselves. This is because the most valuable predictor for the development of subsequent MS is the presence of white matter abnormalities. In various studies, 27–70% of patients with isolated optic neuritis show abnormal MRI findings of the brain, as defined by two or more white matter lesions on T2-weighted images.

Treatment

Optic neuritis is treated with intravenous corticosteroids, which hasten recovery by several weeks but has no effect on visual function at 1 to 3 years. Also, intravenous steroids have no effect on recurrence of optic neuritis in the affected eye; they do decrease the risk of attacks of clinical MS in the first 2 years following treatment in patients without clinical MS who have abnormalities on their MRI at the onset of their visual loss. Treatment with interferon beta 1a at the onset of optic neuritis can be beneficial for patients with MRI brain lesions suggesting high risk of MS.

Comprehension Questions

[23.1]   A 28-year-old man complains of loss of vision to his right eye. The examination suggests optic neuritis. Which of the following conditions is most likely to be associated?

A. Sjögren syndrome
B. Influenza A virus infection
C. Diabetes mellitus
D. Syphilis

[23.2]   A 24-year-old man is noted to have optic neuritis and also weakness. A tentative diagnosis of multiple sclerosis is made. Which of the following is associated with an increased risk of developing MS?

A. One lesion on MRI of brain
B. Cerebrospinal fluid (CSF) oligoclonal bands
C. History of ocular trauma
D. Recent history of vaccination

[23.3]   The patient in [23.2] is confirmed to have multiple sclerosis. Which of the following is the best therapy for his condition?

A. Immunoglobulin therapy
B. Interferon beta 1a
C. Hypothermic therapy
D. Corticosteroid therapy

Answers

[23.1]   **A.** Sjögren syndrome is associated with optic neuritis. Guillain Barré, HIV infection are also associated conditions.

[23.2]   **B.** CSF oligoclonal bands are associated with MS.

[23.3]   **B.** Interferon beta 1a started early is optimal therapy for optic neuritis diagnosed in MS and has a beneficial effect on disease course.

CLINICAL PEARLS

❖ Optic neuritis usually presents as an acute monocular compromise of vision, involving either acuity or visual field or both.

❖ The risk of development of multiple sclerosis after an episode of isolated optic neuritis was 30% at 5-year follow-up and 38% at 10-year follow-up.

❖ The prevalence of optic neuritis is highest among white populations of northern European ancestry, and lowest in African, black, or Asian populations.

> ❖ Optic neuritis is usually associated with pain of eye movement.
> ❖ The prognosis for a single event of optic neuritis is fairly good. At issue is whether the patient will develop multiple sclerosis. MRI of the brain (three or more lesions) places the patient at increased risk.

REFERENCES

Brazis PW, Lee AG. Optic neuritis. In: Evans RW, ed. Saunders manual of neurologic practice. Philadelphia, PA: Saunders/Elsevier; 2003;371–374.

Brazis PW, Lee AG. Optic neuropathy. In: Evans RW, ed. Saunders manual of neurologic practice. Philadelphia, PA: Saunders/Elsevier; 2003;375–383.

A 24-year-old medical student was studying late at night for an examination. As he looked at his textbook, he realized that his left arm and left leg were numb. He dismissed the complaint, recalling that 6 or 7 months ago he had similar symptoms. He rose from his desk and noticed that he had poor balance. He queried whether his vision was blurred, and remembered that he had some blurred vision approximately 1 to 2 years earlier, but that this resolved. He had not seen a physician for any of these previous symptoms. He went to bed and decided that he would seek medical consultation the next day.

◆ **What is the most likely diagnosis?**

◆ **What is the next diagnostic step?**

◆ **What is the next step in therapy?**

ANSWERS TO CASE 24: Multiple Sclerosis

Summary: A 24-year-old man developed multiple neurological symptoms and, in retrospect, recognized that he had had multiple symptoms over the past 1 to 2 years.

◆ **Most likely diagnosis:** Multiple sclerosis.

◆ **Next diagnostic step:** See a physician and undergo a careful neurologic assessment. Blood studies, lumbar puncture, brain imaging, and visual evoked responses can be indicated.

◆ **Next step in therapy:** Probably intravenous corticosteroids followed by an immune modulatory therapy directed at improving disease course.

Analysis

Objectives

1. Understand the differential diagnosis of multiple sclerosis.
2. Describe the evaluation for multiple sclerosis.
3. Understand the prognosis of multiple sclerosis.
4. Describe when and how to treat multiple sclerosis.

Clinical Considerations

This is a case of a young man who notes symptoms suggestive of hemisensory deficit and visual disturbance affecting balance. Although the patient has not undergone a medical evaluation, his symptoms suggest involvement of at least two sites of the central nervous system, the spinal cord or brain contralateral to the side of numbness and possibly his optic nerve affecting vision. The case presentation is also significant for similar symptoms in the past that resolved without treatment. In a young, presumably healthy, person with acute onset of symptoms localized to the CNS that are separated by time (acute and past symptoms) and space (optic nerve and brain/cord), multiple sclerosis is the diagnosis until proven otherwise.

APPROACH TO MULTIPLE SCLEROSIS

Definitions

Multiple sclerosis: Multiple sclerosis (MS) is a chronic disease, usually beginning in young adults, characterized by relapsing, remitting, or progressive neurologic deficits. These deficits reflect lesions in scattered areas of the central nervous system that appear and can resolve over time.

Clinical Approach

Epidemiology and Etiopathogenesis

MS is the most common cause of neurologic disability in young adults.
There are between 250,000 and 500,000 patients with MS in the United States.
MS is more common in northern climates in Europe and the United States,
with a prevalence of approximately 1 per 1,000 people in these areas. It is
more common in women by a ratio of two women to one male, with a peak
incidence of 24 years. Symptoms usually begin between the ages of 10 and
60 years. Onset of symptoms outside this range should cause suspicion of disease other than MS. Seventy percent of patients with MS develop their symptoms between ages 21 and 40 years; 12% develop symptoms between ages 16
to 20; 13% develop symptoms between ages 41 and 50.

There are different clinical patterns or types of multiple sclerosis.

1. *Benign, comprising approximately 20% of cases,* is the least severe
   type of MS. It includes a few, mild early attacks with complete clearing
   of symptoms. There is minimal or no disability in this condition.
2. *Relapsing/Remitting* **MS, accounting for approximately 25% of
   cases,** is characterized by frequent, early attacks and less complete
   clearing, but with long periods of stability. Some degree of disability is
   usually present.
3. *Secondary chronic progressive, comprising approximately 40% of diagnosed cases,* is characterized by increasing attacks, with fewer and less
   complete remissions after each attack. The MS can continue to worsen for
   many years and then level off with moderate to severe disability.
4. *Primary progressive, accounting for approximately 15% of cases,* is
   the most disabling form of multiple sclerosis. The onset is quite severe,
   and the course is slowly progressive without any clearing of symptoms. Fortunately it is the least common of the types of MS.

Research studies reveal that the risk of MS is increased in individuals born
or living in temperate zones, but that people born or migrating to low-risk areas
(i.e., nontemperate zones) prior to 15 years of age have decreased risk. This
suggests that exposure to some factor prior to age 15 is important in the gen-
esis of MS. Migration, ethnic, and twin studies suggest that MS is related to
genetic as well as environmental factors. If one member of an identical twin
pair has MS, there is a 30% chance the other twin will have MS. Siblings of
MS patients have a 2.6 percent risk of MS, parents 1.8 %, and children 1.5%.

Clinical Features

The onset of MS symptoms usually occurs over several days and is seldom
sudden. The initial symptoms often relate to motor dysfunction. Patients may

complain of weakness in the legs and, less commonly, their arms. They may also complain of limb or foot drop, causing difficulty walking, or causing them to trip on sidewalks or curbs. Weakness and stiffness in MS can reflect compromise of the corticospinal tract, which can occur in 30–40% of the initial attacks of MS patients and is present in 60% of MS patients with chronic symptoms.

MS patients can also have sensory symptoms, such as tingling, pins and needle sensations, numbness, or a sensation of a band around the torso. Fifty to seventy percent of MS patients will have sensory complaints some time during their illness. Patients can also have cerebellar symptoms. Fifty percent of MS patients have cerebellar signs sometime during the course of their illness. These patients can have limb tremor, ataxia, scanning speech (i.e., cerebellar dysarthria), and titubation of the head or trunk. Charcot's triad, consisting of intention tremor, dysarthria, and nystagmus, is a well recognized syndrome in MS but occurs rarely.

Optic neuritis and retrobulbar neuritis, both of which can cause blurred vision, scotomas, and decreased color perception, can also occur in MS. Optic neuritis is the presenting symptom in 14–23% of patients with MS. Diplopia, exhibited in 12–22% of patients, is generally a result of brainstem compromise. Trigeminal neuralgia, also caused by brainstem compromise, is characterized by very brief, severe, lancinating maxillary or mandibular pains, and occurs in 1% of MS patients. Trigeminal neuralgia can be due to causes other than MS, but when these symptoms occur in a young adult, MS should be highly suspected.

Another brainstem-related symptom is **facial myokymia**, a wormlike movement of muscles that the patient feels but is difficult for an observer to see. This frequently involves the orbicularis oculi muscles. Vertigo occurs in 14% of MS patients and can be associated with diplopia, also caused by brainstem compromise.

Patients with MS may complain of sensations of electricity running down their spine, sometimes extending into the limbs (Lhermitte sign). This symptom is often aggravated by flexing the cervical spine and should raise suspicion of MS or other compromise of the spinal cord. Mood disorders, including depression, bipolar illness, and dysphoria occurs in one-third to one-half of MS patients. There is disagreement whether these emotional/behavioral disturbance reflect the primary process of MS or the patient's reaction to their disease, or both. Regardless, these symptoms need to be addressed and appropriately treated. MS patients can experience sudden and transient neurologic deterioration if their body temperature is elevated. This can occur with fever, increased physical exertion, or taking a hot bath.

Diagnosis

The criteria for diagnosing MS is constantly changing, in part because of increasingly sophisticated brain imaging and immunologic investigations. Briefly, if a patient has symptoms reflecting two or more separate brain lesions

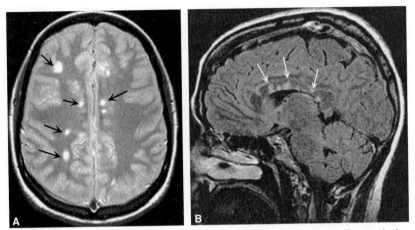

Figure 24–1. T2-weighted MRI brain in multiple sclerosis. (*With permission from Kasper DL, Braunwal E, Fauci A, et al. Harrison's principles of internal medicine, 16th ed. New York: McGraw-Hill; 2004: Figs. 359–3a, 3b.*)

over time, and this is confirmed on MRI brain imaging, MS should be suspected. MRI imaging of the brain and spinal cord, especially with gadolinium infusion, helps diagnose MS. **Typical MS lesions are bright lesions on T2-weighted imaging, especially in the corpus callosum and periventricular regions** (Fig. 24–1). These lesions are usually linear or ovoid and at right angles to the ventricular surface. MRI brain lesions larger than 5 mm or lesions inferior to the tentorium, especially in the cerebellar peduncle, help confirm the diagnosis of MS.

T1-weighted images are usually less sensitive in detecting demyelinating plaques than are T2-weighted images. Newer techniques of brain imaging, such as fluid attenuated inversion recovery (FLAIR) provide increased sensitivity and specificity for MS white matter lesions. FLAIR images detect two to three times the number of lesions observed on T2-weighed images. N-acetylaspartate (NAA) also assists detecting MS lesions. NAA, a marker for neuronal and axonal function, can be measured by magnetic resonance (MR) spectroscopy. NAA levels are decreased in MS plaques and can also be decreased in seemingly unaffected areas of white matter, suggesting axonal damage.

Analysis of cerebrospinal fluid also helps diagnosing MS. Elevated IgG index, presence of oligoclonal bands, and increased myelin basic protein support the diagnosis. Oligoclonal bands occur in more than 90% of patients with MS, but they also occur in 30% of CNS inflammatory and infectious disease patients, and in 5–10% of other noninflammatory neuralgic diseases. Oligoclonal bands by themselves do not diagnose MS. MS is a clinical diagnosis that can be supported by brain imaging and cerebrospinal fluid (CSF) investigations. Increased CSF white cells can be seen in MS; however, CSF leukocyte counts greater than 50 mm^3 of CSF are rare in MS and should prompt the physician to consider other diagnoses.

Visual evoked responses, in which a patient views repeated reversal of light and dark checkerboard stimuli while a computer averages scalp electrode potentials, is useful in evaluating patients for MS. Prolongation of the P100 wave occurs in more than 75% of MS patients. This disturbance reflects compromise of the pathway between the optic nerve and the brain.

The differential diagnosis of MS is broad (Table 24–1). Many different conditions can mimic multiple sclerosis because of primary or secondary demyelination of CNS pathways. However, the clinical history, physical examination, and diagnostic studies are fundamental in distinguishing these conditions from MS.

Treatment

Treatment of patients with MS needs to be individualized for each specific patient, depending on particular problems and needs. The treatment should be focused on the disease itself and on associated symptoms.

The **primary treatment can consist of intravenous steroids**, primarily employed during acute attacks. **Steroids** have **not been shown** to **decrease the risk of future attacks**, or change in the natural history of disease, but are indicated to hasten recovery from the acute attack. **Immunomodulating agents** can be used to modify the course of MS, and thus are used on a chronic, ongoing basis. These include **interferon β-1a** (Avonex, Rebif), **interferon β-1b** (Betaseron), and a synthetic polypeptide of myelin basic protein, **glatiramer acetate** (Copaxone). These medications are injected subcutaneously or intramuscularly and are usually well tolerated. These agents can impact on the relapse rate, slow down progression of disability and prevent the accumulation of MRI lesion load. Moreover, two formulations of interferon-beta delayed conversion into clinically definite MS in patients with clinically isolated syndromes suggestive of MS. Because axonal damage leading to irreversible neurologic disability is already present early at the onset of the disease, immunomodulatory therapy should start as soon as possible.

Intravenous mitoxantrone, an antineoplastic immunomodulatory agent, also has been shown to improve neurologic disability and delayed progression of MS in patients with worsening relapsing-remitting or secondary-progressive disease. Other immunosuppressive agents, including cyclophosphamide, methotrexate, and cyclosporine, have been shown to be of clinical benefit in patients with worsening disease.

Symptomatic Therapy

Symptomatic therapy for MS can include physical and emotional rest, physical therapy, amantadine, or modafinil for fatigue, anticholinergic medication for bladder dysfunction, and medication for mood disorders (e.g., antidepressants).

Table 24–1
DIFFERENTIAL DIAGNOSIS OF MULTIPLE SCLEROSIS

1. Polyneuropathies
   a. Guillain-Barré syndrome, including Miller Fisher syndrome
   b. Chronic inflammatory demyelinating polyradiculoneuropathy

2. Infections
   a. Bacteria: syphilis, tuberculosis, Lyme disease, *Bartonella henselae* (cat-scratch fever), mycoplasma, Whipple disease, brucellosis, beta-hemolytic streptococcus, meningococcus
   b. Fungi: aspergillus, histoplasmosis, Cryptococcus
   c. Rickettsia (e.g., Q fever, epidemic typhus)
   d. Protozoa (e.g., toxoplasmosis)
   e. Parasites (e.g., toxocariasis, cysticercosis)
   f. Viruses (e.g., adenovirus, hepatitis A, B, cytomegalovirus (CMV), coxsackie B, rubella, chickenpox, herpes zoster, herpes simplex virus I, Epstein-Barr (infectious mononucleosis), measles, mumps, influenza, human T-cell leukemia virus 1 (HTLV-1), Creutzfeldt-Jacob disease
   g. Human immunodeficiency virus (HIV) or acquired immunodeficiency syndrome (AIDS)-related
      i. Primary HIV-related optic neuritis
      ii. Syphilis
      iii. Cat-scratch disease (*Bartonella henselae*)
      iv. Cryptococcus
      v. Histoplasmosis
      vi. CMV
      vii. Herpes zoster
      viii. Hepatitis B
      ix. Toxoplasmosis
   h. Postvaccination (e.g., smallpox, tetanus, rabies, influenza, hepatitis B, Mantoux tuberculin skin test, Bacille Calmette-Guérin (bCG), trivalent measles-mumps-rubella vaccine
   i. Focal infection or inflammation
      i. Paranasal sinusitis
      ii. Postinfectious
      iii. Malignant Otis externa

3. Systemic inflammation and disease
   a. Behçet disease
   b. Inflammatory bowel disease
   c. Reiter syndrome3
   d. Sarcoidosis
   e. Systemic lupus erythematosus
   f. Sjögren syndrome
   g. Mixed connective tissue disease
   h. Rheumatoid arthritis

(Continued)

Table 24–1
DIFFERENTIAL DIAGNOSIS OF MULTIPLE SCLEROSIS (*Continued*)

4. Miscellaneous
   a. Familial Mediterranean fever
   b. Bee or wasp sting
   c. Snakebite
   d. Postpartum optic neuritis
   e. Neuromyelitis optica (Devic disease)
   f. Recurrent optic neuromyelitis with endocrinopathies
   g. Other

Comprehension Questions

[24.1] Multiple sclerosis is characterized by which of the following diagnostic findings?

    A. Oligoclonal bands in cerebrospinal fluid
    B. Increased N-acetyl aspartate with MR spectroscopy
    C. Abnormal peripheral nerve conduction by electromyograph (EMG)/nerve conduction velocity (NCV) studies
    D. Meningeal enhancement on contrast MRI of brain

[24.2] A 33-year-old man is noted to have exacerbations of weakness. He is diagnosed with MS. Which of the following findings is consistent with the diagnosis?

    A. The diagnosis of MS is based on clinical lesions separated by time and space
    B. Oligo bands in the CSF are specific for multiple sclerosis
    C. Steroids are effective in improving the course of disease
    D. This is a genetic disorder well characterized on chromosome 11

[24.3] The same patient in case 24.2 is noted to have significantly progressive disease. Which of the following is likely to be helpful for his symptoms of weakness?

    A. Mitoxantrone
    B. Corticosteroid therapy
    C. Plasmapheresis
    D. Immunoglobulin therapy

Answers

[24.1] **A.** Oligoclonal bands are present in the CSF of up to 90% of MS patients.

[24.2] **A.** Clinical exacerbations separated by time and space are the hallmark of the diagnosis of MS.

[24.3] **A.** Mitoxantrone is helpful for secondary progressive disease.

CLINICAL PEARLS

❖ Earlier age of disease onset is usually associated with benign or relapsing remitting forms of MS.

❖ Visual compromise, stiffness, and weakness are frequent presenting symptoms in MS.

❖ MS patients can have lesions on brain MRIs without associated clinical complaints directly related to those lesions.

❖ Oligoclonal bands are also found in systemic lupus erythematosus, neurosarcoidosis, subacute sclerosing panencephalitis (SSPE), subarachnoid hemorrhage, syphilis, and CNS lymphoma.

❖ The symptoms of MS seem to worsen with elevation of temperature or fever.

REFERENCES

Flachenecker P. Disease-modifying drugs for the early treatment of multiple sclerosis. Expert Rev Neurother 2004 May;4(3):455–63.

Minagar A, Sheremata WA. Multiple sclerosis. In: Evans RW, ed. Saunders manual of neurologic practice. Philadelphia, PA: Saunders/Elsevier; 2003:234–240.

Sadiq, SA. Multiple sclerosis. In: Rowland LP, ed. Merritt's neurology, 11th ed. Philadelphia, PA: Lippincott Williams & Wilkins; 2005:941–961.

Scott LJ, Figgitt DP. Mitoxantrone: a review of its use in multiple sclerosis. CNS Drugs 2004;18(6):379–396.

A 20-year-old college student was studying late at night for an examination. Three weeks previously, he had a viral illness but his symptoms had resolved. Suddenly, in the study hall, he developed headache, nausea, confusion, and complained of weakness of both legs. He also could not hold his urine and had urinary incontinence. His roommate carried him to the infirmary for evaluation. On examination, the patient was lethargic, with some slurring of his speech. His vitals were stable, and he was afebrile. General examination was normal. Neurologic examination was significant for weakness in his lower extremities, but he was able to stand. Gait was significantly unsteady, and he required assistance with walking. His reflexes were diffusely increased with bilateral upgoing toes. His sensory examination revealed a subjective sensory level at the level of his navel. The patient was admitted for evaluation and management.

◆ **What is the most likely diagnosis?**

◆ **What is the prognosis for this condition?**

◆ **What is the next step in therapy?**

ANSWERS TO CASE 25: Acute Disseminated Encephalomyelitis

Summary: A 20-year-old man developed multiple neurologic symptoms 3 weeks following a viral illness. He suddenly complained of headache and had symptoms of spinal cord compromise (i.e., weakness in lower extremities, urinary incontinence, sensory level).

◆ **Most likely diagnosis:** Acute disseminated encephalomyelitis.

◆ **Prognosis:** Fairly good.

◆ **Next step in therapy:** Consider intravenous corticosteroids, plasmapheresis, and intravenous immunoglobulin.

Analysis

Objectives

1. Understand the differential diagnosis of acute disseminated encephalomyelitis.
2. Understand the evaluation for acute disseminated encephalomyelitis.
3. Understand the prognosis of acute disseminated encephalomyelitis.
4. Understand when and how to treat acute disseminated encephalomyelitis.

Considerations

Acute disseminated encephalomyelitis (ADEM) is a monophasic illness associated with multiple neurologic symptoms as a result of involvement of the brainstem, spinal cord, optic nerves, cerebrum, and/or cerebellum. ADEM usually follows infection or vaccination, especially in children. One-quarter of patients with ADEM will develop multiple sclerosis (MS), often causing difficulty differentiating the first attack of MS from ADEM. However, ADEM is usually uniphasic and has a favorable long-term prognosis.

APPROACH TO ACUTE DISSEMINATED ENCEPHALOMYELITIS

Definitions

Acute disseminated encephalomyelitis: ADEM is an acute, uniphasic syndrome, probably caused by immune-mediated inflammatory demyelination. It often is associated with immunization, vaccination, or postviral illness.

Acute necrotizing hemorrhagic encephalomyelitis (ANHE): ANHE is a hyperacute form of ADEM, with similar symptoms and cause.

Clinical Approach

Etiologies and Clinical Presentation

ADEM can occur as a postinfectious complication in 1:400 to 1:2,000 patients with measles, 1:600 patients with mumps, 1:10,000 patients with varicella, and 1:20,000 rubella patients. It is a postvaccination complication in 1:63 to 1:300,000 patients with vaccinia and can also occur following other immunizations. ADEM can also occur following diphtheria (tetanus), pertussis, and rubella.

ADEM is a monophasic illness, characterized by multiple neurologic signs and symptoms reflecting compromise of the brainstem, spinal cord, cerebrum, optic nerves, and cerebellum. The symptoms appear suddenly 1 to 3 weeks following the infection and can include headache, nausea, vomiting, confusion, and can progress to obtundation and coma.

In addition to the above-noted symptoms of ADEM, patients can have hemiparesis, hemisensory compromise, ataxia, optic neuritis, transverse myelitis, seizures, myoclonus, and memory loss. When ADEM follows mumps, the disease usually presents with cerebellar ataxia.

ADEM is probably a T-cell–mediated autoimmune disease targeting myelin/oligodendrocyte antigens, possibly myelin basic protein. Viral infection causing subsequent downregulation of CD4+ suppressor T cells, activating myelin-reactive T-helper cells, has been implicated.

Neuropathology of ADEM consists of perivenular inflammatory myelinopathy, with engorgement of veins in the white matter of the brain. There is perivascular edema with significant mononuclear infiltration, primarily lymphocytes and macrophages. The primary finding is perivenular demyelination, with relative sparing of axons.

The diagnosis of ADEM primarily focuses on the clinical presentation of a uniphasic illness. Cerebrospinal fluid (CSF) findings can be abnormal but are not specific for ADEM (e.g., mononuclear pleocytosis, mildly elevated protein). MRI imaging of the brain reveals hyperintense white matter T2-weighted signals and enhancement on T1-weighted images. The lesions vary in size because of the significant associated edema. The lesions described are rather extensive and symmetric or asymmetric and more often located in the peripheral subcortical cerebral white matter. Lesions in the thalami are more often described in ADEM than MS and can be a useful finding that suggests ADEM.

The differential diagnosis of ADEM is the same as that noted in case 24 for MS. The fact that ADEM is monophasic, whereas MS is usually not, and the clear time frame of feeling well for several weeks following a viral illness, respectively, help differentiate ADEM from MS and an acute viral episode.

The prognosis of ADEM is fairly good. However, approximately one-quarter (up to one-third) of these patients will subsequently relapse following the acute illness. If relapse occurs, the physician should suspect MS.

Treatment

There is no specific treatment for ADEM. Management is supportive and symptomatic. In severe cases, it is important to maintain vital functions, maintain fluid and electrolyte balance, and avoid pneumonia, urinary infection, and decubitus ulcers. In some patients with ADEM, physicians prescribe high doses of intravenous corticosteroids to shorten the duration of the disease. There is some controversy about the efficacy of plasmapheresis or intravenous immunoglobulin.

Comprehension Questions

[25.1] Select the combination of signs and symptoms that best help to distinguish ADEM from a first attack MS.

    A. Oligoclonal bands in CSF, recurrent symptoms, positive vaccination history

    B. Positive vaccination history, lesions of the thalami, mental confusion

    C. Pleocytosis in CSF, recurrent symptoms, positive vaccination history

    D. Recent viral exposure, mental confusion, late ataxia

[25.2] A 43-year-old woman is diagnosed with acute lower extremity weakness caused by acute disseminated encephalomyelitis. Which of the following is the best therapy for this condition?

    A. Interferon 1b

    B. Corticosteroid therapy

    C. Amantadine

    D. Immunoglobulin therapy

[25.3] A 33-year-old man has lower extremity weakness and urinary incontinence approximately 2 weeks after a viral illness. Which of the following is most likely to be present?

    A. Sensorineural hearing loss

    B. Ataxia

    C. Facial nerve palsy

    D. Tinnitus

Answers

[25.1] **B.** In the absence of a biologic marker, the distinction between ADEM and MS cannot be made with certainty at the time of first presentation. However certain features are more indicative of ADEM and include a viral prodrome or recent vaccination exposure, early-onset ataxia, high lesion load on MRI, involvement of the deep gray matter, especially thalami, and absence of oligoclonal bands.

[25.2] **B.** Standard of care for patients with MS is interferon beta 1b therapy. Corticosteroids can help to reduce the duration and severity of symptoms in patients with ADEM. Intravenous gammaglobulin therapy remains controversial.

[25.3] **B.** Although ADEM patients can have hemiparesis, hemisensory compromise, ataxia, optic neuritis, transverse myelitis, seizures, myoclonus, and memory loss, sensorineural hearing loss is not a complication of the disease.

CLINICAL PEARLS

❖ **Acute disseminated encephalomyelitis** is a "rare disease" affecting less than 200,000 people in the U.S. population.

❖ The etiopathogenesis of ADEM is **multifactorial.** In a subset of patients who are **genetic**ally susceptible to these disorders, the immune system is triggered to react to myelin by an **environmental** trigger, either by a vaccine or by a virus, and that sets up a cascade of events that causes ADEM.

❖ Episodes of *recurrent ADEM* have been described, which are usually triggered by infections. It is possible that episodes of recurrent ADEM are multiple episodes of MS.

❖ In the absence of a biologic marker, differentiation of ADEM from the initial presentation of MS, at times, may not be possible.

REFERENCES

Minagar A, Sheremata WA. Acute disseminated encephalomyelitis. In: Evans RW, ed. Saunders manual of neurologic practice. Philadelphia, PA: Saunders/Elsevier; 2003:241–243.

Sadiq, SA. Multiple sclerosis. In: Rowland LP, ed. Merritt's neurology, 11th ed. Philadelphia, PA: Lippincott Williams & Wilkins;2005:941–961.

A 28-year-old man presents to the emergency room with a 48-hour complaint of headache. The headache is primarily in the frontal and occipital regions and associated with mild nausea. He has taken various over-the-counter analgesics without any improvement in the headache. The intensity of the headache has gradually increased since it began prompting evaluation as he was no longer able to tolerate it. His only other symptom besides nausea, is a tightness in the shoulders and neck. He is not known to have any medical illnesses, and there is no history of head trauma. On examination, he has a temperature of 32.8°C (100.8°F); blood pressure, 110/68 mmHg; and pulse, of 100 beats/min. He is awake and alert and fully oriented. His Mini Mental Status Examination (MMSE) is normal; however, he feels he is taking too much time to answer the questions. His general examination is notable for the finding of a Kernig sign without evidence of any skin rash. A Brudzinski sign is not present. Cranial nerves are normal except for bilateral horizontal nystagmus. His motor, sensory, and cerebellar examinations are normal. The deep tendon reflexes are hyperreflexic throughout without evidence of a Babinski sign. A CT scan of the head is performed without contrast, which is read as normal. Importantly his headache is worse now than what it was when he presented to the emergency room.

◆ **What is the most likely diagnosis?**

◆ **What is the best diagnostic next step?**

◆ **What is the next step in therapy?**

ANSWERS TO CASE 26: Viral Meningitis

Summary: A 28-year-old man without medical illnesses presents with a 48-hour history of crescendo headache. Associated symptoms include nausea and slowness in responding to questions. The examination is notable for a Kernig sign, horizontal nystagmus, and generalized hyperreflexia.

◆ **Most likely diagnosis:** Viral meningitis

◆ **Best diagnostic step:** Lumbar puncture

◆ **Next step in therapy:** Start IV antibiotics and IV acyclovir

Analysis

Objectives

1. Know the clinical presentation of meningitis.
2. Learn to develop a diagnostic strategy for the diagnosis of meningitis and understand the cerebrospinal fluid (CSF) findings in bacterial and viral meningitis.
3. Know the treatment strategy for meningitis in the emergency room.

Considerations

The presentation of a crescendo headache associated with nausea, fever, and slowness in responding to questions should alert the clinician of meningitis or encephalitis. The presence of neck tightness and a Kernig sign is consistent with meningitis. The lumbar puncture CSF study is the best way to determine the etiology of meningitis allowing one to distinguish between a bacterial versus viral, and so forth. Although CSF studies are key to identifying meningitis, an imaging study with either a CT head scan or MRI brain scan is preferably done prior to the spinal tap. Although the MRI brain scan offers better resolution than a CT head scan, it may not always be ready available. The study of choice between the latter is based on what can be done the quickest. The importance of the imaging studies is to help exclude increased intracranial pressure caused by impaired CSF drainage or a space-occupying lesion. Increased intracranial pressure could potentially lead to cerebral herniation and death of the patient. **Focal neurologic findings or the presence of papilledema mandate an imaging study.** Once it is determined that the risk of herniation is low, a lumbar puncture is performed. Lumbar puncture analysis should include opening and closing pressure, and CSF studies for glucose, protein, cell count with differential, Gram stain, culture, latex particle agglutination, herpes simplex virus (HSV) polymerase chain reaction (PCR), enteroviral (EV) reverse transcriptase (RT)-PCR, Venereal Disease Research Laboratory (VDRL), and hold extra CSF for additional studies. Other tests to consider include chemistry 20, complete blood count (CBC) with differential and platelets, international normalized ratio (INR)/prothrombin time (PT)/partial thromboplastin time (PTT), HIV, blood cultures. However, if there is a delay in obtaining an imaging study, blood cultures are taken from the patient, and empiric IV antibiotics are started immediately until a lumbar puncture is performed. The initial choice of antibiotics is customarily a third-generation cephalosporin such as ceftriaxone or cefotaxime plus vancomycin, IV dexamethasone, IV acyclovir. These should be given after blood and CSF are collected, or even when there is a delay in obtaining a lumbar puncture.

APPROACH TO SUSPECTED MENINGITIS

Definitions

Meningitis: Inflammation of the membranes of the brain and spinal cord (meninges) caused by many different organisms.

Kernig sign: The inability to completely extend the leg when the hip is flexed in the supine position. This is caused by severe stiffness in the hamstrings muscles from inflammation of the lumbosacral roots.

Brudzinski sign: Flexion of the neck causes involuntary flexion of the thighs and the legs.

Latex particle agglutination: A test where an antibody or antigen coats the surface of latex particles (sensitized latex). When a sample containing the specific antigen or antibody is mixed with the milky appearing sensitized latex, visible agglutination is noted. It is used to detect *Haemophilus influenzae* type b, *Streptococcus pneumoniae*, and *Neisseria meningitidis* A, B, and C soluble antigens.

HSV PCR: Polymerase chain reaction is a molecular technique that allows a small amount of DNA to be replicated and amplified. In this case HSV DNA is detected. HSV PCR for CSF has an estimated sensitivity of 95% and specificity of almost 100%.

EV RT-PCR: Enteroviral reverse transcriptase polymerase chain reaction is a technique in which cDNA is made from RNA via reverse transcription. The cDNA is then replicated and amplified through standard PCR protocols. In this particular case various viruses belonging to the enterovirus family can be detected.

Nystagmus: A rapid involuntary oscillatory movement of the eyes.

Clinical Approach

Etiology

Bacterial meningitis is typically more severe and carries a higher morbidity and mortality rate when compared to viral meningitis. The incidence of bacterial meningitis is approximately 3 to 5 per 100,000 people per year in the

United States. Annually 2000 deaths have been reported in the United States from bacterial meningitis. The relative frequency of bacterial species as a cause of meningitis varies with age. During the neonatal period *Escherichia coli, Listeria monocytogenes* and group B streptococci account for most of the causes of neonatal meningitis. Following the neonatal period *H. influenza, S. pneumoniae,* and *N. meningitidis* account for 80% of cases. In 1987 widespread vaccination against *H. influenza* type B led to a marked reduction in this pathogen causing meningitis in children. Streptococcal pneumonia and Neisseria meningitis are now the principal causes of meningitis following the neonatal period.

The most common causes of viral meningitis in the United States are viruses from the enterovirus family. Approximately 75,000 cases of enterovirus meningitis occur in the United States each year. Coxsackie A9, B3–5, and echovirus 4, 6, 7, 8, 11, 18, and 30 are the most common strains. The infection is spread by fecal-oral route although spread through the respiratory route is noted rarely. Outbreaks can be associated with pharyngitis or gastroenteritis and occur in the late summer and early fall. There can be a viral exanthem present. Other viral causes of meningitis include HSV, arboviruses (St. Louis encephalitis virus, West Nile virus, Japanese encephalitis virus, Western equine encephalitis virus, Eastern equine encephalitis, and La Crosse virus), Arenaviruses and retroviruses. The arboviruses are viruses that are transmitted to humans via arthropods, most commonly mosquitoes or ticks.

Clinical Presentation and Evaluation

Typical symptoms of meningitis include the classic triad of headache, fever, and neck stiffness. Other symptoms include photophobia (eye pain or sensitivity to light), nausea, vomiting, myalgia confusion, declining levels of consciousness (from lethargy to coma), seizures, and focal neurologic deficits such as cranial nerve palsies, hemiparesis, or dysphasia, because of ischemic strokes caused by secondary thrombosis or inflammation of cerebral vessels.

In evaluating patients with meningitis it is critical to differentiate between a bacterial and viral or other type of meningitis. Certain findings on clinical examination can point toward a bacterial infection rather than a viral infection. For example, the presence of a very high fever or widespread macular papular rash or the presence of purpura or ecchymosis suggests a bacterial infection such as Neisseria meningitis. CSF studies, however, are more definitive and will allow the differentiation between viral and bacterial meningitis. CSF studies in bacterial meningitis reveal an elevated opening pressure (greater than 200 mm of H_2O), elevated protein 100–500 mg/dL (normal 15 to 45 mg/dL), reduced glucose (less than 40% serum glucose) and pleocytosis (100 to 10,000 white blood cells/μL; normal <5) with 60% or greater polymorphonuclear leukocytes. Sixty percent of bacterial meningitis cases will have a positive Gram stain result with approximately 75% having a positive CSF culture. Blood cultures will pick up the causative organism of bacterial meningitis in

50% of cases emphasizing the fact that bacteremia is present early on and explains why bacterial meningitis is a true medical emergency. Antibiotics administered up to 2 hours before a lumbar puncture do not decrease the sensitivity of CSF culture done in conjunction with latex particle agglutination and blood cultures. Antibiotics administered for longer than 2 hours before a lumbar puncture may decrease the findings of a positive Gram stain or positive culture in the CSF by 5–40%.

CSF studies in viral meningitis also may reveal an elevated opening pressure, normal glucose, elevated CSF cell counts from 200 to >1000 white blood cells /μL with no more than 50% polymorphonuclear cells. However, within the first 24 hours of infection up to 90% of white blood cells can be polymorphonuclear cells. Viral CSF cultures have a relatively low sensitivity and poor ability to grow. Furthermore the clinical utility of this is limited by the amount of time requiring the enterovirus to grow (days to weeks). The EV RT-PCR on CSF has 100% specificity and 95% sensitivity. Results are often available within 4 hours.

Neuroimaging studies in bacterial meningitis are often normal but can also reveal complications such as infarction, venous sinus thrombosis, communicating or noncommunicating hydrocephalus, and increased intracranial pressure. In most cases of viral meningitis the neuroimaging studies are normal, however, a key exception is HSV meningitis in which there can be evidence of hemorrhage in the temporal lobe region.

Treatment

The key in reducing morbidity and mortality in patients with meningitis is rapid recognition so that treatment can be implemented. This means identifying the causative agent as soon as possible. Many tests discussed above take several hours before results are available making it impossible to wait for the results before treatment is instituted. As a result, treatment with antibiotics and/or retrovirals is started while waiting for test results (Fig. 26–1). Penicillin G or ampicillin and a third-generation cephalosporin are typical first-line agents for the treatment of bacterial meningitis. However the drug resistance has started to become a frequent problem, and as a result, treatment recommendations are changing based on local resistance patterns. Ampicillin covers most pneumococcus, meningococcus, and Listeria. Ceftriaxone or cefotaxime, third-generation cephalosporins, cover gram-negative organisms as well as ampicillin-resistant *H. influenza*. Vancomycin is added to third-generation cephalosporins to cover *Staphylococcus aureus* when patients have undergone recent neurosurgical procedures or head trauma. If the sensitivity for *S. pneumoniae* is unknown then adding vancomycin to a third-generation cephalosporin is appropriate. Penicillin G is used to treat gram-negative cocci and gram-positive bacilli. Aminoglycosides are added to treat gram-positive bacilli. Gram-negative bacilli are treated with third-generation cephalosporins and aminoglycosides.

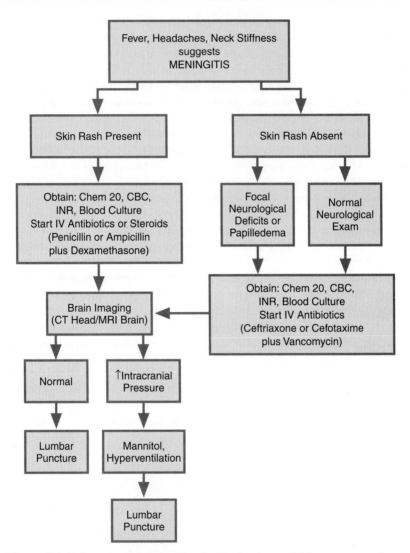

Figure 26–1. Sample Algorithm for the Evaluation and Management of possible meningitis.

Adjuvant therapy with intravenous corticosteroids for bacterial meningitis is clearly indicated in children. In adults, the use of intravenous corticosteroids is not as clear. There is some evidence to suggest that penetration of vancomycin into CSF is reduced by the administration of corticosteroids. Additionally corticosteroids can mask clinical signs for antibody response. However, recent studies have shown the benefit in preventing systemic complications as well as neurologic deficits in adult patients with *S. pneumoniae* meningitis when corticosteroids are given.

As of yet, there is no effective treatment for viral meningitis except if HSV is suspected. The treatment for HSV meningitis is intravenous acyclovir. HSV meningitis is infrequently present in individuals at the time of their first episode of genital herpes. Approximately 11% of men and 36% of women with genital herpes will exhibit symptoms consistent with HSV meningitis. In adults, the prognosis for recovery is excellent, although some patients will have residual headache. Sensorineural hearing loss can occur especially in children. Infants and neonates can have more serious long-term sequelae such as cognitive deficits or learning disabilities. Herpes encephalitis is the most common cause of sporadic viral encephalitis, with the predilection for the temporal lobes. The clinical presentation can range from aseptic meningitis and fever to severe rapidly progressive forms with significant mortality of the latter.

Comprehension Questions

[26.1] A 42-year-old woman presents to the emergency room with fever, neck stiffness, and severe headache. Her examination reveals a widespread macular papular rash. Which of the following is the most appropriate next step in management?

A. Obtain a stat CT scan of the head followed by a lumbar puncture.
B. Perform a stat lumbar puncture without obtaining a CT scan of the head.
C. Obtain a CBC with differential, blood cultures, chemistry 20 and INR and begin IV penicillin G or ampicillin.
D. Obtain a CBC with D-P, blood cultures, chemistry 20, and INR, and begin IV ceftriaxone plus vancomycin.

[26.2] A 21-year-old man is brought in by emergency medical services (EMS) to the emergency room with a severe headache, fever, and confusion. His neurologic examination is notable for a Kernig sign and hyperreflexia. His lumbar puncture reveals a protein of 72 mg/dL, glucose of 50 (serum glucose of 100), 235 white blood cells (WBCs) with 60% lymphocytes and cultures/Gram stain pending. These CSF studies are most consistent with which of the following?

A. Bacterial meningitis
B. Viral meningitis
C. Bacterial and viral meningitis
D. Cannot tell without knowing the result of the cultures and Gram stain

[26.3] A 34-year-old woman is noted to have a stiff neck, fever, and photophobia. Which of the following is the best method to differentiate viral versus bacterial meningitis?

A. Sensorium
B. Nuchal rigidity
C. Lumbar puncture
D. CT scan

Answers

[26.1] **C.** The presence of a macular papular rash should alert the clinician that this patient might have meningococcal meningitis. The treatment initially until a Gram stain and culture results are available is penicillin G and/or ampicillin. Serologic studies including blood cultures are necessary prior to starting antibiotics should there be a delay in obtaining an imaging study while antibiotics have been started. Because of the high morbidity and mortality with meningococcal meningitis, treatment should be started immediately.

[26.2] **B.** The finding of an elevated CSF protein, normal glucose, and the predominance of lymphocytes is consistent with a viral meningitis. Early on a viral meningitis can have a predominance of polymorphonuclear cells making it easy to confuse viral and bacterial meningitis. However a normal CSF glucose is uncommon in bacterial meningitis.

[26.3] **C.** The lumbar puncture with CSF findings is the best method of differentiating bacterial versus viral meningitis.

CLINICAL PEARLS

❖ Meningitis classically presents with the triad of altered mental status, fever, and neck stiffness but is present in only 44% of confirmed cases of meningitis. When headache occurs with one of the other three symptoms the sensitivity improves to 95%.

❖ Meningococcal meningitis is an emergency requiring prompt treatment and can be identified in the emergency room by the presence of a macular papular rash.

❖ The key CSF difference between viral and bacterial meningitis is the predominance of lymphocytes and a normal CSF glucose in viral meningitis.

❖ Nuchal rigidity is assessed in the supine position with both hips and knees flexed. Pain elicited when the knees are passively extended indicates nuchal rigidity and meningitis, **Kernig sign**. In infants, forward flexion of the neck can cause involuntary knee and hip flexion, **Brudzinski sign**.

REFERENCES

Debasi R, Solbrig M, et al. Infections of the nervous system. In: Bradley WG, Daroff, RB, Fenichel G, et al. Neurology in Clinical Practice, 4th ed. Philadelphia, PA: Butterworth-Heinemann; 2003.

Dorland's Illustrated Medical Dictionary, 27th ed. Philadelphia, PA: WB Saunders; 1988.

van de Beek D, de Gans J. Dexamethasone in adults with community-acquired bacterial meningitis. Drugs 2006;66(4):415–427.

van de Beek, et al. Clinical features and prognostic factors in adults with bacterial meningitis. N Engl J Med 2004 Oct 28;351(18):1849–1859.

A 9-month-old baby girl is brought to the emergency room by her parents with a history of constipation, poor feeding, and weak cry over the past 72 hours. The mother notes that the baby has been constipated for at least 1 week prior to the onset of decreased oral intake. She has also noticed that the baby is unable to suck on a bottle as well as before. The baby girl has been irritable and unable to hold up her head. Over the past 24 hours she has developed weakness in her arms, and this morning was found to have weakness in her legs. On physical examination the baby is noted to be hypotensive with a blood pressure of 70/30 mmHg and profoundly hypotonic. She is unable to move her eyes, and she has marked pooling of her oral secretions. Deep tendon reflexes (DTRs) are reduced. Her maternal grandmother saw the housekeeper give the baby honey 1 week ago.

◆ **What is the most likely diagnosis?**

◆ **What is the next step to confirm the diagnosis?**

◆ **What is the next step in therapy?**

ANSWERS TO CASE 27: Infantile Botulism

Summary: A 9-month old baby girl presents with a 1-week history of consti-pation and a 72-hour history of poor feeding and weak cry. She has been noted to have difficulty sucking on a bottle, holding her head up, and moving her arms and legs. Her examination is notable for hypotension, hypotonia, gener-alized hyporeflexia, and weakness of the extraocular muscles. She was given honey 1 week ago.

◆ **Most likely diagnosis:** Infantile botulism

◆ **Next diagnostic to confirm diagnosis:** Stool sample culture for *Clostridium botulinum* and serum sample for *C. botulinum*

◆ **Next therapeutic step:** Admit to the ICU as respiratory depression can ensue in more than 70% of affected infants, give aggressive supportive care including nasogastric feeds and ventilatory support, administer antitoxin human botulism immunoglobulin (intravenously).

Analysis

Objectives

1. Describe the common clinical manifestations of infantile botulism and food-borne botulism.
2. Understand the pathophysiology of botulism.
3. Know how to treat infantile botulism.

Considerations

This 9-month-old infant presents with profound generalized weakness of the peripheral nervous system. This is based on the finding of generalized hypo-tonia, hyporeflexia, and weakness. The history is critical in this case as it describes a **descending weakness** as opposed to an ascending weakness often seen in Guillain-Barré syndrome (GBS). The presence of autonomic dysfunc-tion with hypotension and constipation is a key to diagnosing this infant. Although, dysautonomia may be seen in patients with GBS, the pattern of developing weakness is different (ascending in GBS and descending in botu-lism); additionally, GBS is rare in children younger than 1 year of age. Hypotonia can also be seen in central nervous system diseases such as menin-gitis and encephalitis. However the absence of fever points toward botulism or other processes. Other considerations in the differential diagnosis include toxic causes such as heavy metals, organophosphates, and anticholinergics; metabolic causes such as Reye syndrome (because of irritability and lethargy), hepatic encephalopathy, hypermagnesemia, hypothyroidism, and organic acidurias. Other neuromuscular causes to consider include poliomyelitis,

GBS, congenital myasthenia gravis (excluded by neonatal and maternal history), muscular dystrophy, and spinal muscular atrophy. Poliomyelitis is asymmetric and will have elevated white blood cells (WBCs) in the cerebrospinal fluid, whereas spinal muscular atrophy does not affect the autonomic nervous system.

APPROACH TO INFANT BOTULISM

Definitions

Infantile botulism: A neuroparalytic disease presenting in a subacute manner caused by *C. botulinum* toxin type A and B that typically occurs when ingested spores germinate and colonize in the gastrointestinal tract of the infant.

Electromyograph (EMG) with repetitive nerve stimulation studies: An electrophysiological test that evaluates motor unit action potentials and function at the neuromuscular junction. When performed at different frequencies it is helpful in differentiating a presynaptic neuromuscular junction transmission disorder such as botulism from a postsynaptic neuromuscular junction transmission disorder such as acquired myasthenia gravis.

Dysautonomia: Dysfunction of the autonomic nervous system manifested by tachycardia, bradycardia, hypotension, hypertension, hyperthermia, hypothermia, blurred vision, xerostomia, constipation, diarrhea, bladder urgency, bladder hesitancy, erectile dysfunction, hyperhidrosis, or anhidrosis.

Clinical Approach

Infantile botulism is caused by a neurotoxin produced by *C. botulinum*, a spore forming anaerobic gram-positive bacilli found in soil. There are seven distinct types (A–G) described based on different types of toxins produced. Infantile botulism is specifically caused by types A and B. Type E is also associated with disease in humans, whereas type C and D cause disease in birds and fish as well as other nonhuman mammals.

In adults, normal intestinal flora prevents colonization of *C. botulinum* in the gut. However in infants, normal intestinal flora has not developed, and as such intestinal colonization of *C. botulism* can take place. Colonization typically occurs in the cecum. Toxins are produced and absorbed throughout the intestinal tract after colonization occurs. The toxin irreversibly binds to presynaptic cholinergic receptors at motor nerve terminals and is then internalized. Inside the cell, the toxin acts as a protease, damaging membrane proteins, inhibiting the release of acetylcholine and disrupting exocytosis. Thus, the **inhibition of acetylcholine release** results in disruption of neurotransmission between the **nerve and end plate on the muscle.**

In the United States, 95% of infantile botulism occurs in patients younger than 6 months of age. Approximately 60 cases are reported each year; infantile botulism is the most common form of botulism in the United States. Nearly 50% of all cases are reported from California. The two most commonly recognized sources of botulinum spores are honey and soil contamination. A history of honey consumption is seen in almost 15% of cases reported to the Centers for Disease Control (CDC). Thus, **honey should not be given to infants** younger than 1 year of age. The typical incubation period is anywhere from 3 to 30 days.

Foodborne botulism accounts for almost 1000 reported annual cases worldwide. Type B contamination is most commonly seen in Europe, whereas type A is more commonly seen in China. Outbreaks in Alaska, Canada, and Japan have been reported with type E. The majority of cases in the United States occur from home canned vegetables.

The clinical presentation of infantile botulism includes **constipation, hypotonia, respiratory difficulties, cranial nerve abnormalities, and hyporeflexia.** The most common signs and symptoms at the time of hospital admission include weakness, poor feeding, constipation, lethargy, weak cry, irritability, and respiratory distress. Constipation is often the first symptom and can precede the other symptoms by several weeks. Dysautonomia can occur early in the disease prior to signs of weakness. Ptosis, lack of ocular motility, facial weakness, and mydriasis can also be noted. Weakness occurs in a descending fashion beginning in the head and working its way down the limbs. **Respiratory distress** is a late sign in the disease but can quickly result in a respiratory arrest. Poor anal sphincter tone is also described.

The clinical presentation for foodborne botulism includes **progressive symmetric descending weakness or paralysis** affecting the muscles of the head followed by those of the neck and then the limbs. Sensation and cognitive function are normal. Respiratory distress occurs from diaphragmatic weakness and airway obstruction. Half of affected patients have dilated or unreactive pupils. Other symptoms include dysphagia, dysarthria, diplopia, dry mouth, dysphonia, and diminished gag. **Gastrointestinal symptoms** such as nausea, vomiting, and diarrhea often precede the neurologic symptoms.

Fecal specimens from infants are the best way to diagnose infantile botulism. A minimum of 25 to 50 g of feces is required to detect *C. botulinum* and its toxin. Enema fluids can be required in constipated individuals. A passed stool sample is preferred. The collected sample should be placed in a sterile container and refrigerated. Confirmation of the organism and/or the toxin has been reported in up to 75% of cases. Laboratory confirmation via mouse bioassay is performed by the CDC or state health departments. Additional studies for the toxin can be obtained by serum, however, the frequency of detection is quite low. **EMG** with repetitive nerve stimulation study aids in early confirmation. The finding of decreased amplitude in two muscle groups, tetanic and posttetanic facilitation (>120% of baseline), and absence of post-tetanic exhaustion are the three findings diagnostic for infantile botulism.

Treatment

Treatment is with **antitoxin**. The botulinum immunoglobulin in infants has been shown to shorten the hospital stay and cost of hospitalization. Additionally it has been shown to reduce the severity of illness. **Human botulinum immunoglobulin is directed toward type A and B.** Supportive care is vital. Patient should be carefully monitored in an ICU setting for impending respiratory distress. Additionally, tube feedings and care for the prolonged immobility and stress ulcers are needed. The case fatality rate is less than 2%; on average, infants will spend 44 days in the hospital. Rare cases of relapse have been reported with no known predictors identified. Most relapses occur within 2 weeks of being discharged from the hospital.

Comprehension Questions

[27.1] A 2-month-old baby boy presents with a history of poor suck, irritability, decreased oral intake, ptosis, head drop, and weakness in the arms and legs. The baby is in foster care, and there is not a good way to obtain a history. While evaluating the baby he develops respiratory distress. Key findings on his examination include external ophthalmoplegia, reactive pupils, ptosis, facial weakness, and weakness in the arms and legs. His DTRs and tone appear to be normal. What is the likely diagnosis?

A. Infantile botulism
B. Neonatal myasthenia gravis
C. Guillain-Barré syndrome
D. Meningitis

[27.2] In cases of suspected infantile botulism which of the following is the most helpful in evaluating the patient?

A. Serum test for botulinum toxin
B. CSF studies for botulinum toxin
C. EMG with repetitive nerve stimulation studies
D. Pharyngeal culture for botulinum toxin

[27.3] A 73-year-old man presents to the emergency room complaining of diplopia, blurred vision, dysphagia, and xerostomia. His examination reveals ptosis, impaired ocular motility, dilated pupils, symmetrical weakness in the arms and legs, and normal cognitive function. Which of the following would be most consistent with his presentation?

A. Antecedent gastrointestinal disease with nausea, vomiting, and diarrhea
B. Loss of sensation in a glove and stocking distribution
C. A history of eating honey from California
D. Normal EMG with repetitive nerve stimulation studies

Answers

[27.1] **B.** The presence of reactive pupils and normal deep tendon reflexes points away from infantile botulism. Likewise the presence of normal deep tendon reflexes is unlikely in GBS. The absence of fever makes it unlikely that this is meningitis.

[27.2] **C.** Fecal cultures and not pharyngeal cultures are the best way to diagnose infantile botulism. EMG with repetitive nerve stimulation studies are key in making the diagnosis of infantile botulism.

[27.3] **A.** This case is illustrative of foodborne botulism, which is known to have normal sensation and normal cognitive function. EMG with repetitive nerve stimulation studies will be abnormal. Botulism from spores in honey occur primarily in infants.

CLINICAL PEARLS

❖ Infantile botulism is the most common cause of botulism in the United States.

❖ Infantile botulism is commonly acquired from spores in soil or in honey.

❖ Classic presentation for infantile botulism includes antecedent constipation with the ascending paralysis, ptosis, dilated or unreactive pupils, and weakness in the arms and legs.

❖ The best way to test for infantile botulism is through stool samples via a mouse bioassay.

❖ More than 70% of these infants with botulism will eventually require mechanical ventilation.

REFERENCES

Arnon SS, Schecter R, Maslanka SE, et al. Human botulism immune globulin for the treatment of infant botulism. N Engl J Med 2006 Feb 2;354(5):462–471.

Cherington M. Clinical spectrum of botulism. Muscle Nerve 1998;21:701–710.

Schreiner M, Field E, Ruddy R. Infant botulism: a review of 12 years experience at the Children's Hospital of Philadelphia. Pediatrics 1991;87:159–165.

A 52-year-old man is referred for further evaluation of mild forgetfulness, poor concentration, and withdrawal from friends. His wife who has accompanied him feels that he is clumsier noting that he is often times tripping. The patient has also noticed that he is clumsier and that he is more forgetful and is having difficulty focusing at work. He also notes a reduction in libido. His physical examination is notable for a normal Mini Mental Status Examination (MMSE) but with slowness in answering questions. Cranial nerves and motor strength are normal. Mild fine hand movements are awkward, and there is mild ataxia noted. Deep tendon reflexes are slightly increased. He is concerned because he has been losing weight and is currently awaiting the results of a second HIV test. A previous HIV test 4 weeks ago was positive.

◆ **What is the most likely diagnosis?**

◆ **What is the next diagnostic step?**

ANSWERS TO CASE 28: HIV-Associated Dementia

Summary: A 52-year-old man with weight loss has been experiencing mild forgetfulness, poor concentration, clumsiness, difficulty focusing at work, reduced libido, and withdrawal from friends. His examination shows normal cognitive function by MMSE but mental slowness in answering questions. Mild ataxia and poor coordination of his hands are noted. Additionally he has mild hyperreflexia. His HIV test 4 weeks ago is positive.

◆ **Most likely diagnosis:** Dementia/HIV-associated dementia (HAD)

◆ **Next diagnostic step:** Neuropsychologic testing, obtain results of his last HIV tests, MRI of the brain, lumbar puncture for cerebrospinal fluid (CSF) studies

Analysis

Objectives

1. Be familiar with the diagnosis of HIV associated dementia (HAD).
2. Know how to diagnose and treat HAD.
3. Describe the differential diagnosis of HAD.

Considerations

This 52-year-old man with a positive HIV test presents with poor concentration, mild forgetfulness, difficulty focusing, withdrawal from friends, clumsiness, and reduced libido. The classic findings of behavioral changes, difficulty with coordination, and mild impaired intellect in the setting of a positive HIV test is likely to be **HIV associated dementia (HAD)**. Depression could also present this way; however, one would not expect there to be problems with coordination. Encephalitis, neurosyphilis, frontal temporal dementia, and HIV-1 associated opportunistic infections are also in the differential diagnosis. These can be distinguished from HAD by performing an MRI of the brain, lumbar puncture, and neuropsychologic testing. Neurologic complications from HIV can be seen from opportunistic infections, drug-related complications, tumors secondary to HIV, and HIV itself. The pathophysiology of HAD is likely multifactorial. First, there is invasion of HIV into the central nervous system. HIV-infected monocytes are thought to enter the brain and infect microglia, astrocytes, neurons, and oligodendrocytes. Additionally, the HIV virus may replicate in the cells. Viral toxins or HIV proteins may be directly toxic to neurons or may cause damage by activating macrophages, microglia, and astrocytes, which in turn release chemokines, cytokines, or neurotoxic substances. A cytokine called *oncostatin M* may be the most damaging of the cytokines, although it acts in concert with other cytokines. Finally, there is evidence to support oxidative stress and increases in excitatory amino acids and intracellular calcium.

APPROACH TO HIV-ASSOCIATED DEMENTIA

Definitions

Ataxia: Unsteady motion of the limbs or trunk or a failure of muscular coordination.

Dementia: A disorder characterized by a general loss of intellectual abilities involving memory, judgment, abstract thinking, and changes in personality.

Neuropsychological testing: A battery of tests used to evaluate cognitive impairment. It is an extension of the MMSE.

HAART: Highly active antiretroviral therapy.

Clinical Approach

HAD has an incidence of 10.5 cases per 1000 person-years in the United States. This incidence has decreased since HAART was introduced as before HAART (before 1992) the incidence was 21 cases per 1000 person-years. Older patients with HIV have a higher likelihood of having HAD. A poor prognosis has been associated with low CD4 counts, high HIV RNA levels, low body mass index, lower educational levels, and anemia. Most patients with HAD have developed an AIDS-defining systemic illness. A few patients, however, present with only immunosuppression by laboratory criteria.

The earliest symptoms of HIV-associated dementia include difficulty with concentration, attention, and slowness of thinking. The forgetfulness is present early on, and patients have increasing difficulty performing complex tasks. Personality changes begin to appear such as apathy, social withdrawal, and quietness. Dysphoria and psychosis are rare. Psychomotor dysfunction manifested by poor balance and lack of coordination follows cognitive dysfunction, although rarely it can be the initial symptom of HAD. **Tripping or falling** along with poor handwriting are the more common motor symptoms. As the disease progresses, the ataxia worsens and can become disabling. Myoclonic jerks, postural tremor, and bowel and bladder dysfunction can be present in the later stages of the disease. Patients at end stage of the disease are unable to ambulate, have incontinence, and are almost in a vegetative state. Importantly focal neurologic deficits tend to be absent.

Early in the disease course, **neuropsychologic testing can be normal**; however, as time progresses there is evidence of a subcortical dementia. Typical abnormalities include difficulty in concentration, motor manipulation, and motor speed. Mild problems with word finding and impaired retrieval can be present. Eventually, severe psychomotor slowing and language impairment occur. Initially, the neurologic examination is normal, and at this time, subtle impairment in rapid limb and eye movements can be found. As the disease progresses, hyperreflexia, spasticity, and frontal release signs can be found. Additionally **apraxia** (inability to perform previously learned tasks) and **akinetic mutism** (severely decreased motor-verbal output) can develop.

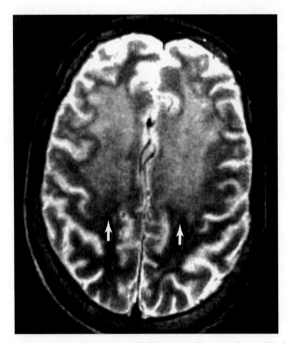

Figure 28–1. T2-weighted MRI in AIDS dementia complex. (*With permission from Aminoff MJ, Simon RR, Greenberg D. Clinical neurology, 6th ed. New York: McGraw-Hill/Lange Medical Books; 2005: Fig. 1–16.*)

Neuroimaging (MRI brain) studies are essential in evaluating patients with AIDS and cognitive impairment. **Diffuse cerebral atrophy is typical in HAD.** Some patients have white matter changes and abnormalities in the thalamus and basal ganglia (Fig. 28–1). Other conditions which can mimic or cause dementia can be excluded by MRI. CSF studies are nonspecific and are performed primarily to exclude other diagnoses. These nonspecific findings include a mildly elevated CSF protein (60% of cases) and mild mononuclear pleocytosis (25%). Quantitative HIV polymerase chain reaction (PCR) that evaluates CSF in viral load is the best parameter that relates to HAD. Improvement in CSF viral load leads to improvement in the clinical status of HAD.

Differential Diagnosis

1. Cerebral lymphoma
2. Progressive multifocal leukoencephalopathy
3. CNS infections such as cryptococcal meningitis, toxoplasmosis, cytomegalovirus encephalitis, neurosyphilis, histoplasmosis, and coccidioides
4. Toxic metabolic states such as vitamin B_{12} deficiency, thyroid disease, alcoholism, medication effect, illicit drug abuse
5. Metastatic malignancy

Histopathologic findings include atrophy in the frontotemporal distribution with diffuse myelin pallor. Some cortical neuronal loss is noted in 25% of cases. Activated glial cells are twice as frequent as in brains of controls.

The management of HAD depends on viral suppression by means of HAART. HAART not only protects against but also induces the remission of HAD. Selective retroviral drugs that enter the CSF can be helpful and include zidovudine, indinavir, and lamivudine.

Comprehension Questions

[28.1] A 29-year-old male with a history of illicit drug abuse in the past presents with complaints of mild forgetfulness, social withdrawal, and difficulty concentrating. He has a good appetite and has not experienced alteration in his sleep cycle. His neurologic examination including his MMSE is completely normal. His girlfriend has commented that she has seen him stumble more frequently. What is the next step in evaluating this individual?

    A. Obtain neuropsychologic testing to evaluate for personality disorder

    B. Obtain an MRI of the brain

    C. Obtain a stat lumbar puncture for CSF studies to exclude meningitis/encephalitis

    D. Clinically observe and follow the patient

[28.2] Which of the following have been associated with a poor prognosis in HAD?

    A. A history of multiple AIDS defining illnesses with high CD4 counts

    B. Low CD4 counts, high HIV RNA, and low body mass index

    C. Head trauma with loss of consciousness prior to becoming HIV positive

    D. Low CD4 counts, anemia, and low HIV RNA

[28.3] A 32-year-old HIV positive man is noted to have forgetfulness, gait disturbance, and confusion. A lumbar puncture is performed, and the India ink preparation is positive. Which of the following is the most likely diagnosis?

    A. HIV-associated dementia

    B. Cryptococcal meningitis

    C. Toxoplasmosis

    D. CNS lymphoma

Answers

[28.1] **B.** The first test to request in evaluating this patient is in imaging study. This will determine whether or not there is increased intracranial pressure so that a lumbar puncture can be safely performed. Although neuropsychologic testing is required, it is not meant to evaluate solely for a personality disorder.

[28.2] **B.** A history of multiple AIDS defining illnesses would be seen with low CD4 counts and thus would be a poor prognostic factor for HAD. The answer in the question, however, states a high CD4 count.

[28.3] **B.** India ink positive stain is highly suggestive of cryptococcal meningitis.

CLINICAL PEARLS

❖ HIV-associated dementia is typically associated with forgetfulness, difficulty concentrating, slowness in thinking, and loss of coordination.

❖ HIV-associated dementia is more commonly seen in individuals with low CD4 counts, high HIV RNA, low body mass index, anemia, and low levels of education.

❖ The best way to prevent and reduce the severity of HAD is by using HAART.

❖ AIDS dementia complex (ADC) is divided into two clinical categories: (1) severe form-HIV-associated dementia complex, and (2) less severe form- HIV-associated minor cognitive/motor disorders.

❖ Patients with mild HIV dementia commonly present with depression and anxiety. Therefore, HIV-infected individuals with depression should be screened for early HIV dementia.

REFERENCES

Dorland's Illustrated Medical Dictionary, 27th ed. Philadelphia, PA: WB Saunders; 1988.

Gibbie T, Mijch A, Ellen S, et al. Depression and neurocognitive performance in individuals with HIV/AIDS: 2-year follow-up. HIV Med 2006 Mar;7(2): 112–121.

Kaul M, Lipton SA. Mechanisms of neuronal injury and death in HIV-1 associated dementia. Curr HIV Res 2006 Jul;4(3):307–318.

McArthur JC. HIV dementia: an evolving disease. J Neuroimmunol 2004 Dec; 157(1–2):3–10.

A 53-year-old female presents with loss of balance, mood swings, and memory loss. She had not noticed these symptoms until her coworkers and family pointed it out to her. Although these symptoms presented 4 months ago, she did not seek medical attention until now when they began interfering with her daily activities. Her ataxia has progressed to the point that she is stumbling and falling. She has noticed difficulty with problem solving, and her boss has witnessed inappropriate behavior. Her family reports that over the past month her memory has quickly deteriorated to the point that she is unable to recognize friends, is unable to drive, is not able to work, and forgets if she has eaten. She has also developed slurred speech and has been witnessed to "jerk" during the day. Your neurologic examination reveals an Mini Mental Status Examination (MMSE) score of 17/30 having difficulty with orientation, object recall, calculations, naming, concentration, and drawing the intersecting polygons. There is horizontal nystagmus with moderate dysarthria and anomia noted. Her strength appears to be normal; however, she has dysmetria and a wide-based gait. Her deep tendon reflexes (DTRs) are hyperreflexic, and she has evidence of myoclonus. A CT scan of the brain is performed and shows no abnormalities.

◆ **What is the most likely diagnosis?**

◆ **What is the next diagnostic step?**

◆ **What is the next step in therapy?**

ANSWERS TO CASE 29: Sporadic Creutzfeldt-Jakob Disease

Summary: A 53-year-old woman presents with a 4-month history of rapidly progressive memory loss, ataxia, mood swings, inappropriate behavior, and dysarthria. Her examination is notable for a markedly abnormal MMSE with global abnormalities, moderate dysarthria, and anomia. She additionally has nystagmus, dysmetria, ataxia, myoclonus, and hyperreflexia.

◆ **Most likely diagnosis:** Sporadic Creutzfeldt-Jakob disease.

◆ **Next diagnostic step:** Serologic studies including chemistry 20, complete blood count (CBC), HIV, erythrocyte sedimentation rate (ESR), thyroid-stimulating hormone (TSH), thyroxine (T_4), triiodothyronine (T_3), vitamin B_{12}, rapid plasma reagin (RPR), international normalized ratio (INR), MRI of the brain, lumbar puncture for protein, glucose, cell count with differential, Gram stain and cultures and 14–3-3 protein. Additionally an electroencephalograph (EEG) may be requested.

◆ **Next step in therapy:** Supportive therapy.

Analysis

Objectives

1. Be familiar with the clinical presentation of sporadic Creutzfeldt-Jakob disease and its variants.
2. Know the differential diagnosis for Creutzfeldt-Jakob disease.
3. Know how to diagnose Creutzfeldt-Jakob disease.

Considerations

This 53-year-old woman presents with a rapidly progressive set of neurologic symptoms including memory loss, ataxia, behavioral changes, poor coordination, and myoclonus. These abnormalities are consistent with a rapidly progressive dementia atypical for Creutzfeldt-Jakob disease (CJD). At first, patients experience problems with muscular coordination; personality changes, including impaired memory, judgment, and thinking; and impaired vision. The CT scan rules out stroke or brain tumor; most other causes of dementia are of slower onset. Nevertheless, in this patient, potentially treatable causes of dementia are sought with the laboratory and MRI tests.

Clinical Approach

Clinical Features and Epidemiology

Creutzfeldt-Jakob disease (CJD) is a rare, degenerative, invariably fatal brain disorder. It affects approximately one person in every one million people per year worldwide; in the United States there are approximately 200 cases per year. CJD usually appears in later life and runs a rapid course. Typically, onset of symptoms occurs approximately at 60 years of age, and approximately 90% of patients die within 1 year. In the early stages of disease, patients can have failing memory, behavioral changes, lack of coordination, and visual disturbances. As the illness progresses, mental deterioration becomes pronounced, and involuntary movements, blindness, weakness of extremities, and coma can occur.

There are three major categories of CJD:

- In **sporadic CJD**, the disease appears even though the person has no known risk factors for the disease. This is by far the most common type of CJD and accounts for at least 85% of cases.
- In **hereditary CJD**, the person has a family history of the disease and/or tests positive for a genetic mutation associated with CJD. Approximately 5–10% of cases of CJD in the United States are hereditary.
- In **acquired CJD**, the disease is transmitted by exposure to brain or nervous system tissue, usually through certain medical procedures. There is no evidence that CJD is contagious through casual contact with a CJD patient. Since CJD was first described in 1920, fewer than 1% of cases have been acquired CJD.

CJD belongs to a family of human and animal diseases known as the transmissible spongiform encephalopathies (TSEs). Spongiform refers to the characteristic appearance of infected brains, which become filled with holes until they resemble sponges under a microscope. CJD is the most common of the known human TSEs. Other human TSEs include kuru, fatal familial insomnia (FFI), and Gerstmann-Straussler-Scheinker disease (GSS). Kuru was identified in people of an isolated Cannabalistic tribe in Papua, New Guinea, and has now almost disappeared. FFI and GSS are extremely rare hereditary diseases, found in just a few families around the world. Other TSEs are found in specific kinds of animals. These include bovine spongiform encephalopathy (BSE), which is found in cows and is often referred to as "mad cow" disease; scrapie, which affects sheep and goats; mink encephalopathy; and feline encephalopathy. Similar diseases have occurred in elk, deer, and exotic zoo animals.

CJD is characterized by rapidly progressive dementia. Initially, patients experience problems with muscular coordination, personality changes, including impaired memory, judgment, and thinking, and impaired vision. Affected patients also can experience insomnia, depression, or unusual sensations. CJD does not cause a fever or other flu-like symptoms. As the illness progresses, the patients' mental impairment becomes severe. They often develop involuntary muscle jerks called **myoclonus**, and they may go blind. They eventually lose the ability to move and speak and enter a coma. Pneumonia and other infections often occur in these patients and can lead to death.

There are several known variants of CJD. These variants differ somewhat in the symptoms and course of the disease. For example, a variant form of the disease–called *new variant* or *variant* (nv-CJD, v-CJD), described in Great Britain and France–begins primarily with psychiatric symptoms, affects younger patients than other types of CJD, and has a longer than usual duration from onset of symptoms to death. Another variant, called the *panencephalo-pathic* form, occurs primarily in Japan and has a relatively long course, with symptoms often progressing for several years. Scientists are trying to learn what causes these variations in the symptoms and course of the disease. Some symptoms of CJD can be similar to symptoms of other progressive neurologic disorders, such as Alzheimer or Huntington disease. However, CJD causes unique changes in brain tissue that can be seen at autopsy. It also tends to cause more rapid deterioration of a person's abilities than Alzheimer disease or most other types of dementia.

Etiology and Pathogenesis

Some researchers believe an unusual "slow virus" or another organism causes CJD. However, a virus or other organism in affected individuals has not been isolated. Furthermore, the agent that causes CJD has several characteristics that are unusual for known organisms such as viruses and bacteria. It is difficult to kill, it does not appear to contain any genetic information in the form of nucleic acids (DNA or RNA), and it usually has a long incubation period before symptoms appear. In some cases, the incubation period can be as long as 40 years. The leading scientific theory at this time maintains that CJD and the other TSEs are caused by a type of protein called a *prion.*

Prion proteins occur in both a normal form, which is a harmless protein found in the body's cells, and in an infectious form, which causes disease. The harmless and infectious forms of the prion protein have the same sequence of amino acids (the "building blocks" of proteins) but the infectious form of the protein takes a different folded shape than the normal protein. Sporadic CJD may develop because some of a person's normal prions spontaneously change into the infectious form of the protein and then alter the prions in other cells in a chain reaction. Once they appear, abnormal prion proteins aggregate, or clump together. Investigators think these protein aggregates may lead to the neuron loss and other brain damage seen in CJD. However, they do not know exactly how this damage occurs.

Approximately 5–10% of all CJD cases are inherited. These cases arise from a mutation, or change, in the gene that controls formation of the normal prion protein. Although prions themselves do not contain genetic information and do not require genes to reproduce themselves, infectious prions can arise if a mutation occurs in the gene for the body's normal prion protein. If the prion protein gene is altered in a person's sperm or egg cells, the mutation can be transmitted to the person's offspring. Several different mutations in the prion gene have been identified. The particular mutation found in each family affects how frequently the disease appears and what symptoms are most noticeable. However, not all people with mutations in the prion protein gene develop CJD.

CJD cannot be transmitted through the air or through touching or most other forms of casual contact. Spouses and other household members of sporadic CJD patients have no higher risk of contracting the disease than the general population. However, exposure to brain tissue and spinal cord fluid from infected patients should be avoided. In some cases, CJD has spread to other people from grafts of dura mater (a tissue that covers the brain), transplanted corneas, implantation of inadequately sterilized electrodes in the brain, and injections of contaminated pituitary growth hormone derived from human pituitary glands taken from cadavers. Since 1985, all human growth hormone used in the United States has been synthesized by recombinant DNA procedures, which eliminates the risk of transmitting CJD by this route.

The appearance of the new variant of CJD (nv-CJD or v-CJD) in several younger people in Great Britain and France has led to concern that BSE may be transmitted to humans through consumption of contaminated beef. Although laboratory tests have shown a strong similarity between the prions causing BSE and v-CJD, there is no direct proof to support this theory. Many people are concerned that it may be possible to transmit CJD through blood and related blood products such as plasma. Some animal studies suggest that contaminated blood and related products may transmit the disease, although this has never been shown in humans. If there are infectious agents in these fluids, they are probably in very low concentrations. Scientists do not know how many abnormal prions a person must receive before he or she develops CJD, so they do not know whether these fluids are potentially infectious or not. They do know that, even though millions of people receive blood transfusions each year, there are no reported cases of someone contracting CJD from a transfusion. Even among people with hemophilia, who sometimes receive blood plasma concentrated from thousands of donors, there are no reported cases of CJD.

Although there is no evidence that exposure to blood from people with sporadic CJD is infectious, prions from BSE and vCJD can accumulate in the lymph nodes, the spleen, and the tonsils. These findings suggest that blood transfusions from people with vCJD might transmit the disease. Thus, in the United States, prospective blood donors are disqualified if they have resided for more than 3 months in a country or countries where BSE is common.

Transmissible spongiform encephalopathies, such as CJD, are known to affect various animal species including sheep, goats, mink, mule deer, cows, and recently cats. Scrapie, a disorder of sheep and goats, has been known for more than 300 years and is endemic in the British Isles. In 1938 experimental transfer of scrapie from one sheep to another by inoculation provided evidence of an infective etiology. However, there is no evidence of transmission of scrapie from sheep to man.

Diagnosis

There is currently no single diagnostic test for CJD. When a doctor suspects CJD, the first concern is to rule out treatable forms of dementia such as encephalitis (inflammation of the brain) or chronic meningitis. Standard diagnostic tests will include a spinal tap to rule out more common causes of dementia, and an EEG to record the brain's electrical pattern often shows periodic sharp wave complexes, which has a sensitivity for CJD of 66% and a specificity of 74% (Fig. 29–1). **Computerized tomography of the brain can help rule out the possibility that the symptoms result from other problems such as stroke or a brain tumor.** MRI brain scans also can reveal characteristic patterns of brain degeneration that can help diagnose CJD.

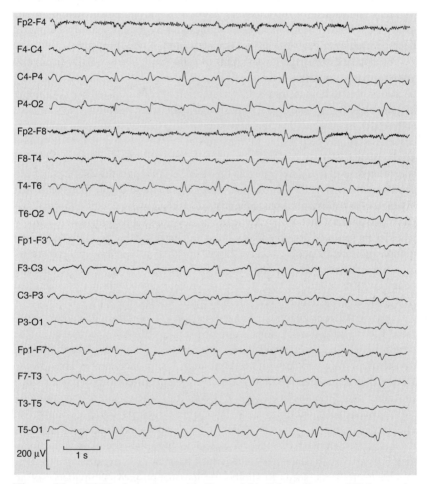

Figure 29–1. EEG of a patient with Creutzfeldt-Jakob disease. (*With permission from Aminoff MJ, Simon RR, Greenberg D. Clinical neurology, 6th ed. New York: McGraw-Hill/Lange Medical Books; 2005: Fig. 1–13.*)

The **only way to confirm a diagnosis of CJD is by brain biopsy or autopsy.** Because a correct diagnosis of CJD does not help the patient, a brain biopsy is discouraged unless it is needed to rule out a treatable disorder. In an autopsy, the whole brain is examined after death. Both brain biopsy and autopsy pose a small but definite risk that the surgeon or others who handle the brain tissue can become accidentally infected by self-inoculation. Special surgical and disinfection procedures can minimize this risk. A fact sheet with guidance on these procedures is available from the National Institute of Neurological Disorders and Stroke (NINDS) and the World Health Organization.

Investigations are being conducted to create laboratory tests for CJD. One such test, developed at NINDS, is performed on a person's CSF and detects a protein marker, 14–3-3 protein, which indicates neuronal degeneration. 14–3-3 proteins in the CSF have been found to correlate with the clinical diagnosis in 94% (sensitivity) and a specificity of 84%. The protein assay in combination with EEG findings further increases the sensitivity but decreases the specificity. However, these tests can help diagnose CJD in people who already show the clinical symptoms of the disease. CSF analysis for the protein is much easier and safer than a brain biopsy. The false positive rate is approximately 5–10%. Scientists are working to develop this test for use in commercial laboratories. They are also working to develop other tests for this disorder.

Treatment and Prevention

There is no treatment that can cure or control CJD. Researchers have tested many drugs, including amantadine, steroids, interferon, acyclovir, antiviral agents, and antibiotics. Studies of a variety of other drugs are now in progress. However, so far none of these treatments has shown any consistent benefit in humans. Current treatment for CJD is aimed at alleviating symptoms and making the patient as comfortable as possible. Opiate drugs can help relieve pain if it occurs, and the drugs clonazepam and sodium valproate can help relieve myoclonus. During later stages of the disease, changing the person's position frequently can keep him or her comfortable and helps prevent bedsores. A catheter can be used to drain urine if the patient cannot control bladder function, and intravenous fluids and artificial feeding also can be used.

To reduce the already very low risk of CJD transmission from one person to another, people should never donate blood, tissues, or organs if they have suspected or confirmed CJD, or if they are at increased risk because of a family history of the disease, a dura mater graft, or other factor. Normal sterilization procedures such as cooking, washing, and boiling do not destroy prions. Caregivers, healthcare workers, and undertakers should take the following precautions when they are working with a person with CJD:

- Wash hands and exposed skin before eating, drinking, or smoking.
- Cover cuts and abrasions with waterproof dressings.
- Wear surgical gloves when handling a patient's tissues and fluids or dressing the patient's wounds.

- Avoid cutting or sticking oneself with instruments contaminated by the patient's blood or other tissues.
- Use face protection if there is a risk of splashing contaminated material such as blood or cerebrospinal fluid.
- Soak instruments that have come in contact with the patient in undiluted chlorine bleach for 1 hour or more, then use an autoclave (pressure cooker) to sterilize them in distilled water for at least 1 hour at 132–134°C (269–273°F).

Comprehension Questions

[29.1] Which of the following is characteristic of the agent that causes CJD?

A. Easy to kill

B. Contain any genetic information in the form of nucleic acids (DNA or RNA)

C. Short incubation period

D. Associated with prion protein

[29.2] A 30-year-old worker at a meat processing plant is very nervous about the prospect of developing CJD. Which of the following is the best method in preventing developing the disease?

A. Sterilization with bleach is effective at neutralizing the prion protein

B. Heating the containers to at least 180°F is effective

C. There is no treatment that can cure or control CJD

D. Scrubbing the containers with hexachloride is effective

[29.3] A 47-year-old woman is noted to have progressive dementia. Which of the following methods is the most accurate method of diagnosing CJD?

A. Serum serology

B. Serum PCR

C. Serum viral culture

D. Brain biopsy

Answers

[29.1] **D.** The agent that causes CJD is difficult to kill, does not seem to contain genetic information in the form of nucleic acids, has a long incubation period, and is associated with prion protein.

[29.2] **C.** There is no effective way of preventing CJD.

[29.3] **D.** Brain biopsy and histologic analysis is the only definitive method of diagnosis.

CLINICAL PEARLS

❖ Ninety percent of patients diagnosed with CJD die within 1 year.
❖ The annual rate of CJD is approximately 3.4 cases per million. In recent years, the United States has reported fewer than 300 cases of CJD a year.
❖ H. G. Creutzfeldt is credited with the first description of the disorder in 1920. A year later another German neurologist, A. Jakob, described four cases, at least two of whom had clinical features suggestive of the entity we recognize as CJD.

REFERENCES

National Institute of Neurological Disorders and Stroke. Creutzfeldt-Jakob disease fact sheet. Available at: http://www.ninds.nih.gov/disorders/cjd/detail_cjd.htm.
Zerr I, Pocchiari M, Collins S, et al. Analysis of EEG and CSF 14-3-3 proteins as aids to the diagnosis of Creutzfeldt–Jakob disease. Neurology 2000;55:811–815.

A 58-year-old man is referred for evaluation of severe lancinating pain in the legs and loss of balance over a period of 3 years. He has recently developed impotence, and his grandchildren have started to tease him about how his eyes are looking droopy. He reports that his balance is worse in darkness or when he closes his eyes. He has a history of gastroesophageal reflux disease and migraine headaches. He is only taking over-the-counter famotidine (Pepcid) and a multivitamin each day. He has been married for 35 years and is a retired structural engineer. He has not been exposed to toxins, does not smoke, or drink alcohol. The only other pertinent information is that he served as a natural disaster relief volunteer overseas before getting married and contracted a "venereal disease." He thinks he contracted syphilis and received oral antibiotics. The neurologic examination reveals a Mini Mental Status Examination (MMSE) score of 30/30 with intact cranial nerves except for Argyll Robertson pupils and ptosis bilaterally. His strength is normal; however, he has impaired proprioception in the toes with diminished temperature sensation in the legs. Additionally he has loss of pinprick sensation in a glove-and-stocking distribution. A Romberg sign is present. Cerebellar examination is normal; however, his deep tendon reflexes are diminished (1+/2) in the legs. His gait is wide-based with marked ataxia.

◆ **What is the most likely diagnosis?**

◆ **What is the next step to confirm diagnosis?**

◆ **What is the treatment plan?**

ANSWERS TO CASE 30: Tabes Dorsalis

Summary: A 58-year-old man with a history of syphilis more than 20 years ago, gastroesophageal reflux disease, and migraine headaches presents with a 3-year history of lancinating pain in the legs, loss of balance, and recent impotence and ptosis. His examination is notable for cranial nerve impairment with Argyll Robertson pupils and ptosis. Other findings included impaired posterior column function with loss of proprioception in the feet and impaired lateral spinothalamic tract function (loss of temperature and pinprick). His deep tendon reflexes are diminished in the legs, and he has a sensory ataxia. The Romberg test is positive.

◆ **Most likely diagnosis:** Tabes dorsalis (spinal form of syphilis).

◆ **Confirm the diagnosis:** Lumbar puncture for Venereal Disease Research Laboratory (VDRL).

◆ **Next therapeutic step:** High-dose intravenous aqueous penicillin G at a dose of 2-million to 4-million units every 4 hours for 10 to 14 days. If there is a penicillin allergy then doxycycline at a dose of 200 mg twice a day for 28 days and ceftriaxone at a dose of 2 g intravenously per day for 14 days are administered.

Analysis

Objectives

1. Be familiar with the clinical presentation of tabes dorsalis and other neurologic syndromes caused by syphilis.
2. Know how to diagnose tabes dorsalis and differentiate it from other late forms of neurosyphilis.
3. Know how to treat tabes dorsalis.

Considerations

Any individual with a history of syphilis that presents with neurologic symptoms should alert the clinician to possible neurosyphilis. Other etiologies need to be excluded and other sexually transmitted diseases such as HIV or hepatitis B or C can also cause similar neurologic symptoms. Lancinating pain with associated sensory ataxia, cranial nerve abnormalities, and impotence or bowel and bladder dysfunction is a classical presentation for tabes dorsalis. In this particular case tabes dorsalis is the most likely diagnosis, however, to diagnose it, confirmation from laboratory studies must be obtained. The most common serologic studies requested are a rapid plasma reagin (RPR) assay or VDRL test. These are quite sensitive for primary and secondary syphilis; however, they are less sensitive for neurosyphilis. A negative RPR does not exclude neurosyphilis.

Importantly the RPR assay can frequently have a false positive results. If these tests are positive, proceed in confirming the diagnosis in cerebral spinal fluid (CSF). The following indicates the typical CSF findings of neurosyphilis:

◆ **Elevated CSF protein up to 200 mg/dL**

◆ **Lymphocytic pleocytosis <400/μL**

◆ **CSF VDRL positivity in most individuals**

◆ **Elevated IgG synthesis**

If however the RPR or VDRL studies are negative and neurosyphilis is still clinically suspected, serum studies for *Treponema pallidum*-specific antibodies should be performed. These include fluorescent treponemal antibody absorbed (FTA-ABS) test, *T. pallidum* hemagglutination (TPHA) test, or microhemag-glutination assay-*T. pallidum* (MHA-TP). These studies are much more expensive than the reaginic assays but are much more sensitive for neurosyphilis. In fact if these studies are nonreactive, neurosyphilis is excluded.

Detection of *T. pallidum* by polymerase chain reaction in the CSF is quite low. Importantly, the serologic studies cannot distinguish between syphilis, pinta, and yaws due to cross reactivity. HIV or hepatitis B and C can present with very similar symptoms of sensory ataxia, cranial mononeuropathies, and pain. A distinguishing feature between these infections and neurosyphilis is the type of pain. The classical lancinating pain is seen with neurosyphilis, whereas a burning type pain is associated with the others. Nevertheless, laboratory studies are the only way to distinguish these conditions.

APPROACH TO TABES DORSALIS

Definitions

Argyll Robertson pupils: Small pupils that constrict when focusing but fail to constrict when exposed to bright light (accommodate but do not react).

Electromyograph (EMG)/nerve conduction studies: An electrophysiological examination that evaluates the integrity of the peripheral nerve and evaluates various electrical muscle properties allowing the clinician to determine the presence of either a muscle or nerve disorder. This test is useful in evaluating primarily the peripheral nervous system.

H reflex: The H reflex is the electrical equivalent—to a mono-synaptic stretch reflex. It often reflects pathology along the afferent and efferent fibers and/or the dorsal root ganglion.

Lancinating pain: A sensation of piercing, stabbing or cutting.

Ptosis: Droopiness of the eyelids.

Romberg sign: Falling over when a person is standing with eyes closed, feet together, and hands in the outstretched position.

Clinical Approach

Neurosyphilis is an infection of the nervous system by the spirochete *T. pallidum*, the organism responsible for syphilis. It is estimated that up to 10% of patients with primary syphilis that have not received treatment will develop neurosyphilis. In the HIV population the percentage of this is higher. Risk factors for syphilis include drug consumption, sexual habits, and social background. Importantly, syphilis is a risk factor for acquiring HIV. It is well recognized that HIV patients with syphilis are at increased risk for developing neurosyphilis and may do so earlier than HIV-negative individuals. Neurosyphilis is twice as common in men as it is in women.

T. pallidum can first be detected clinically approximately 3 weeks after infection by the presence of a primary lesion on the skin or mucous membranes (primary syphilis). Secondary syphilis results from a second bacteremic stage with generalized mucocutaneous lesions. Although neurosyphilis (tertiary syphilis) may not present until many years after a primary infection, *T. pallidum* enters the central nervous system at the same time that individuals develop primary and secondary syphilis. Pathogenic changes consist of endarteritis of terminal arterioles with resultant inflammatory and necrotic changes. In the central nervous system, *T. pallidum* causes meningeal inflammation, arteritis of small and medium-sized vessels with subsequent fibrotic occlusion, and eventually direct neuronal damage.

The **clinical features of neurosyphilis are dependent on the time period after infection (see Table 30–1). Hyporeflexia** is the **most common finding** on clinical examination with up to 50% of patients with neurosyphilis having this finding. Other clinical findings include sensory impairment (48%), pupillary changes (43%) including Argyll Robertson pupils, cranial neuropathy (36%), dementia or psychiatric symptoms (35%), and positive Romberg test (24%). **The Argyll Robertson pupil is almost pathognomonic for neural syphilis.** Tabes dorsalis is caused by the syphilitic involvement of the spinal cord, leading to intermittent pain of the arms and legs, ataxia and gait disturbance as a result of loss of position sense, and impaired vibratory and position sense.

The diagnosis of neurosyphilis is made on clinical grounds and confirmed by CSF serology (RPR or VDRL). Usually the CSF protein and cell count are abnormal. The differential diagnosis of neurosyphilis is based on the clinical features. For example, the differential for gummatous neurosyphilis consists of the differential diagnosis for space occupying lesions (metastatic brain tumors, primary brain tumors, etc.). Meningovascular syphilis presenting like a stroke merits the differential diagnosis of cerebral vascular accident (vasculitis, hemorrhage, etc.). Three disorders should be considered in the differential diagnosis of tabes dorsales: subacute combined degeneration from vitamin B_{12} deficiency, multiple sclerosis, and Lyme disease. Other less common diagnoses in the differential include sarcoidosis, herpes zoster, and diffuse metastatic disease. The finding of an Argyll Robertson pupil is highly suggestive of tabes dorsalis but can also be seen with multiple sclerosis, diabetes mellitus,

Table 30–1
NEUROLOGIC FORMS OF SYPHILIS

CLINICAL SYNDROME	TIME PERIOD AFTER INITIAL INFECTION	CLINICAL FEATURES
Syphilitic meningitis	1–2 years	Cranial mononeuropathies, hydrocephalus, and focal hemispheric signs
Cerebrovascular and meningovascular disease	5–7 years	Ischemia particularly along the middle cerebral artery territory and meningeal inflammation. Can also present with stroke in evolution.
General paresis	10 years	Impairment of higher cortical functions, dementia, frontotemporal encephalitis, pupillary abnormalities, cerebellar dysfunction, optic atrophy, pyramidal tract dysfunction and features suggesting psychiatric illness
Tabes dorsalis	10–20 years	Lancinating pain, sensory ataxia, bowel dysfunction, bladder dysfunction, or cranial nerve abnormalities
Gummatous neurosyphilis	Any time after infection	Features are directly related to the location of the gummas causing compression
Asymptomatic neurosyphilis	Any time after infection	Absence of symptoms despite abnormal CSF findings seen with neurosyphilis

CSF, cerebrospinal fluid.

sarcoidosis, Lyme disease, and Wernicke encephalopathy. Tabes dorsalis is a slow and progressive disease that causes demyelination in the posterior columns and inflammatory changes in the posterior roots of the spinal cord. Nerve conduction studies can show impaired sensory nerve conduction studies with normal motor nerve conductions. EMG is normal, but absent H reflexes are common due the damage of the dorsal root ganglion. Abnormalities in motor nerve conduction studies should raise doubt on the diagnosis of tabes dorsalis.

The **treatment of neurosyphilis** consists of **high-dose intravenous aqueous penicillin** G at a dose of 2 million to 4 million units every 4 hours for 10 to 14 days. If there is a penicillin allergy then doxycycline at a dose of 200 mg twice a day for 28 days and ceftriaxone at a dose of 2 g intravenously per day for 14 days are administered. Although there are alternate regimens that have been tried in treating patients with neurosyphilis, they have not been found to be as effective as the use of aqueous penicillin G. Use of intramuscular procaine penicillin at a dose of 2.4 million units intramuscularly every day plus oral probenecid for 10 to 14 days has been tried in those individuals that cannot receive intravenous preparations. This has typically been combined with intramuscular Benzathine penicillin G at a dose of 2.4 million units weekly for 3 weeks. If treatment fails to improve symptoms (for early neurosyphilis) or there is continued progression of symptoms (late neurosyphilis) retreatment should be considered. Cerebrospinalfluid (CSF) studies should be reexamined after the completion of therapy with an improved drop in white blood cell count, protein, and IgG synthesis.

Comprehension Questions

[30.1] A neurologist performs an examination on a 19-year-old man and believes that he has diagnosed an Argyll Robertson pupil. Which of the following statements is most likely to be accurate?

A. The pupil likely constricts to light
B. The patient has multiple sclerosis
C. The pupils fail to constrict when focusing up close.
D. The patient is diagnosed with subacute combined degeneration

[30.2] All of the following are true regarding neurosyphilis except:

A. *Treponema pallidum* infects the central nervous system at the time of the primary infection
B. HIV-positive individuals are at increased risk for developing neurosyphilis
C. Tabes dorsalis occurs 10 years after initial infection
D. Stroke-like symptoms may occur any time after infection
E. General paresis may present as a psychiatric illness

[30.3] The differential diagnosis of tabes dorsalis consists of all of the following except:

A. Toxoplasmosis
B. Lyme disease
C. Sarcoidosis
D. Multiple sclerosis
E. Subacute combined degeneration

[30.4] A 30-year-old man who abuses IV drugs presents to your office complaining of left-sided weakness for the past 6 weeks. His examination is notable for Argyll Robertson pupils, hyporeflexia in the legs and left hemiparesis. He is healthy otherwise except for having developed syphilis while serving in the military at age 27. His last HIV test was 18 months ago. Which of the following is most accurate?

A. He does not have neurosyphilis as the time period from primary infection to symptoms is too short
B. He has definite tabes dorsalis
C. He has neurosyphilis and you are going to write him up in a medical journal as a novel case presenting after a short incubation time following primary infection
D. Obtain an HIV test and RPR, and if positive, begin treatment with intravenous aqueous penicillin G

Answers

[30.1] **C.** Argyll Robertson pupils means accommodation but no light reflex. It is seen with multiple sclerosis. Subacute combined degeneration has not been reported to cause Argyll Robertson pupils.
[30.2] **D.** Stroke-like symptoms occur 5–7 years after the initial infection in individuals who are HIV negative.
[30.3] **A.** Toxoplasmosis usually presents with symptoms suggesting an intracranial mass lesion.
[30.4] **D.** HIV-positive individuals are known to develop signs and symptoms of neurosyphilis much earlier than individuals that are HIV negative. His presentation is not novel and merits treatment as soon as possible. Although patients with tabes dorsalis may have an Argyll Robertson pupil, they present with lancinating pain and not hemiparesis; thus, an MRI of the brain is indicated.

CLINICAL PEARLS

❖ Tabes dorsalis classically presents with lancinating pain, sensory deficits, ataxia, and hyporeflexia.

❖ HIV-positive individuals can present with neurosyphilis at a much earlier time then HIV negative individuals.

❖ The treatment of choice for neurosyphilis remains intravenous aqueous penicillin G. Alternative treatments consisting of intramuscular doses of penicillin have not been found to be as effective.

❖ Individuals that present with neurologic symptoms and have a history of syphilis should be considered to have neurosyphilis until proven otherwise.

❖ There are four different forms of neurosyphilis: asymptomatic, meningovascular, tabes dorsalis, and general paresis.

❖ Syphilitic aseptic meningitis occurs as a chronic infection and can involve headaches, cognitive changes, and cranial nerve abnormalities.

REFERENCES

Dacso CC, Bortz DL. Significance of the Argyll Robertson pupil in clinical medicine. Am J Med 1989 Feb;86(2):199–202.

Dorland's Illustrated Medical Dictionary, 27th ed. Philadelphia, PA: WB Saunders; 1988.

Golden MR, Marra CM, Holmes KK. Update on syphilis: resurgence of an old problem. JAMA 2003 Sep 17;290(11):1510–1514.

Clinical Effectiveness Group. National guideline for the management of late syphilis: Clinical Effectiveness Group (Association of Genitourinary Medicine and the Medical Society for the Study of Venereal Diseases). Sex Transm Infect 1999 Aug;75(suppl 1):S34–37.

Stevenson J, Heath M. Syphilis and HIV infection: an update. Dermatol Clin 2006 Oct;24(4):497–507.

A 25-year-old man is brought to the emergency room after experiencing a generalized tonic-clonic seizure. He was getting ready for work when he apparently fell to the floor and had the seizure. His mother who witnessed the event states that he lost consciousness and "shook all over." The seizure lasted approximately 30 seconds and was associated with tongue biting as well as bladder incontinence. He returned to his baseline within 20 minutes and refused to come to the emergency room. Over the past 6 months he has been complaining of headaches and had two previous generalized tonic-clonic seizures. He has also lost approximately 6.8 kg (15 lb) over 1 month. He has been healthy otherwise, and the only other pertinent history is that he has been sexually promiscuous and experimented with intravenous cocaine. His last HIV test was 12 months ago, and he did not wait for the result. On physical examination he is afebrile with a blood pressure of 130/68 mmHg and a heart rate of 88 beats/min. He is awake and alert and oriented to person, time, location, and situation. His cranial nerves, sensory examination, cerebellar examination, and deep tendon reflexes are normal. His motor examination is notable for increased tone on the right with intact motor strength. His gait shows decreased arm swing on the right but otherwise is unremarkable. A CT scan of the head without contrast shows that he has a solitary mass lesion measuring 15 mm over the left motor strip region with surrounding edema. Additionally there is a 12-mm lesion in the left basal ganglia. With the administration of IV contrast, these lesions enhance.

◆ **What is the most likely diagnosis?**

◆ **What is the best way to confirm the diagnosis?**

◆ **What is the next step in therapy?**

ANSWERS TO CASE 31: Intracranial Lesion (Toxoplasmosis)

Summary: A 25-year-old previously healthy man presents to the emergency room after experiencing a generalized tonic-clonic seizure that lasted 30 seconds. He has been experiencing headaches over the past 6 months but no other associated symptoms. His mother states she has witnessed him to have two previous seizures. The history is notable for being sexually promiscuous and using intravenous illicit drugs. The result of his last HIV test is unknown. On neurologic examination he is noted to have increased tone on the right and decreased right arm swing when walking. The remainder of his neurologic examination is normal. A CT scan of the head with contrast reveals that he has a ring-enhancing lesion measuring 15 mm over the left motor strip region and a 12-mm ring-enhancing lesion in the left basal ganglia.

◆ **Most likely diagnosis:** Cerebral toxoplasmosis.

◆ **Tests to confirm diagnosis:** Serum IgM and IgG titers for *Toxoplasmosis gondii*, and lumbar puncture to evaluate for polymerase chain reaction (PCR) *T. gondii*.

◆ **Treatment plan:** Start anticonvulsants to prevent further seizures and then start treatment for toxoplasmosis. Therapy consists of a combination of medications including pyrimethamine, sulfadiazine, and folinic acid.

Analysis

Objectives

1. Know a diagnostic approach to toxoplasmosis including the use of imaging studies and cerebrospinal fluid studies.
2. Describe the clinical features of toxoplasmosis.
3. Describe how to treat toxoplasmosis and what precautions are necessary.

Considerations

This 25-year-old healthy man has been experiencing headaches for the past 6 months and just experienced his third generalized tonic-clonic seizure. His examination suggests a left-sided brain lesion as he has right-sided motor findings (decreased right arm swing and increased tone on the right). The fact that he seems to have constitutional symptoms of weight loss and has risk factors for an HIV infection narrows the differential diagnosis significantly. This individual is most likely now HIV positive. This is based on the fact that he has been experiencing weight loss and has continued to participate in behavior placing him at high risk for HIV infection. Primary CNS lymphoma, syphilitic gummas, tuberculomas, abscesses, neurocysticercosis, or metastatic brain tumors should be considered in the differential diagnosis. The presentation of headache, weight loss, generalized tonic-clonic seizures, and a focal neurologic examination suggests an intracranial lesion. An individual that is young and HIV positive should be considered to have toxoplasmosis, primary CNS lymphoma, syphilitic gummas, tuberculomas, or brain abscesses. A CT scan of the head with and without contrast usually confirms the clinical suspicion but cannot differentiate each entity. Serologic studies in addition to cerebrospinal fluid studies will help best determine the diagnosis. Besides the diagnostic tests described above, other cerebrospinal fluid (CSF) studies include protein, glucose, cell count with differential, Gram stain, cytology, Venereal Disease Research Laboratory (VDRL). Other serological studies including chemistry 20, CBC, HIV, erythrocyte sedimentation rate (ESR), rapid plasma reagin (RPR), international normalized ratio (INR).

APPROACH TO INFECTIONS IN IMMUNOCOMPROMISED HOSTS: TOXOPLASMOSIS

Definitions

Generalized tonic-clonic seizure: It is often referred to as a *grand mal seizure* and involves loss of consciousness, violent muscle contractions, and rigidity.

Folinic acid: The reduced form of folic acid that does not require reduction reaction by enzyme for activation.

Radiculomyelopathy: A process affecting the nerve root and spinal cord.

Ring-enhancing lesion: A lesion that shows peripheral enhancement with central hypodensity after being administered contrast. This is in contrast to a disk enhancement lesion where there is uniform enhancement with contrast.

Clinical Approach

Toxoplasmosis is caused by the single-celled parasite, *T. gondii*, which is found throughout the world. It was discovered in 1908 in the *gondi*, a small rat-like animal from North Africa, and causes CNS toxoplasmosis in immunocompromised hosts. Toxoplasmosis has multiple hosts including humans, **cats,** and other warm-blooded animals. **Toxoplasmosis is a common opportunistic infection in the HIV population.** In fact, it is the leading cause of focal central nervous system disease in AIDS and is most frequently seen during the later phases of the disease. It is a fairly common infection with approximately 33% of all humans having come in contact with this parasite during their lifetime. In immunocompetent adults, exposure to toxoplasmosis is asymptomatic; however, in immunocompromised patients it can lead to severe disease and death. Toxoplasmosis acquired in pregnancy can cause various congenital anomalies in the fetus including hydrocephalus, intracerebral calcification, retardation, chorioretinitis, hearing loss, and even death.

Toxoplasmosis is frequently seen in advanced AIDS when the CD4+ counts are <200cells/mm^3. Up to 5% of patients initially diagnosed with AIDS in the United States will present with toxoplasmosis. Fortunately, the incidence of toxoplasmosis has significantly declined since the use of highly active anti-retroviral therapy (HAART). In Africa and Europe as many as 50% of patients with AIDS will develop CNS toxoplasmosis.

Transmission

There are three primary ways of transmission: by ingesting uncooked meat containing tissue cysts, by ingesting food and water contaminated with oocysts from infected cat feces, and by vertical transmission. The parasite can also be transmitted by transplantation of organs and blood transfusions. Although CNS toxoplasmosis occasionally results from a primary infection, it is more commonly caused by hematogenous spread of a previous infection.

Clinical Presentation and Diagnosis

The most common clinical presentation in HIV-infected patients is encephalitis as a result of multiple brain lesions (Table 31–1). Usually, the patient experiences a deterioration in mentation over days to weeks, including headaches, seizures, or cognitive impairment; motor or sensory deficits can also be seen. *T. gondii* can also affect other organs such as the eyes or lungs.

Diagnostic studies used to help diagnose CNS toxoplasmosis include *T. gondii* IgG and IgM titers. An IgM antibody response is associated with newly acquired toxoplasmosis. **However, antibody levels can be very low in AIDS patients.** It has been reported that up to 22% of patients diagnosed with toxoplasmosis by histologic confirmation had absent antibody levels. If there are no signs of increased intracranial pressure, then a lumbar puncture

Table 31–1
CLINICAL FEATURES OF INTRACRANIAL TOXOPLASMOSIS

Clinical Features (Signs and Symptoms)
  Headache and constitutional symptoms early on
  Confusion, drowsiness, focal weakness, aphasia, and seizures later on in the course
  Coma can ensue within days to weeks if no treatment is started
  Radiculomyelopathy can occasionally be present
  Other features: ataxia, cranial nerve palsies, hemianopia, personality changes

may be obtained. Cerebrospinal fluid studies show an elevated protein level consistently. There is a great degree of variability when it comes to other CSF studies. PCR for *T. gondii* in the CSF has moderate sensitivity and high specificity.

The typical findings on CT scan or MRI of the brain are single or **multiple hypodense lesions in the white matter** and occasionally in the basal ganglia with mass effect. Lesions are usually **ring enhancing.** Typically, patients will present with multiple rather than solitary lesions (see Fig. 31–1). In fact a solitary lesion favors CNS lymphoma over toxoplasmosis.

Brain biopsy, revealing the organism, should only be performed if there is no response to empiric treatment within 2 weeks or if there is a solitary lesion and negative serological studies. Microscopic examination is notable for lymphocytic vasculitis, microglial nodules, and astroglial nodules. Cases that show marked increased intracranial pressure and herniation are best handled with the aid of neurosurgeons.

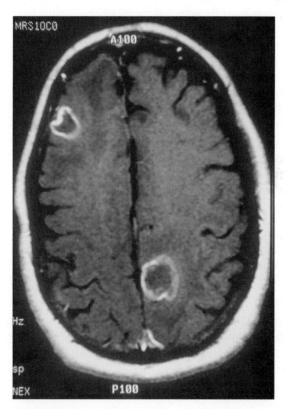

Figure 31–1. CT brain image with ring-enhancing Toxoplasmosis. (*With permission from Knoop KJ, Stack LP, Storrow AB: Atlas of Emergency Medicine; 2nd ed. New York:McGraw-Hill; 2006: Fig 20–7, p 656.*)

Treatment

The main treatment for CNS toxoplasmosis consists of pyrimethamine at a dose of 100 mg orally twice a day on the first day followed by 25–100 mg per day. Due to its selective activity against dihydrofolate reductase it is imperative that folic acid be given concomitantly. This is often in the form of folinic acid. Sulfadiazine, which acts synergistically with pyrimethamine, should also be concomitantly given at a dose of 1–2 g orally four times a day. If there is significant edema corticosteroids such as dexamethasone (Decadron) should be given. Almost 75% of patients will improve within 1 week of receiving antibiotic therapy. The prognosis for full recovery is guarded as there may be frequent relapses as a result of requiring larger doses of medication.

Prophylaxis

Trimethoprim/sulfamethoxazole is effective prophylaxis against *T. gondii*, and indicated for HIV-infected individuals with CD4 counts less than 200 cells/mm^3. Precautions include cooking meats completely, hygiene when handling uncooked or undercooked meat, and avoiding exposure to cat feces, such as cleaning litter boxes.

Comprehension Questions

[31.1] A 22-year-old man is suspected to be infected by *T. gondii*. Which of the following routes is he most likely to have been infected?

   A. Ingesting uncooked vegetables
   B. Congenital
   C. Fecal oral route
   D. Inhalation of spores

[31.2] Which of the following is a clinical feature of CNS toxoplasmosis?

   A. Bladder retention
   B. Aortic dilation
   C. Argyll Robertson pupil
   D. Hemiparesis

[31.3] Which of the following is true regarding CNS toxoplasmosis?

   A. Brain biopsy is the only reliable method of diagnosis
   B. It is frequently seen in early cases of AIDS
   C. Treatment consists of penicillin
   D. Multiple ring-enhancing lesions as opposed to solitary lesions are suggestive of CNS toxoplasmosis

Answers

[31.1] **C.** Spores are not part of the life cycle of *T. gondii.*

[31.2] **D.** Argyll Robertson pupil has not been reported with CNS toxoplasmosis. Bladder incontinence, although uncommon, is part of an underlying myelopathy.

[31.3] **D.** Brain biopsies are deferred unless patients are not responsive to empiric therapy or if serologic studies are negative, and there is a solitary lesion on imaging studies.

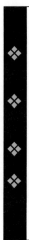

CLINICAL PEARLS

❖ Imaging studies suggestive of CNS toxoplasmosis are those with multiple ring-enhancing lesions as opposed to a solitary ring-enhancing lesion, which speaks more for CNS lymphoma.

❖ The diagnosis of CNS toxoplasmosis can be made by positive serologic studies, although these may be undetectable in AIDS patients.

❖ One-fourth to one-half of the world's population is infected, and infection is most common in places with warm moist climates.

❖ Infection in the unborn child, called congenital toxoplasmosis, is the result of an acute usually asymptomatic infection acquired by the mother in pregnancy and transmitted in utero.

REFERENCES

Garcia LS, Bruckner DA. Diagnostic medical parasitology, 3rd ed. Washington, DC: American Society of Microbiology; 1997:111–121; 423–424; 577–589.

Jones JL, Kruszon-Moran D, Wilson M, et al. *Toxoplasma gondii* infection in the United States: seroprevalence and risk factors. Am J Epidemiol 2001;154: 357–365.

Remington JS, Thulliez P, Montoya JG. Recent developments for diagnosis of toxoplasmosis. J Clin Microbiol 2004 Mar;42(3):941–945.

Steinmetz H, Arendt G, Hefter H. Focal brain lesions in patients with AIDS: aetiologies and corresponding radiological patterns in a prospective study. J Neurol 1995 Jan;242(2):69–74.

You are paged stat to the emergency room (ER) to evaluate a 17-year-old young woman who was hit in the head by a joystick while playing a video boxing game. She did not lose consciousness but has experienced a headache in the right frontal region since her injury. Over the past 2 hours, the severity of the headache has significantly increased. She has not experienced nausea, vomiting, weakness, confusion, memory loss, numbness, blurred vision, diplopia, loss of vision, anosmia, or loss of balance. She took acetaminophen, which did not help her headache. On her parents' insistence, she presented to the emergency room for further evaluation. Her friend who has accompanied her to the emergency room placed a bag of ice over her right forehead, which has started to alleviate the pain. The emergency room physician has completed a thorough evaluation and has found that she has tenderness to palpation over the right forehead but no laceration, swelling, or bruising. The Glasgow Coma Scale is 15, and the neurologic examination is normal except for a right pupil that is unreactive. A CT scan of the brain without contrast done on an emergent basis is normal. The emergency room physician is concerned that this young woman has suffered significant trauma because her right pupil is not reactive.

 What is the most likely diagnosis?

 What is the next diagnostic step?

ANSWERS TO CASE 32: Unreactive Pupil

Summary: A 17-year-old female presents to the emergency room with a right frontal headache after being hit by a joystick from a video game. She did not lose consciousness and does not have other associated symptoms with a headache. Acetaminophen has not helped her headache; however, an ice bag over the frontal region of the head has helped improve the pain. Her Glasgow Coma Scale is 15, and the neurologic examination is completely normal except for an unreactive right pupil. A CT scan of the head is normal.

◆ **Most likely diagnosis:** Holmes-Adie pupil.

◆ **Next diagnostic step:** Perform the neurologic examination to confirm the findings by the ER physician. Pay special attention to the pupillary response on near effort as there is often slow constriction with prolonged near effort and slow redilation after near effort. Apply 0.1% pilocarpine to the right pupil to see if it constricts. If there is pupillary constriction after application of 0.1% pilocarpine, the diagnosis of Holmes-Adie pupil has been confirmed

Analysis

Objectives

1. Know a diagnostic approach to an unreactive pupil including the role of CT scan of the head.
2. Understand the physiology of pupillary reaction and the effects of the sympathetic and parasympathetic nervous system on the pupil.
3. Be familiar with the workup for an unreactive pupil and common etiologies for unreactive pupils such as Holmes-Adie pupil, third nerve palsy, and pharmacologic blockade.

Considerations

This 17-year-old woman was found to have an unreactive right pupil following head trauma without loss of consciousness. The most immediate concern is ensuring that she does not have severe head injury. Most closed head injuries are mild with only approximately 3% of these mild injuries progressing to more serious ones. It is highly unlikely that an individual will suffer significant head trauma without loss of consciousness. Nonetheless, a thorough evaluation with a good history and neurologic examination is crucial in determining the severity of head trauma. The lack of associated symptoms with a headache, normal neurologic examination including normal mental status, and normal CT scan of the head makes it highly unlikely for significant head trauma to be present. The solitary finding of an unreactive pupil in this particular setting suggests a benign process.

Conversely, closed head injuries associated with nausea, vomiting, dizziness, confusion, unusual behavior, or seizures are at high risk of being severe head injury. The finding of a unilateral unreactive pupil in this setting despite a normal neurologic examination or normal CT of the head should alert the clinician of serious brain trauma. Bilateral unreactive pupils in the setting of severe head injury carry a grave prognosis. Unilateral unreactive pupils indicate structural lesions of the oculomotor nerves or midbrain. They can also be present in the setting of pharmacologic blockade with atropine or scopolamine (parasympatholytic drugs). Lastly, unreactive pupils can be associated with peripheral neuropathies including autonomic neuropathies or be present in healthy individuals (Holmes-Adie syndrome).

A CT scan of the head without contrast is the gold standard in evaluating patients with head injuries as it is reliable, readily available, and is easy and quick to perform. Information obtained from this study includes the skull anatomy, cerebral hemisphere anatomy, and whether or not there is hemorrhage present (subdural hematomas, epidural hematomas, subarachnoid hemorrhage, or intracerebral hemorrhage). MRI of the brain is able to detect diffuse axonal injury and small contusions much better than CT scans. However, in the acute setting an MRI has a limited role as it takes longer to acquire the study and is often difficult to obtain in individuals who are severely ill.

APPROACH TO UNRESPONSIVE PUPILS

Definitions

Glasgow Coma Scale (GSC): The GCS was developed to delineate categories of head injury and levels of consciousness in patients with traumatic brain injury. The scale is divided into three categories consisting of eye-opening (E), verbal response (V), and motor response (M). The maximum score is 15, and the minimum score is 3. GCS = E + M + V (Table 32–1).

Epidural hematoma: A collection of blood between the inner table of the skull and dura. It is considered to be an extra-axial hematoma and appears to have a biconvex shape on CT scan of the head.

Subdural hematoma: Also considered to be an extra-axial hematoma. It is a collection of blood between the brain and the dura. It appears as a concave shape on CT scan of the head.

Unreactive pupil: Absence of pupillary constriction when exposed to light.

Table 32–1
GLASGOW COMA SCALE

GLASGOW COMA SCORE

Eye Opening (E)	Verbal Response (V)	Motor Response (M)
4 = Spontaneous	5 = Normal conversation	6 = Normal
3 = To voice	4 = Disoriented conversation	5 = Localizes to pain
2 = To pain	3 = Words, but not coherent	4 = Withdraws to pain
1 = None	2 = No words—only sounds	3 = Decorticate posture
	1 = None	2 = Decerebrate
		1 = None
		Total = E + V + M

Clinical Approach

Assessing the pupillary response requires the use of a strong light source. The pupils are tested individually with a normal examination consisting of bilateral reactive pupils that constrict to direct and consensual stimulation. There are factors that can alter pupillary examination including eye surgery; the use of narcotics, which causes miosis (pupillary constriction); and sympathomimetic drugs that cause mydriasis (pupillary dilation).

The size of the pupil depends on a balance between parasympathetic and sympathetic tone. Each of these branches of the autonomic nervous system interface with antagonistic muscles, which determine the size of the pupil. The first muscle, the sphincter muscle, is innervated by the parasympathetic nervous system, and its activation results in pupillary constriction or myosis. The second muscle, the dilator muscle, is innervated by the sympathetic nervous system, and its activation results in pupillary dilation otherwise known as mydriasis.

The cell bodies for the parasympathetic preganglionic neurons are located in the Edinger-Westphal nucleus of the upper midbrain. These axons join with the ipsilateral oculomotor nuclei motor fibers and form the third cranial nerve. Throughout the course of the oculomotor nerve the parasympathetic fibers are situated immediately internal to the epineurium (superficially) and are susceptible to compressive injury. The parasympathetic axons eventually synapse in the ciliary ganglion. The ciliary ganglion houses the cell bodies of the postganglionic neurons, which emerge to form the short ciliary nerves. These in turn innervate the sphincter muscle.

Sympathetic innervation starts in the ipsilateral posterolateral hypothalamus and terminates in the ciliospinal center of Budge-Waller (intermediolateral gray matter of cord segments C8–T2). These preganglionic neurons (second-order) ascend in the sympathetic chain and synapse in the superior cervical ganglion.

These postganglionic neurons travel superficially on the internal carotid artery until reaching the cavernous sinus when the nerve joins the ophthalmic division of the trigeminal nerve and then enters the orbit with the nasociliary nerve to innervate the dilator muscle via the long ciliary nerves (Fig. 32–1).

An abnormally small pupil is a sign of a lesion in the sympathetic nervous system whereas a large pupil suggests a lesion affecting the parasympathetic nervous system. Parasympathetic dysfunction can occur from one of four possibilities: the first being injury to the third nerve, the second one being damage to the iris itself, the third occurring from pharmacologic effects (atropine, scopolamine, etc.), and the last resulting from damage to the ciliary ganglion or the short ciliary nerves. Lesions to the third nerve or injury to Edinger-Westphal nucleus cause pupillary

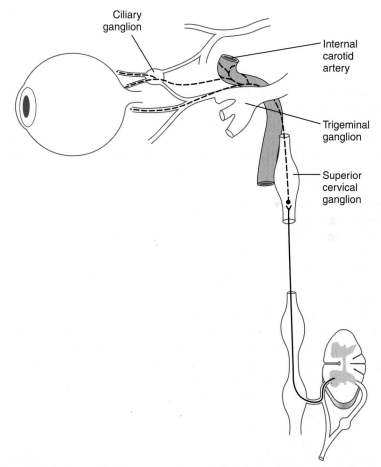

Figure 32–1. Sympathetic nerve pathway of the eye. (*With permission from Tintinalli JE, Kelen GD, Stapczynski JS (eds). Emergency medicine: a comprehensive study guide, 6th ed. New York: McGraw-Hill; 2003: Fig. 238–21.*)

dilation. Compression of the third nerve by the uncus of the temporal lobe or by a posterior communicating artery aneurysm presents with unilateral dilation and unresponsiveness. Extraocular muscle function is typically intact.

Dysfunction of the ciliary ganglion or the short ciliary nerves gives rise to a tonic pupil. This is characterized by absent reaction of the pupil to light but a slow constriction to prolonged near effort focusing (light-near dissociation). Redilation after constriction to near stimuli is slow and tonic. On slit lamp examination segmental palsy of the iris sphincter can be seen as evident by segmental vermiform movements of the iris borders. These movements represent physiologic pupillary unrest that becomes noticeable in areas where the sphincter muscle still reacts. This reaction is most likely from collateral sprouting to the sphincter after damage to the ciliary ganglion or short ciliary nerves. Cholinergic supersensitivity of the innervated iris sphincter may be demonstrated with agents such as 1% pilocarpine. Autonomic peripheral neuropathy can cause damage to the ciliary ganglion or short ciliary nerves. However, healthy individuals are also known to have tonic pupils. A syndrome known as Holmes-Adie syndrome consists of a unilateral or in some cases bilateral tonic pupils (unresponsive pupils), impaired corneal sensation, and absent or depressed deep tendon reflexes in the legs. It is idiopathic with a female predilection and tends to occur in young adults (20–40 years of age). This syndrome can present with sudden blurring of vision, photophobia, or without symptoms as an incidental finding. Pain is not associated with this syndrome. There are other rare causes of tonic pupils including orbital injuries, orbital tumors, retinal cryotherapy, herpes zoster, amyloidosis, and other autonomic neuropathies. Treatment for Holmes-Adie syndrome is often only reassurance that it is a benign condition. If treatment is necessary because of blurred vision the use of a contact lens with an artificial pupil may be of help.

Comprehension Questions

[32.1] On clinical examination, how can you differentiate a third nerve palsy from Holmes-Adie pupil?

  A. Associated symptoms such as weakness of the extraocular muscles support a third nerve palsy
  B. Light responses are absent in both conditions; however, in a third nerve palsy normal accommodation is present
  C. Light responses are normal in Holmes-Adie pupil but absent in the third nerve palsy
  D. Deep tendon reflexes are absent in a third nerve palsy but present in Holmes-Adie pupil.

[32.2] Holmes-Adie pupil can be confirmed by the following:

  A. Instilling the pupil with scopolamine
  B. Obtaining a CT scan of the eye
  C. Instilling the pupil with 0.1% pilocarpine
  D. Instilling the pupil with morphine

[32.3] Which of the following statements is false regarding evaluation of unresponsive pupils?

    A. In the acute setting an MRI of the brain is the study of choice

    B. The history including associated symptoms is critical in determining severity

    C. Additional clinical findings are useful in differentiating the various causes of unresponsive pupils

    D. There are benign causes for unresponsive pupils

Answers

[32.1] **A.** Light responses are abnormal in both a third nerve palsy and in Holmes-Adie pupil; however, constriction of the pupil on accommodation is seen with the latter only.

[32.2] **C.** Instilling a normal pupil with 0.1% pilocarpine does not affect the pupil.

[32.3] **A.** A CT scan of the head is the study of choice in the acute setting as it is quick and reliable.

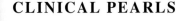

CLINICAL PEARLS

❖ An unresponsive pupil in an individual that is awake and otherwise has a normal neurologic examination is a benign process.

❖ A simple way to differentiate a tonic pupil from a third nerve palsy is to check for pupillary response on accommodation.

❖ Holmes-Adie syndrome is typically seen in young women and associated with a unilateral unresponsive pupil and depressed deep tendon reflexes in the legs.

REFERENCES

Dorland's Illustrated Medical Dictionary, 27th ed. Philadelphia, PA: WB Saunders; 1988.

Jennett B, Snoek J, Bond MR, et al. Disability after severe head injury, observations on the use of the Glasgow Outcome Scale. J Neurol Neurosurg Psychiatry 1981;44:285–293.

Loewenfeld, IE. The pupil: anatomy, physiology and clinical applications. Ames, IA: Iowa State University Press and Detroit, MI: Wayne State University Press; 1993.

A 26-year-old woman presents to the emergency room with severe headache and blurred vision. She has been experiencing headaches over the past 2 –3 weeks. Her headaches are described as an aching type sensation encompassing the entire head. The severity of the headache has been such that she has been able to do all activities of daily living until today when the headache acutely worsened to the point she could not function. She has taken acetaminophen without improvement in her symptoms. She has not experienced nausea, vomiting, or other symptoms besides visual impairment. Over the past 2 weeks, she has experienced transient graying-out of her vision most noticeably when she gets up from a chair. As the emergency room physician you notice the following on examination: temperature (T), 37.2°C (98.9°F); blood pressure (BP), 134/72 mmHg; heart rate (HR), 78 beats/min; weight, 108.8 kg (240 lb); height, 155 cm (5 ft 1 in). There are no cranial bruits, and her cardiovascular examination is normal. Her neurologic examination is notable for bilateral papilledema with intact visual acuity and intact extra-ocular muscles. She appears to have constriction of the visual fields on initial examination, however on retesting, her visual fields are normal. She has normal color perception. The remainder of her neurologic examination including mental status is completely normal. Serologic studies including a comprehensive metabolic panel, complete blood count (CBC) with differential, and urinalysis are normal.

◆ **What is the most likely diagnosis?**

◆ **What is the next diagnostic step?**

◆ **What is the next step in therapy?**

ANSWERS TO CASE 33: Papilledema

Summary: A 26-year-old woman presents with blurred vision and severe headache. She provides a history of experiencing transient graying out of her vision over the past 2–3 weeks. She has no other associated symptoms. Her physical examination is notable for normal blood pressure and heart rate, obesity, bilateral papilledema, and decreased color perception. The serum laboratory tests and urinalysis are normal.

◆ **Most likely diagnosis:** Increased intracranial pressure.

◆ **Next diagnostic step:** CT of the head without contrast, lumbar puncture, and ophthalmologic evaluation with formal visual field testing.

◆ **Next step in therapy:** If pseudotumor cerebri is diagnosed, then high-volume lumbar puncture should be done.

Analysis

Objectives

1. Describe a diagnostic approach to papilledema.
2. Describe the differential diagnosis of papilledema.
3. Be familiar with emergent treatment of papilledema.

Considerations

The presentation of headache with blurred vision and papilledema is a medical emergency. Papilledema denotes a serious neurologic problem, and most commonly occurs bilaterally. When acute, vision for the most part is well preserved. By definition, **papilledema is swelling of the optic disk from elevated intracranial pressure** (Fig. 33–1). It can be a sign of an underlying **brain mass**, which even if benign can cause increased intracranial pressure, placing patients **at risk for irreversible neurologic dysfunction or even death**. Depending on the size of the brain mass and the extent of its associated edema, patients are at risk for herniation syndromes, which eventually can lead to death. In general, **all patients with increased intracranial pressure with papilledema require emergent neuroimaging studies**. The study of choice in emergent situations remains a CT scan of the head with contrast. Conditions that cause papilledema include meningitis, hydrocephalus, space occupying lesions, dural sinus thrombosis, and pseudotumor cerebri (idiopathic intracranial hypertension). Pseudotumor cerebri tends to affect women of childbearing age who are somewhat obese and is a diagnosis of exclusion.

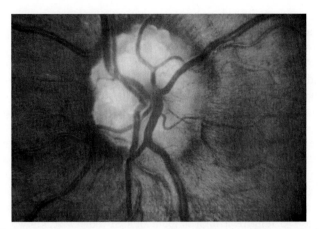

Figure 33–1. Funduscopic examination of papilledema. (*With permission from Kasper DL, Braunwal E, Fauci A, et al. Harrison's principles of internal medicine, 16th ed. New York: McGraw-Hill; 2004: Fig. 25–12.*)

APPROACH TO PAPILLEDEMA

Definitions

Papilledema: Disk edema from raised intracranial pressure; commonly bilaterally.

Increased intracranial pressure: Cerebrospinal fluid (CSF) pressures above 200 mm of water in a nonobese patient or greater than 250 mm of water in obese patients.

Herniation syndromes: A downward displacement of brain tissue when intracranial pressure in the supratentorial compartment reaches a certain level.

Hydrocephalus: Abnormal excessive accumulation of cerebral spinal fluid in the brain.

Lumbar puncture: A test that evaluates cerebral spinal fluid. It is performed under local anesthesia and involves placing a needle into the spinal canal typically at L4–L5 for collection of spinal fluid.

Clinical Approach

The finding of papilledema on clinical examination in the setting of recent neurologic symptoms such as headaches or visual disturbances should alert the clinician of a possible space occupying lesion in the brain. The history and physical examination can help localize the mass lesion if any. For example, right-sided weakness associated with headaches, papilledema, and visual disturbances would place the mass lesion in the left cerebral hemisphere. However, the etiology of this space-occupying lesion cannot be determined by examination alone.

A CT scan of the head with and without contrast is helpful in trying to determine if this mass lesion is a tumor, hemorrhage, abscess, and so forth. Importantly, it will assist in diagnosing associated cerebral edema and impending cerebral herniation. A CT scan of the head is often adequate for evaluating patients with increased intracranial pressure, however, an MRI of the brain can be useful in excluding dural sinus venous thrombosis. Typically neuroimaging studies are normal in patients with pseudotumor cerebri. However, enlarged optic nerve sheaths, small slit-like ventricles or an empty sella may be seen.

In the absence of a mass lesion, a lumbar puncture is the next step taken to evaluate the cause of increased intracranial pressure. Opening pressure of the CSF is made and recorded with the patient in the recumbent position. Lumbar punctures performed in an upright position do not allow for accurate pressure measurements. If the cerebral spinal fluid pressure is elevated, the clinician can choose to remove a high amount of CSF otherwise known as a high-volume tap. The CSF should be analyzed for protein, glucose, cell count with differential, cytology, and culture. Additionally, a note should be made of the color and clarity of the fluid. This analysis will help evaluate for conditions such as meningitis or other infections, hemorrhage, or inflammation. Normal studies are associated with pseudotumor cerebri.

Physiology of Papilledema

Papilledema results from axoplasmic flow stasis in the slow axoplasmic transport system. Increased intracranial pressure is transmitted to the subarachnoid, which in turn encompasses the entire optic nerve and is continuous with the optic nerve sheath. As intracranial pressure increases the pressure in this sheath also increases resulting in a blockage at the nerve preventing normal axoplasmic transport. The collection of components involved in axonal transport leads to mark distension of optic axons, which in turn results in edema of the nerve and optic disk. Disk edema can be caused from many different etiologies including inflammation, tumors, infections, and ischemia. However papilledema refers only to the disk edema caused by increased intracranial pressure.

Symptoms of Papilledema

Visual dysfunction can present in a variety of ways. One of the more common presentations is **transient visual obscuration or graying out/dimming of vision.** Quite often this can occur after bending over. Other visual disturbances include sudden visual loss from intraocular hemorrhage as a result of neovascularization from chronic papilledema; blurring and distortion of central vision, and progressive loss of peripheral vision (often beginning in the nasal inferior quadrant). Loss of color perception and loss of central visual fields can occur later on.

Pseudotumor Cerebri

Pseudotumor cerebri is often referred to as idiopathic intracranial hypertension or benign intracranial hypertension. It is often seen in young obese women and has an incidence rate in the United States of approximately 1 per 100,000 in the general population. The incidence is slightly higher in women who are overweight. The diagnosis is one of exclusion and requires the findings of increased intracranial pressure (papilledema), nonfocal neurologic signs (with the exception of a possible sixth cranial nerve palsy), normal imaging studies (except for slit-like ventricles), and normal CSF studies except for an elevated opening pressure. Although this can present at any age, most patients present in the third decade of life. It is unclear as to why there is an increased incidence in obese women, however, it has been suggested that obesity leads to increased intra-abdominal pressure, which raises cardiac filling pressures, which in turn leads to impaired venous return from the brain. This in turn leads to an elevation in intracranial venous pressure.

The pathophysiology of pseudotumor cerebri is unclear; however, it is presumed that there is a resistance to absorption of CSF across the arachnoid villi. Others believe that the cerebral circulation is abnormal and that cerebral venous outflow is impaired, which results in increased water content in the brain. Whatever the cause, the resultant increased intracranial pressure is relayed to anatomical structures in the brain cavity resulting in neurologic signs and symptoms. The most severe of these is papilledema, which in turn can lead to irreversible optic nerve damage. Typical signs for pseudotumor cerebri include headache, transient visual obscuration, dizziness, nausea, vomiting, tinnitus, and horizontal diplopia from a sixth nerve palsy. The classic headache associated with pseudotumor cerebri is diffuse, worsens in the morning, and worsens by Valsalva maneuver. The most common abnormality on clinical examination is bilateral disk edema. Disk edema can be asymmetric, and there can be associated subretinal hemorrhages.

Risk factors for pseudotumor cerebri include obesity, recent weight gain, female gender, especially in the reproductive age group, and menstrual irregularity. Some cases have been found to be associated with abnormalities such as hypothyroidism, Cushing disease, adrenal insufficiency, chronic renal failure, systemic lupus erythematosus, corticosteroid use, lithium, tamoxifen, tetracycline, cimetidine, and isotretinoin (Accutane) use. Although pregnancy was previously thought to be a risk factor, there is no evidence-based medicine that supports this.

In the evaluation process, **imaging studies** should be performed to exclude mass lesions, infections, and hemorrhages. If imaging studies are normal, a **lumbar puncture** is performed to evaluate opening pressure. CSF studies for protein, glucose, and cell count as described above should be performed. **In pseudotumor cerebri all CSF studies are normal except for an elevated opening pressure.** Additionally, visual fields should be evaluated by an ophthalmologist to clearly document any subtle abnormalities.

Treatment of pseudotumor cerebri includes a high-volume lumbar puncture performed at the time of the initial evaluation. This, however, is only temporary. Long-term treatment includes the use of acetazolamide, a carbonic anhydrase inhibitor, which lowers the intracranial pressure. If progressive visual loss ensues then optic nerve sheath fenestrations are used. This involves cutting patches in the dura surrounding the optic nerve allowing the efflux of cerebral spinal fluid, which in turn reduces pressure. If medical management is insufficient then a lumbar peritoneal shunt or ventriculoperitoneal shunt is performed by neurosurgeons. Ultimately, the treatment of these patients involves not only a neurologist but also an ophthalmologist and neurosurgeon. If patients are obese, recommendations for weight reduction are made to assist in treatment.

Comprehension Questions

[33.1] An emergency room physician has found what appears to be papilledema in a 40-year-old woman. The intracranial pressure is noted to be normal. Which of the following conditions is most likely to be causative?

A. Metastatic breast cancer
B. Intracerebral hemorrhage
C. Hydrocephalus
D. Idiopathic intracranial hypertension
E. Optic nerve trauma

[33.2] Which of the following is a risk factor for pseudotumor cerebri or idiopathic intracranial hypertension?

A. Thin physique
B. Hyperthyroidism
C. Recent weight loss
D. Female gender

[33.3] A 25-year-old woman is diagnosed with increased intracranial pressure and pseudotumor cerebri. Which of the following is the best next step in therapy?

A. Acetazolamide
B. Optic nerve ablation
C. CSF saline infusion
D. Oral hypoglycemic therapy

Answers

[33.1] **E.** Optic nerve trauma can cause optic disk swelling; however, papilledema refers to optic disc swelling occurring from increased intracranial pressure.

[33.2] **D.** Female gender places the patient at higher risk for benign intracranial hypertension.

[33.3] **A.** Acetazolamide decreases the intracranial pressure and is a treatment for pseudotumor cerebri.

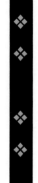

CLINICAL PEARLS

❖ Papilledema associated with visual dysfunction is a medical emergency requiring immediate neuroimaging studies.

❖ The neurologic examination in patients with benign intracranial hypertension is normal except for visual loss (loss of color perception, loss of visual fields, transient visual obscuration) and a sixth nerve palsy.

❖ Most adult brain tumors present without papilledema, however, most children with brain tumors present with papilledema.

❖ Papilledema is a term that should only be used for optic disc swelling secondary to increased intracranial pressure.

REFERENCES

Allen ED, Byrd SE, Darling CF, et al. The clinical and radiological evaluation of primary brain tumors in children. Part I: clinical evaluation. J Natl Med Assoc 1993;85:445–451.

Brazis PW, Lee AG. Elevated intracranial pressure and pseudotumor cerebri. Curr Opin Ophthalmol 1998 Dec;9(6):27–32.

Miller NR, Newman NJ. Pseudotumor cerebri (benign intracranial hypertension). In: Miller NR, Newman NJ, Biousse V, et al. Walsh and Hoyt's clinical neuro-ophthalmology, vol. 1, 6th ed. Philadelphia, PA: Lippincott Williams & Wilkins; 2004:523–538.

A 65-year-old man with a history of hypertension, coronary artery disease, and early Alzheimer disease presents with a complaint of double vision since yesterday. He has not experienced chest pain, chest palpitations, nausea, light-headedness, vertigo, headache, facial weakness, hemisensory loss, hemiparesis, loss of balance, hearing loss, tinnitus, visual loss, ptosis, or proptosis. He has noticed that covering up either eye corrects his double vision. He has resorted to wearing an eye patch since yesterday so that he can see and walk without falling. In fact he was able to drive on his own on the freeway to your office much to his family's dismay. On further questioning you elicit the history that his double vision occurs only on horizontal gaze and not vertical gaze. He has been com-pliant with his medications for hypertension and coronary artery disease. On examination, his blood pressure (BP) is 124/72 mmHg with a heart rate (HR) of 88 beats/min. He is afebrile and has a regular rate and rhythm without murmurs on cardiac examination. There are no carotid bruits, and his peripheral pulses are normal. His neurologic examination is notable for intact orientation and intact motor strength. His cranial nerve examination is remarkable only for a right lat-eral rectus palsy. Sensory examination is normal, and his deep tendon reflexes are 2+ throughout. Plantar responses are flexor. His gait is normal. Review of his daily blood pressure log shows stable pressures of 130/70 mmHg.

◆ **What is the most likely diagnosis?**

◆ **What is the neurologic deficit?**

ANSWERS TO CASE 34: Sixth Nerve Palsy (Ischemic Mononeuropathy)

Summary: A 65-year-old man with hypertension, coronary artery disease, and early Alzheimer disease presents with a 24-hour history of binocular horizontal diplopia (double vision). He has not experienced associated symptoms such as chest pain or headache. His examination is significant for a normal blood pressure and heart rate and the findings of the isolated right sixth nerve palsy.

 Most likely diagnosis: Sixth nerve palsy secondary to ischemic mononeuropathy

 Likely neurological deficit: Sixth nerve palsy

Analysis

Objectives

1. Understand the diagnostic approach in evaluating diplopia.
2. Describe the difference between monocular and binocular diplopia.
3. Know the differential diagnosis of a sixth nerve palsy.

Considerations

This 65-year-old man with known risk factors for cerebral vascular disease (hypertension and coronary artery disease) presents with an acute episode of binocular diplopia. The history suggests binocular diplopia as he tells you that covering up an eye resolves the diplopia. You are given the history that he has diplopia only on horizontal gaze. In this particular case you are told that the patient's blood work and MRI brain is normal. Given the history of hypertension and coronary artery disease he is at risk for cerebrovascular disease and ischemia. In this setting, the most likely cause of this man's diplopia is an ischemic mononeuropathy to the abducens nerve. In this particular case the patient has a completely normal examination except for a sixth nerve palsy. This makes it easy to pinpoint the location of the abnormality as the only location for an isolated abducens nerve palsy is in the nucleus. Table 34–1 shows locations where the sixth nerve can be affected and its associated clinical findings.

Table 34–1
CLINICAL FINDINGS

LOCATION	ASSOCIATED CLINICAL FINDINGS	ETIOLOGIES
Nuclear	Horizontal gaze palsy, sixth nerve dysfunction or other brainstem signs	Ischemia, demyelinating, inflammatory, trauma, vascular (aneurysm or other vascular malformations), neoplastic, congenital, metabolic
Fascicle	Contralateral hemisensory loss, contralateral hemiparesis, central Horner syndrome	Ischemia, inflammatory, vascular, neoplastic, trauma, demyelinating
Subarachnoid space	Signs of increased intracranial pressure (e.g., headache, papilledema) or other cranial neuropathies	Inflammatory, infectious, toxic, vascular, neoplastic, cervical traction, myelogram, infiltrative
Petrous apex	Facial pain or fifth, seventh, or eighth cranial nerves dysfunction	Traumatic, infectious, inflammatory (sarcoid), neoplastic (meningioma)
Cavernous sinus	Sixth nerve palsy with any combination of third, fourth or ophthalmic division of the fifth cranial nerve dysfunction; Horner syndrome	Ischemic, neoplastic, inflammatory, infectious, vascular, fistula, or thrombosis
Orbit/superior orbital fissure	Can have proptosis or optic nerve atrophy/edema	Traumatic, infectious, inflammatory, neoplastic

APPROACH TO BINOCULAR DIPLOPIA

Definitions

Ptosis: Drooping of the eye lids
Proptosis: Abnormal protrusion of the eyeball
Diplopia: Double vision
Ischemic mononeuropathy: Isolated nerve injury from inadequate blood flow to the nerve

Clinical Approach

Sixth nerve palsy has a variety of causes, and clinical examination usually leads to an accurate diagnosis. The abducens nucleus is located in the lower dorsal pons. The motor neurons of this nucleus send axons that course anteriorly in the pons and travel near the corticospinal tract and emerge in the sulcus between the pons and medulla. The abducens nerve exits the pons ventrally and ascends in the prepontine cistern via the subarachnoid space. It then rises over the petrous apex of the temporal bone and enters the cavernous sinus laying between the carotid artery and the ophthalmic branch of the trigeminal nerve laterally. It finally passes into the orbit through the superior orbital fissure.

Etiology of Sixth Nerve Palsy

After the localization of the sixth nerve lesion, the next step is to determine the etiology of the abnormality. Table 34–1 shows there are various causes for a nuclear abducens abnormality. The evaluation includes serologic studies including an erythrocyte sedimentation rate, antinuclear antibody (ANA), complete blood count (CBC), glycosylated hemoglobin, and if appropriate a 2-hour glucose tolerance test. An MRI of the brain without contrast should be ordered concomitantly. An erythrocyte sedimentation rate (ESR) and ANA can help exclude inflammatory causes such as vasculitis; glycosylated hemoglobin can exclude diabetes mellitus, and a CBC can exclude infectious processes. An MRI brain and orbits can exclude vascular abnormalities such as an aneurysm and can exclude mass lesions that are inflammatory (sarcoid), demyelinating, neoplastic, or traumatic. An ischemic process may not be readily visualized on imaging studies and is often a diagnosis of exclusion.

Evaluation of Diplopia

Diplopia results from lack of visual fusion. The first step in evaluating a patient with diplopia is to determine whether it is binocular or monocular. **Binocular diplopia is usually caused by an underlying primary neurologic problem. Monocular diplopia,** conversely, is primarily caused by an **ophthalmologic disorder** such as abnormalities of the lens, cornea, vitreous humor, or iris. Rarely, monocular diplopia can be caused by occipital lobe disease or seizures. Binocular diplopia denotes double vision arising from misalignment of both eyes. Covering up one eye resolves the double vision. Monocular diplopia, however, arises from a primary problem within one eye. This type of diplopia does not resolve when an eye is covered.

The next step in evaluating someone with binocular diplopia is to determine if it is horizontal or vertical. Different eye muscles are involved in moving the eyes horizontally or vertically. There are only two muscles in each eye responsible for horizontal gaze and those are the medial rectus, which is innervated by the third nerve, and the lateral rectus, which is innervated by the sixth nerve. Worsening diplopia on near vision suggests a problem with the medial rectus, whereas diplopia that worsens when viewing distant and lateral objects suggest a problem with the lateral rectus.

The other four eye muscles (superior rectus, inferior rectus, inferior oblique, and superior oblique) move the eyes vertically. Individuals that present with vertical binocular diplopia are experiencing weakness in one or several of these muscles. Vertical diplopia that worsens on near vision suggests a problem with either the inferior oblique or superior oblique. At this point in the evaluation, it must be differentiated whether or not the patient's binocular diplopia is secondary to a medial rectus or a lateral rectus problem. Examining extra-ocular muscles in the nine cardinal fields of gaze can readily point out which of the two muscles is affected. For example, if the right eye cannot cross the midline and look out laterally, the lateral rectus is affected. Conversely, if the right eye cannot cross the midline and turn inward, the medial rectus is affected.

One of these tests is called the alternate cover test and is performed by asking the patient to fixate on an object in each position of gaze. As the patient moves the eyes in each position, deviations in the eye as each one is alternately covered may be seen. The second test often used for evaluating binocular diplopia is the red lens test. In this test, a red lens is placed over an eye, most commonly the right eye, and the patient is asked to look at the nine positions of a cardinal gaze. The key to performing this test is to understand the following: (1) image separation will be greatest in the direction of the weak muscle and (2) the image that is the furthest away from the midline is a false image and corresponds to the eye with impaired motility.

Evaluating other aspects of the cranial nerve examination will help determine where the diplopia is arising from. Special attention should be given to the eyelid, pupillary responses, symmetry of the pupillary size, abnormalities of cranial nerves V, VII, and VIII. For example, ptosis or droopiness of the eyelid can suggest a third nerve problem. Likewise, pupillary asymmetry suggests a third nerves problem. Fatigue of the eyelid can suggest myasthenia gravis. Patients who have a head tilt can also provide you with clues as to where the problem may lie. For example, someone with a right superior oblique palsy may have a leftward tilt of the head.

Treatment

Treatment of the underlying disorder of sixth nerve palsy is indicated when significant and persistent. An isolated and presumed ischemic-related sixth nerve palsy can be observed for improvement for 1 to 3 months. Patching of the involved eye can help alleviate diplopia symptoms temporarily. Prism therapy can also be used. Some suggest using botulinum toxin as a temporizing measure. However if these measures fail, surgery may be the only way to correct this problem.

Comprehension Questions

[34.1] Which of the following is most accurate regarding diplopia?

    A. Binocular diplopia refers to double vision occurring from intrinsic problems in both eyes

    B. Monocular diplopia most commonly occurs because of extrinsic eye problems

    C. The green lens test is a way of evaluating binocular diplopia

    D. The key in evaluating diplopia is to start by determining if it is monocular or binocular

[34.2] A 33-year-old woman has a 3-minute seizure episode caused by her epilepsy. There are no underlying medical disorders or brain structural lesions. Which of the following indicates a more complicated underlying neurologic problem?

    A. Urinary incontinence with seizure

    B. Confusion and lethargy after seizure

    C. Headache after the seizure

    D. Sixth nerve palsy after seizure

[34.3] A 58-year-old woman suffers from an ischemic-related sixth nerve palsy which occurred 6 months ago. Various methods have been tried with limited success, and the patient still has diplopia. Which of the following is most likely to be helpful at this stage?

    A. Surgery

    B. Eye patch

    C. Prisms

    D. Prednisone at a dose of 10 mg per day

    E. Botulinum toxin

Answers

[34.1] **D.** The key to evaluating diplopia is to assess unilateral versus bilateral. Binocular diplopia arises from misalignment of the eye muscles on a target.

[34.2] **D.** Seizures have not been reported to cause sixth nerve dysfunction and thus, its presence indicates a more complex situation.

[34.3] **A.** Surgery is the best option for persistent symptoms that have not resolved. Prednisone has not been used for sixth nerve palsies from ischemia. It can be used for inflammatory causes of sixth nerve abnormalities.

CLINICAL PEARLS

❖ Binocular diplopia occurs from misalignment of the eye muscles on a target and commonly denotes an underlying primary neurologic problem within the brain parenchyma.

❖ Younger patients with sixth nerve palsies more often have malignant etiologies, whereas older patients usually have more benign etiologies.

❖ Monocular diplopia results from intrinsic eye problems, including ocular muscles and neuromuscular junction.

❖ MRI of the brain is critical in evaluating patients with binocular diplopia as it allows for the detection of vascular or demyelinating processes.

REFERENCES

Dorland's Illustrated Medical Dictionary, 27th ed. Philadelphia, PA: WB Saunders; 1988.

Patel SV, Mutyala S, Leske DA, et al. Incidence, associations, and evaluation of sixth nerve palsy using a population-based method. Ophthalmology 2004; 111:369–375.

Quah BL, Ling YL, Cheong PY, et al. A review of 5-years experience in the use of botulinum toxin A in the treatment of sixth cranial nerve palsy at the Singapore National Eye Centre. Singapore Med J 1999;40:405–409.

Savino PJ. Diplopia and sixth nerve palsies. Semin Neurol 1986;6:142–146.

A 68-year-old woman presents with right facial paralysis. She states she was well until approximately 3 days ago when she began to have right ear pain. She has not taken any pain medication and has not had any fever. Today, she awoke with right facial paralysis. She feels slightly dizzy and notices that she has right-sided hearing loss. She denies any past history of ear infections. Her medical history is unremarkable. She does have a past history of chicken pox as a child. Her physical examination shows a 68-year-old woman with obvious right facial paralysis involving her forehead and mouth. She is afebrile but is anxious because of the loss of facial function. There is no motion in any of the branches of the right facial nerve. Her head and neck examination finds small blisters on an erythematous base in the right conchal bowl of the external ear. The examination of the ear canal is painful to her, but the tympanic membrane is intact. No pus is seen in the ear canal. The left ear canal is normal. The Weber tuning fork test lateralizes to the left ear. The Rinne test is normal in both ears. The examination of the nose, oral cavity, throat, and neck are normal. The cranial nerve (CN) examination is normal except for the right VII and VIII nerve problems listed above. The remaining physical examination is normal.

◆ **What is the most likely diagnosis?**

◆ **What is the next diagnostic step?**

◆ **What is the next step in therapy?**

ANSWERS TO CASE 35: Facial Paralysis

Summary: A 68-year-old woman presents with right facial paralysis, a 3-day history of right ear pain, and right-sided hearing loss. There is no motion in any of the branches of the right facial nerve. There are small blisters on an erythematous base in the right conchal bowl of the external ear. The examination of the ear canal is painful to her, but the tympanic membrane is intact. The Weber tuning fork test lateralizes to the left ear. The Rinne test is normal in both ears. The cranial nerve examination is normal except for the right VII and VIII nerve problems listed above.

◆   **Most likely diagnosis:** Herpes zoster oticus (Ramsay Hunt syndrome)

◆   **Next diagnostic test step:** Tzanck smear, audiogram, consider facial nerve electrodiagnostic studies and diagnostic imaging, if indicated

◆   **Next therapeutic step:** anti-herpes virus medication

Analysis

Objectives

1. Describe the clinical presentation and diagnostic approach to facial weakness.
2. Be familiar with the differential diagnosis of facial weakness.
3. Know the treatment for Ramsey Hunt syndrome.

Considerations

This elderly woman has a history of chicken pox, blisters on her ear, hearing abnormalities, and unilateral facial paralysis. Her entire right facial muscles are affected, suggestive of a peripheral facial nerve palsy; a central defect usually spares the forehead. The Weber and Rinne tests are consistent with a sensorineural hearing loss rather than a conductive disorder. This constellation of findings is most consistent with Ramsey Hunt syndrome, which is reaction of the herpes zoster affecting both CNs VII and VIII. A diligent history and physical examination should be performed to exclude other possibilities such as central nervous system disorders, cholesteatomas, facial neuromas, and tumors of the parotid. Corticosteroid and antiviral therapy are recommended, with the probability of good recovery.

APPROACH TO FACIAL NERVE PARALYSIS

Definitions

Audiogram: A test that measures the level of hearing in each ear.
Bell palsy: An idiopathic form of facial paralysis, thought to be caused by herpes simplex virus reactivation.

Cholesteatoma: A benign tumor composed of epithelial debris from the tympanic membrane that becomes trapped in the middle ear.

Facial nerve electromyograph (EMG): Like EMG performed for other nerves, a needle electrode is inserted into the facial muscles, and the patient is asked to perform maximal facial motion effort. The electromyographer looks for compound muscle action potentials, abnormal waves, or fibrillation potentials. Evoked potentials, such as the blink reflex, can also be performed with EMG. An absence of motor unit potentials signifies severe damage or loss or nerve continuity. Fibrillation potentials are signs of a lack of facial nerve input, and are a particularly bad prognostic sign.

Facial nerve electroneurogram (ENoG): An electrical test that evokes a compound muscle action potential (cMAP) by stimulating the facial nerve. The ENoG uses surface electrodes rather than needles to measure the cMAP. Each side is stimulated at the stylomastoid foramen, and the responses from muscle groups are measured and compared. Significant nerve damage is indicated by a 90% or greater reduction in the cMAP.

Otorrhea: Drainage from the ear.

Postherpetic neuralgia: Neuropathic pain resulting from resolved herpes infection.

Tzanck smear: A test that looks for intracytoplasmic particles due to viral infection.

Vesicles: Small fluid-filled blisters on an erythematous base.

Clinical Approach

Approach to Facial Paralysis

Facial function can be characterized in many different ways. A distinction is made between paresis, which indicates weakness, but function is still present; and paralysis, which indicates total lack of function despite maximal effort. The American Academy of Otolaryngology has adopted a system for grading facial nerve function called the House-Brackmann score. Evaluation of patients with facial paralysis is performed systematically by considering the anatomy of the facial nerve's pathway. The facial nerve emerges from the brainstem at the pons to traverse the cerebellopontine angle and then through the temporal bone. The bony course through the temporal bone is the longest course of any nerve through bone. It emerges at the stylomastoid foramen to pass through the substance of the parotid gland and divide into branches that innervate the various parts of the face. Additionally, the facial nerve contains general sensation to the ear canal and pinna, special sensation of taste from the anterior two-thirds of the tongue, and secretomotor function of parasympathetics to the submandibular gland, the lacrimal gland, and the nasal mucosa.

As a point of departure, isolated unilateral facial paralysis will be discussed. **Facial paralysis of central origin**, that is, caused by stroke, is marked by **forehead sparing.** The paralysis affects the lower half of the face, but forehead movement remains normal. This is caused by the bilateral cortical connections to the facial nucleus in the brainstem. In such a circumstance, the examining physician should inquire about risk factors for stroke and look for other signs that might indicate a stroke. **Facial paralysis associated with hearing loss and/or dizziness, vertigo, or imbalance suggests cerebellopontine angle and internal auditory canal disorders.** In this circumstance, an audiogram might show a sensorineural type of hearing loss. Further evaluation will include contrast enhanced MRI and possibly CT.

Because the facial nerve passes through the middle ear and temporal bone, examination of the ear canal and tympanic membrane is of paramount importance. Otitis media and cholesteatoma can be associated with facial paralysis. The ear examination will clearly disclose these abnormalities when present. Acute bacterial otitis media produces a purulent middle ear effusion, which can often produce a spontaneous tympanic membrane perforation. In these cases, a preexisting history of otitis media is not always present, although the history and physical examination might indicate an upper respiratory tract infection or inflammation (as from allergic rhinitis). The physical examination will clearly show the abnormal findings in the middle ear. Acute otitis media is probably the most common cause of isolated facial paralysis in children.

Cholesteatoma is a benign tumor of epithelial debris that is produced when the squamous layer of the eardrum is trapped and cannot exfoliate properly. Cholesteatoma usually occurs in patients that have preexisting ear problems. The physical examination in cholesteatoma will show either cheesy epithelial debris in the ear canal or a pearly white tumor behind the ear drum. Generally, patients with cholesteatoma will have a pre-existing history of hearing loss and often a long history of intermittent foul-smelling, purulent otorrhea. Cholesteatomas grow slowly, and sometimes can be present for years without causing many symptoms. Neglected cholesteatomas can produce destruction of the ossicles, the inner ear or the facial nerve. Complications of cholesteatomas can include sigmoid sinus thrombosis, brain abscess, and meningitis. CT scanning of the temporal area is helpful prior to surgical excision. Referral to an otologist-neurootologist is recommended.

Facial neuromas (schwannomas of the facial nerve) are rare, and their occurrence is roughly 1:1,000,000 persons per year. These are benign tumors of the facial nerve that grow slowly and produce a slowly progressive (over several months, not days) form of facial paralysis. When these tumors occur in the middle ear portion of the facial nerve, they produce a conductive hearing loss. When they occur in the internal auditory canal, they can produce a sensorineural form of hearing loss. Again, an audiogram and MRI with contrast will be necessary to diagnose and discover these tumors. Referral to a neurootologist is recommended.

Tumors of the parotid and skull base can produce facial paralysis. Paralysis of an isolated branch of the facial nerve is caused by malignancy until proven otherwise. Malignant tumors of the skin or parotid gland can produce facial paralysis either by compression or perineural invasion. Skull base tumors (meningiomas, carcinomas, sarcomas, etc.) can produce facial paralysis, however, this facial paralysis is usually found along with other CN findings consistent with a skull base location (e.g., loss of CN IX, X, XI, or XII). A careful history and physical examination of the involved area will usually uncover this pathology when present. Imaging studies, such as enhanced MRI or CT, are helpful in identifying neoplasms that affect the facial nerve. Other special considerations in facial paralysis involve its bilateral occurrence. **Bilateral facial paralysis** has a limited number of causes, principally **Lyme disease** or **Guillain-Barré syndrome**. Herpes zoster oticus (or Ramsay Hunt syndrome) is a frequently encountered form of facial paralysis.

Ramsey Hunt Syndrome

The *sine qua non* of Ramsay Hunt syndrome are vesicles in the ear associated with facial paralysis. It is caused by reactivation of varicella-zoster virus (VZV), the virus that causes chicken pox and shingles. This virus lingers in sensory ganglia until reactivated. The sensory ganglion of the facial nerve is the geniculate ganglion. Reactivation of the virus produces vesicles in its area of sensory innervation. For the facial nerve, this can include the posterior ear canal, conchal bowl, or even postauricular skin. (In segmental nerves, the dorsal ganglia contains the dormant virus, a dermatomal distribution of vesicles is often found when it is reactivated). Reactivation can result from being immunocompromised or in some other way "stressed." The pain from herpes zoster might be described as burning and can be intensely painful. This pain can linger for up to 1 year, despite resolution of the active infection, and is called postherpetic neuralgia.

Treatment of Ramsay Hunt syndrome involves use of **anti-herpes virus medication** for 7 to 10 days. Traditionally acyclovir was used; its IV form might still be indicated for severe infections in severely immunocompromised patients. Because of its poor oral absorption, its oral form requires five doses daily and is difficult for patients to maintain. Newer antiviral medications, such as ganciclovir and valacyclovir, have better oral absorption and less frequent dosing schedules. These medications are most often used for limited episodes of Ramsay Hunt syndrome. Topical acyclovir cream might help to speed healing of vesicles. Patients are contagious and can spread the virus to susceptible individuals as long as vesicles are present.

Steroids are frequently prescribed for patients with facial paralysis. Often doses of prednisone, 1 mg/kg/day for 10 to 14 days are given. Use of steroids during an active infection such as Ramsay Hunt syndrome must be weighed carefully. Although steroids might reduce the pain and might improve the chance for facial recovery, the possible risks of worsening an immunocompromised state or of dissemination of the herpes infection to the brain (herpes encephalitis) or eye (ocular herpes) must be considered.

Hearing loss and vestibular symptoms can occur in patients with **Ramsay Hunt syndrome**. This will produce **ipsilateral sensorineural hearing loss** and vestibular weakness. It is unclear if the virus spreads from one ganglion to another (i.e., from the geniculate to the spiral or Scarpa ganglion), or if edema and inflammation produce the associated cochleovestibular symptoms. Nevertheless, patients with facial paralysis who complain of hearing loss should have an audiogram.

Bell Palsy

Bell palsy is likely caused by viral infection. Herpes simplex virus has been implicated and has been isolated from cases of Bell palsy when the facial nerve was decompressed. For this reason, the recommendations for treating Bell palsy include antiviral medications (ganciclovir or valacyclovir) and **oral steroids** (prednisone 1 mg/kg/day for 10–14 days). The use of both forms of medications (antiviral and steroids) has been shown to improve return of facial function compared to either medication alone or to placebo. Although spontaneous rates of recovery are high, especially in patients with mild weakness, treatment should not be withheld on the expectation of speedy and normal recovery. Surgical treatment for Bell palsy has a checkered past. Facial nerve decompression has been advocated for Bell paralysis for several reasons: (1) the facial nerve has the longest bony course of any nerve, peripheral or cranial; (2) this bony confinement does not allow the nerve to swell; (3) this swelling in a confined space produces ischemia of the nerve; (4) poor regeneration occurs once ischemia takes place; and (5) very limited and unsatisfactory methods are available to rehabilitate the paralyzed face. Surgery is only indicated for cases of facial paralysis where ENoG and EMG both show absence of facial function.

Regardless of cause, patients with facial paralysis need special care of the eye on the affected side to avoid permanent vision loss. Because of the loss of the blink reflex and decreased lacrimation, the affected eye can dry out causing exposure keratitis, which can lead to loss of vision in the affected eye. Simple eye care consisting of **artificial tears every hour** while awake and ocular lubricant (Lacri-Lube) ointment at night with eye taping can avoid permanent loss of vision. Ophthalmologic consultation should be sought for any patient with facial paralysis and is mandatory in patients who complain of eye pain, irritation, or loss of vision. Most cases of facial nerve weakness can be fully evaluated and managed by primary care physicians. These patients demand close attention and should be seen once or twice a week until resolution is seen. Bell palsy and Ramsay Hunt syndrome should respond relatively rapidly (over 2 to 3 weeks) to the treatment outlined, but **the greater the weakness, the longer the recovery.**

Consultation with a neurologist should be sought when the diagnosis is in doubt. Also, consider referring patients that have (1) rapid progression (over 3 days) to complete paralysis; (2) evidence of middle ear, inner ear, or skull base disease; (3) an initial improvement in facial weakness to have recurrence a few weeks or months later, or (4) no return of function despite appropriate therapy.

Comprehension Questions

[35.1] What is the most common cause of unilateral facial weakness in an adult?

A. Lyme disease
B. Varicella zoster reactivation
C. Acoustic neuroma
D. Herpes simplex virus reactivation
E. Noncaseating granulomas

[35.2] What is the key indicator of herpes zoster oticus (Ramsay Hunt syndrome)?

A. Vesicles on an erythematous base found in the external ear
B. Noncaseating granulomas on lower lip biopsy
C. Circulating antibodies to *Borrelia burgdorferi*
D. Uveitis and parotid gland swelling
E. Loss of taste on the ipsilateral tongue

[35.3] A 69-year-old man complains of right facial weakness. A close examination of his facial movements indicates loss of the nasolabial fold and inability to raise the upper lip on that side. His blink, forehead, and lower lip movement are normal. What is the most likely cause of his facial paralysis?

A. Bell palsy
B. Herpes zoster oticus
C. Malignant parotid gland tumor
D. Acoustic neuroma
E. Lyme disease

Answers

[35.1] **D.** By far the most common cause of acute facial weakness in an adult is Bell palsy. This disorder is caused by reactivation of herpes simplex virus. However, this is a diagnosis of exclusion as no accurate serologic tests have been discovered that confirm the diagnosis.

[35.2] **A.** The pathognomonic feature of herpes zoster oticus (Ramsay Hunt syndrome) is a vesicular eruption on an erythematous base in an area of facial nerve sensory distribution (external ear). This disorder is caused by reactivation of varicella-zoster virus and is treated with antiviral medications and steroids. Inadequately treated zoster infections can lead to poor recovery of facial function and postherpetic neuralgia.

[35.3] **C.** An isolated facial nerve branch paralysis is caused by malignancy until proven otherwise. Bell palsy, herpes zoster oticus, and Lyme disease affect the entire nerve. Acoustic neuromas can cause facial paralysis when they are very large, but this is very rarely seen in the modern area. Their location in the cerebellopontine angle would produce whole face weakness, and not an isolated branch weakness as described.

CLINICAL PEARLS

❖ Bell palsy is the most common cause of acute, unilateral facial weakness in adults.

❖ The diagnosis of Bell palsy is a diagnosis of exclusion.

❖ Facial paralysis with vesicles on an area of facial nerve sensation is pathognomonic for herpes zoster oticus (Ramsay Hunt syndrome).

❖ An isolated facial nerve branch weakness is a sign of malignant tumor involving the facial nerve until proven otherwise.

❖ Patients with facial paralysis or paresis should be given instructions regarding eye care and moisturization to avoid exposure keratopathy.

❖ Steroid and antiviral medications should be given to patients with either Bell palsy or Ramsay Hunt syndrome.

REFERENCES

Ahmed A. When is facial paralysis Bell palsy? Current diagnosis and treatment. Cleve Clin J Med 2005;72(5):398–401, 5.

Alberton DL, Zed PJ. Bell's palsy: a review of treatment using antiviral agents. Ann Pharmacother 2006;40(10):1838–1842.

Austin JR, Peskind SP, Austin SG, et al. Idiopathic facial nerve paralysis: a randomized double blind controlled study of placebo versus prednisone. Laryngoscope 1993;103(12):1326–1333.

Gilden DH, Cohrs RJ, Hayward AR, et al. Chronic varicella-zoster virus ganglionitis—a possible cause of postherpetic neuralgia. J Neurovirol 2003;9(3):404–407.

House JW, Brackmann DE. Facial nerve grading system. Otolaryngol Head Neck Surg 1985;93(2):146–147.

Kuhweide R, Van de Steene V, Vlaminck S, et al. Ramsay Hunt syndrome: pathophysiology of cochleovestibular symptoms. J Laryngol Otol 2002;116(10):844–848.

Ohtani F, Furuta Y, Aizawa H, et al. Varicella-zoster virus load and cochleovestibular symptoms in Ramsay Hunt syndrome. Ann Otol Rhinol Laryngol 2006;115(3):233–238.

Overell JR, Willison HJ. Recent developments in Miller Fisher syndrome and related disorders. Curr Opin Neurol 2005;18(5):562–566.

Redaelli de Zinis LO, Gamba P, Balzanelli C. Acute otitis media and facial nerve paralysis in adults. Otol Neurotol 2003;24(1):113–117.

Sweeney CJ, Gilden DH. Ramsay Hunt syndrome. J Neurol Neurosurg Psychiatry 2001;71(2):149–154.

A 30-year-old female plastic surgery resident presents with a 1-month history of intermittent ptosis (droopiness of the eyelids) and fatigue. She has been on call every third night over the past 2 months and has been attributing her fatigue to her hectic call schedule. However she became concerned when she acutely developed ptosis last month after being on call. She went home and went to sleep, and by morning her ptosis had resolved. Her 6-year-old triplets have pointed out to her that she can't keep up with them when they're riding their bicycles. She has experienced three more episodes of ptosis over the past month. They all have occurred while she has been post call and have improved by the morning. Today for the first-time she developed ptosis while perform-ing a complicated facial lift. Her attending asked her to stop assisting in sur-gery and to immediately seek medical evaluation. She has not experienced diplopia, dysarthria, dysphagia, difficulty walking up stairs, difficulty blow drying her hair, or shortness of breath. She had always been healthy until now.

Her neurologic examination is notable for normal mental status and speech. Her cranial nerve examination reveals bilateral ptosis on primary gaze, which worsens with sustained upward gaze for 90 seconds. Extraocular muscles are intact as is her facial strength. Her motor strength is normal with the exception of 4+/5 in the deltoid muscles bilaterally. On repetitive testing of the right iliopsoas muscle fatigability is elicited, which improves after 2 minutes of rest. Her sensory examination and deep tendon reflexes are normal.

◆ **What is the most likely diagnosis?**

◆ **What is the best test to confirm the diagnosis?**

◆ **What is the next step in therapy?**

ANSWERS TO CASE 36: Ptosis (Myasthenia Gravis)

Summary: A 30-year-old healthy female presents with a 2-month history of fatigue and a 1-month history of intermittent ptosis. She has not experienced proximal muscle weakness, dysarthria, shortness of breath, or dysphagia. Her examination is notable for ptosis on primary gaze, which worsens with sustained upward gaze, weakness of the deltoid muscles, and fatigability of the iliopsoas muscle, which improves with rest.

◆ **Most likely diagnosis:** Myasthenia gravis

◆ **Best confirmatory test:** Antiacetylcholine receptor antibodies

◆ **Next step in therapy:** Acetylcholinesterase inhibitors (pyridostigmine) and immunosuppression

Analysis

Objectives

1. Know a diagnostic approach to ptosis and understand how associated symptoms are helpful in determining the etiology.
2. Be familiar with the differential diagnosis of ptosis.
3. Understand the basic pathophysiology of myasthenia gravis and the rationale for treatment.

Considerations

This 30-year-old woman developed fatigue and ptosis over a short period of time. The most concerning symptom is ptosis as it has already interfered with her ability to perform her duties as a resident. In this particular case, the patient complained only of fatigue in addition to the ptosis and findings on examination are notable for fatigability and proximal muscle weakness. Based on this the cause of ptosis can be pinpointed to either a neuromuscular junction transmission disorder or myopathy. Electromyograph (EMG)/nerve conduction study (NCS) will help differentiate between the two, and if indicative of a neuromuscular junction issue, then the diagnosis of myasthenia gravis is most likely. Forced vital capacity is very important in evaluating patients with suspected neuromuscular disease associated with diaphragmatic weakness. In this particular case the patient does not complain of shortness of breath; however, the history of fatigue and having difficulty keeping up with her children while bike riding should raise the concern. Forced vital capacity is a simple bedside test that can provide further information on the respiratory status of an individual.

APPROACH TO PTOSIS

Definitions

Anti-MuSK antibodies: Muscle-specific receptor tyrosine kinase antibodies. MuSK is a surface membrane enzyme critical for aggregating acetylcholine receptors during neuromuscular junction development. It is often seen in individuals who are seronegative for acetylcholine receptor antibodies.

Dysarthria: Speech disorder arising from weakness, paralysis, or incoordination of speech musculature.

Dysphagia: Difficulty swallowing.

Forced vital capacity: Total amount of air exhaled during a forced breath with maximal speed and effort.

Myogenic: A disorder of muscle or muscle tissue.

Neurogenic: A disorder affecting either anterior horn cell, nerve root, plexus, or peripheral nerve.

Mitochondrial cytopathies: A diverse group of diseases affecting the mitochondria.

Clinical Approach

Ptosis is a symptom associated with multiple conditions. As noted in Table 36–1, the differential diagnosis will be based on the patient's symptoms and the clinical findings. Ptosis is also known as blepharoptosis and results from the levator palpebrae superioris muscle weakness. Ptosis can occur unilaterally or bilaterally, with the upper eyelid barely covering the upper cornea. If the upper eyelid falls below this position it is considered to be ptosis. In some instances the upper eyelid may only cover up part of the pupil, and in others it may cover up the entire pupil resulting in impaired vision. Acquired ptosis is a sign of an underlying neurologic problem that requires urgent medical evaluation.

The etiologies of ptosis include local mechanical lid abnormalities, myopathy, diseases of the neuromuscular junction such as myasthenia gravis, oculosympathetic lesions, third nerve palsy, third nuclear pathology, and supranuclear lesions in the contralateral hemisphere along the territory of the middle cerebral artery (see Table 36–1).

Associated clinical findings such as miosis, hemiparesis, or other cranial nerve abnormalities will indicate if this is a supranuclear problem, nuclear problem, oculosympathetic problem, third nerve dysfunction, neuromuscular junction transmission disorder, myopathic disorder, or local infiltrative process.

The associated symptoms and findings on neurologic examination are critical in trying to establish the cause of ptosis. Isolated ptosis without other symptoms suggests local mechanical factors as a cause. Conversely, symptoms of proximal muscle weakness (difficulty climbing up stairs, difficulty arising from a chair, difficulty blow drying hair, difficulty reaching over the head)

Table 36–1
ETIOLOGIES OF PTOSIS

LOCATION OF LESION	ETIOLOGIES
Local mechanical lid abnormalities	Thyroid disease, ocular surgery, infiltrative processes (sarcoid, amyloid), orbital cellulitis, primary or metastatic tumors
Myopathy	Mitochondrial cytopathies (Kearns-Sayre), congenital myopathies (centronuclear myopathy), oculopharyngeal muscular dystrophy
Neuromuscular junction	Myasthenia gravis, botulism
Oculosympathetic	Horner syndrome; associated miosis
Third nerve palsy	Ischemic, metabolic (diabetes mellitus), uncal herniation syndrome, posterior communicating artery aneurysm, cavernous sinus; associated with other cranial nerve abnormalities
Third nucleus	Ischemic
Supranuclear	Midbrain neoplasms (bilateral ptosis), contralateral middle cerebral artery ischemia

with ptosis suggest an underlying myopathy. Fatigability of muscle (repetitive use of the same muscle leads to loss of strength) with improvement after a short period of rest associated with ptosis suggests an underlying neuromuscular junction transmission disorder. Contralateral hemiparesis or hemitremor accompanying ptosis suggests ischemic lesions in the midbrain affecting the third nerve. Ptosis from a third nerve palsy associated with other cranial nerve dysfunction such as IV, V, and VI are seen with cavernous sinus syndrome. The history and clinical examination is key to evaluate patients with ptosis. In this particular case, the patient gives a history of fatigue and ptosis; and her examination is notable for ptosis, proximal muscle weakness, and fatigability. These features are suggestive of an underlying neuromuscular junction transmission disorder or less likely a myopathy.

The evaluation of someone who presents with ptosis can be guided by associated symptoms and findings on clinical examination. Serologic studies consisting of a comprehensive metabolic panel and complete blood count (CBC) with differential are helpful in ascertaining metabolic processes such as diabetes mellitus, hypokalemia, infections, or even malignancies. Vasculitis screen with antinuclear antibody (ANA) and erythrocyte sedimentation rate (ESR) can be helpful in evaluating for inflammatory processes such as systemic lupus erythematosus. Thyroid function studies evaluate for thyroid disease whereas serum creatine phosphokinase (CPK) is helpful in evaluating for myopathies. Serum lactate can be helpful in screening for mitochondrial cytopathies. Acetylcholine receptor antibodies are used to evaluate for myasthenia gravis.

An MRI of the brain is requested if there are multiple cranial nerves involved or if there is evidence of contralateral hemiparesis. These findings are suggestive of abnormalities in the cavernous sinus or brainstem. Ptosis associated with a third nerve palsy should always raise the concern of the posterior communicating artery aneurysm for which an MRI of the brain and magnetic resonance (MR) angiogram of the brain are indicated.

An electromyograph/nerve conduction study (EMG/NCS) is one of the most important studies in evaluating patients with suspected neuromuscular diseases. It is helpful in differentiating between a neurogenic process, myogenic process, and a disorder of the neuromuscular junction. Additionally it provides information as to the severity and chronicity of the process. It is a two-part study consisting of nerve conduction studies and electromyography. Nerve conduction studies evaluate conduction velocity of a nerve between two different points. It evaluates both motor and sensory nerves. Electromyography evaluates the electrical properties of the muscle at rest and on contraction. This test should only be performed in patients who have ptosis and are suspected of having either a myopathy, peripheral neuropathy, or underlying neuromuscular junction transmission disorder. EMG/NCS is not helpful in evaluating diseases of the central nervous system.

Myasthenia Gravis

Myasthenia gravis is an uncommon autoimmune disorder affecting the neuromuscular junction postsynaptically. It is characterized by skeletal muscle weakness and fatigability. The prevalence of myasthenia gravis in the United States is approximately 14.2 cases per 100,000. It is estimated that the annual incidence of myasthenia gravis in United States is 2:1,000,000. Women are affected more than men at a ratio of 3:2. Although myasthenia gravis can occur at any age it tends to peak in females during the second and third decade of life and in males during the sixth and seventh decade of life. Women have also been noted to have a second peak during their eighth decade of life.

The classic symptoms are those of skeletal muscle weakness affecting the ocular, facial, bulbar, respiratory, and limb muscles. The weakness quickly fluctuates and worsens throughout the day. Importantly there is fatigability of the muscles with recovery to the baseline strength after a short period of rest. Approximately 75% of patients will present with ocular disturbances including ptosis and diplopia. Up to 90% of patients with myasthenia gravis will eventually experience ocular symptoms. Ptosis can be bilateral or unilateral and can shift quickly from one eye to the other. Weakness of the extraocular muscles causing diplopia can be asymmetrical.

Other common complaints include dysphagia, dysarthria, shortness of breath, fatigue with chewing, difficulty holding head up, limb weakness, and torso weakness. Limb weakness is most commonly proximal and presents as having difficulty raising arms above the head, having difficulty climbing up stairs, and having difficulty arising from a chair. Commonly affected muscles include the neck flexors, deltoids, triceps, finger extensors, wrist extensors, hip flexors, and foot dorsiflexors. Fatigability is frequently observed on physical examination. Fatigability is defined as incremental weakness with repetitive testing of a muscle's strength.

Weakness of the pharyngeal and tongue muscles results in impaired speech and swallowing. Speech can have a nasal quality to it or be slurred. This is most noticeable when the patient continues to talk for prolonged periods of time. A snarling expression on attempted smile can be present denoting facial weakness. Additionally, weakness of the orbicularis oculi muscles can be present on examination when the eyelids are separated against forced eye closure. Patients do not often complain of facial weakness.

Shortness of breath results from weakness of the intercostal and diaphragm muscles. This can become a medical emergency requiring emergent intubation. A good way of evaluating the status of respiratory muscle weakness is to perform a forced vital capacity. Significant precautions should be undertaken when patients are evaluated in the emergency room as they can decompensate very quickly requiring immediate intubation.

Physiology of Myasthenia Gravis

Normally, an excitatory postsynaptic end-plate potential is generated at the neuromuscular junction when acetylcholine (ACh) is released into the synaptic cleft and diffuses to the postsynaptic membrane to bind to nicotinic ACh receptors. Once the threshold for depolarization is reached, an action potential will be generated and spread across muscle leading to contraction. Acetylcholinesterase clears ACh from the synaptic cleft. However, it is not the only mechanism that clears ACh because the presynaptic membrane might also remove ACh by reuptake.

In myasthenia gravis, an action potential is not generated at the postsynaptic membrane, and there is neuromuscular transmission failure that results in weakness. Failure to generate an action potential is caused by the inability of excitatory postsynaptic endplate potentials to reach threshold for depolarization. This is caused by a diminished amount and availability of postsynaptic receptors. If ACh fails to bind to a sufficient number of postsynaptic ACh receptors, the endplate potentials generated are not enough to reach threshold for depolarization. This in essence fails to generate an action potential and thus prevents muscle contraction causing weakness. Circulating antibodies (ACh receptor antibodies) bind to the ACh receptor and prevent ACh from binding. This in turn allows for cross-linking of receptors, which leads to degradation and eventually receptor internalization. Postsynaptic membrane damage can also occur via complement activation. The number of ACh receptors diminishes over time because of these changes (Fig. 36–1).

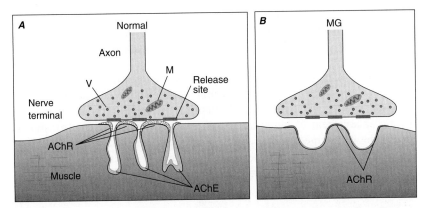

Figure 36–1. End plate from a patient with **myasthenia gravis, electron microscopy.** (*With permission from Ropper AH, Brown RH. Adams and Victor's principles of neurology, 8th ed. New York: McGraw-Hill; 2005: Figs. 36–2, 53–1, Diagrams of (A) normal and (B) myasthenic neuromuscular junctions. With permission from Kasper DL, Braunwal E, Fauci A, et al. Harrison's principles of internal medicine, 16th ed. New York: McGraw-Hill; 2004: Fig. 366–1.*)

Diagnostic Testing for Myasthenia Gravis

Laboratory studies for ACh receptor antibodies are the most specific and sensitive test for myasthenia gravis. There are three antibodies described against the ACh receptor: binding, blocking, and modulating. Up to 90% of patients with generalized myasthenia gravis (affecting more than the ocular muscles) will have a positive test for one of these antibodies. The antibody test most commonly used to screen for myasthenia gravis is the binding ACh receptor antibody. Recently, anti-MuSK antibodies have been associated with myasthenia gravis in individuals who do not have ACh receptor antibodies. The Tensilon test has historically been described as the classic diagnostic test. Importantly thyroid function studies should always be performed as concomitant thyroid disease is often seen in myasthenia gravis.

A simple bedside test that can be used in patients with ptosis is the ice test. Ice is placed over the ptotic eyelid for 2 minutes. If the ptosis improves after removing the ice a diagnosis of an underlying neuromuscular junction transmission disorder can be made. Cooling improves neuromuscular junction transmission whereas heat worsens it. This is the reason that many patients with myasthenia gravis worsen during the summer months.

Electrodiagnostic studies with EMG/NCS can be performed to evaluate patients with myasthenia gravis. Classically nerve conduction studies are normal. EMG can be normal or can show myopathic features. Repetitive nerve stimulation, a part of EMG/NCS, consists of repeatedly stimulating a nerve and recording the compound muscle action potential obtained. This test is usually performed at 2 or 3 Hz. The ulnar, spinal accessory and facial nerves most commonly evaluated. Greater than 10% decrement in the amplitude of the compound muscle action potential is considered an abnormal response and suggestive of a neuromuscular junction transmission disorder. A more specialized study, single fiber EMG, is the most sensitive test available for myasthenia gravis; however, it is not very specific, nor commonly available.

A CT scan or MRI of the mediastinum should be performed to exclude thymic enlargement or more importantly a thymoma. **Thymectomy should always be performed in those individuals that have thymoma.** It is currently controversial as to whether or not thymectomy is of any benefit in those individuals with myasthenia gravis that merely have thymic hyperplasia or a normal thymic size.

Treatment of Myasthenia Gravis

The mainstay of treatment for myasthenia gravis is **immunosuppressive agents.** These include corticosteroids, cyclosporine azathioprine, mycophenolate mofetil, intravenous immunoglobulin, and plasmapheresis. Although most experts believe that corticosteroids are the first line of treatment there is no general consensus as to how to administer it and at what dose. There is no general agreement among experts regarding the timing or use of the other immunosuppressive treatments. **Anti-cholinesterase inhibitors** such as pyridostigmine treat only the symptom but not the disease. However, this is routinely used in patients with myasthenia gravis especially if the only symptoms are ocular. The typical dose of this is 60 mg orally four times a day.

Comprehension Questions

[36.1] A 60-year-old man in the ICU is noted to have a brain pathology and ptosis. Which of the following conditions is the most likely cause for ptosis?

   A. Pituitary necrosis
   B. Uncal herniation
   C. Central herniation
   D. Arterio-venous (AV) malformation

[36.2] A critical difference between myogenic processes and disorders of the neuromuscular junction is:

   A. The finding of fatigability with improvement after rest in neuro-muscular junction transmission disorders
   B. Weakness of the ocular muscles only in neuromuscular junction transmission disorders
   C. Low CPK levels in myogenic processes
   D. Elevated CPK in neuromuscular junction transmission disorders
   E. Myogenic findings on EMG

[36.3] Individuals presenting with ptosis and multiple cranial nerve abnormalities should have which study performed first?

A. MRI of the brain with magnetic resonance angiography (MRA)
B. EMG/NCS
C. Serologic studies for CPK
D. ACh receptor antibodies
E. Thyroid function studies

Answers

[36.1] **B.** Central herniation causes compression of the diencephalon flattening the mid brain and pons whereas uncal herniation compresses the third cranial nerve causing ptosis.

[36.2] **A.** Fatigability of muscles with improvement after rest is a hallmark of neuromuscular junction transmission disorders.

[36.3] **A.** The presence of multiple cranial abnormalities including ptosis speaks for a process in the central nervous system particularly the brainstem or cavernous sinus.

CLINICAL PEARLS

❖ The etiology of ptosis is best determined by recognizing associated symptoms that patients present with and discerning clinical findings on examination.

❖ Ptosis associated with central nervous system signs and symptoms mandates an MRI of the brain.

❖ Fatigability of muscle with improvement after a brief period of rest is seen only with neuromuscular junction transmission disorders.

❖ Up to 90% of patients with myasthenia gravis will eventually have ocular symptoms.

❖ Local cooling of the eye can improve function in a ptotic eyelid, similar to a Tensilon test, and is a rapid, simple, and inexpensive test for myasthenia gravis.

REFERENCES

Dorland's Illustrated Medical Dictionary, 27th ed. Philadelphia, PA: WB Saunders; 1988.

Keesey JC. Clinical evaluation and management of myasthenia gravis. Muscle Nerve 2004 Apr;29(4):484–505.

Saperstein DS, Barohn RJ. Management of myasthenia gravis. Semin Neurol 2004 Mar;24(1):41–48.

A 63-year-old man presents with a 3-month history of dizziness. His dizziness comes and goes, but usually lasts for about 10 to 15 seconds. He notices that his dizziness is worse when he rolls over in bed or when he gets out of bed. One time, he became very dizzy while trying to reach for an object on a high shelf. He does not have any nausea or vomiting associated with it. When it occurs, it is very strong, and he has tried to avoid sleeping on his left side. He does not have any hearing loss or tinnitus. He denies aural pressure and headache. His past medical history is otherwise unremarkable. He is not on any medications.

On physical examination, he is a healthy appearing 63-year-old man. His temperature is 37.1°C (98.8°F); pulse, 64 beats/min; and blood pressure, 124/74 mmHg. There are no lesions or masses on his face or head. His voice is normal, and his speech is fluent. His facial nerve function is normal. His ear canals and tympanic membranes are normal appearing. His remaining head and neck examination is normal. The cranial nerve examination is normal. The remaining physical examination is normal.

◆ **What is the most likely diagnosis?**

◆ **What is the next diagnostic step?**

◆ **What is the next step in therapy?**

ANSWERS TO CASE 37: Vertigo, Benign Paroxysmal Positional

Summary: A 63-year-old man with brief episodes of dizziness that are brought on by different positions, not associated with hearing loss, tinnitus, aural pressure, or headache.

◆ **Most likely diagnosis:** Benign paroxysmal positional vertigo

◆ **Next diagnostic step:** Perform a Dix-Hallpike maneuver

◆ **Next therapeutic step:** Canalith repositioning maneuver, habituation exercises, and/or symptomatic pharmacologic therapy

Analysis

Objectives

1. Learn the most common forms of vertigo.
2. Learn to discern the prominent symptoms of vertigo.
3. Learn about the important physical examination findings in patients with vestibular disorders.
4. Learn about ancillary tests that can be performed to evaluate vertigo.
5. Learn about the appropriate treatments for vertigo.

Considerations

This patient has brief (<30 sec) episodes of vertigo that are brought out by position changes. This vertigo is not associated with any other inner ear symptom or other neurologic symptoms. His physical examination does not indicate any evidence of middle ear disease. His remaining physical examination, including neurologic assessment, does not show any other abnormality. The Dix-Hallpike maneuver is pathognomonic for this disorder. This disorder is caused by otoliths (calcium stones) that have congregated within the posterior semicircular canal and that move like a piston in response to position changes. The treatment involves moving the patient, and by extension the misplaced otoliths, through a series of maneuvers that will place the otoliths back into the otolith organs. Failing this maneuver, other therapies use a strategy that disperses the misplaced otoliths and permits desensitization to the sensation of vertigo.

APPROACH TO VERTIGO

Definitions

Dizziness: A disturbed sense of relationship to space; a sensation of unsteadiness with a feeling of movement within the head; giddiness; lightheadedness; disequilibrium.

Vertigo: An illusion of movement; a sensation as if the external world were revolving around the patient or as if he himself were revolving in space.

Benign paroxysmal positional vertigo: Recurrent vertigo and nystagmus occurring when the head is placed in certain positions, usually not associated with lesions of the central nervous system.

Nystagmus: An involuntary, rapid, rhythmic movement of the eyeball, which may be horizontal, vertical, rotatory, or mixed.

Electronystagmogram (ENG): A recording of eye movements that provides objective documentation of induced and spontaneous nystagmus. These tests include recordings of the following: spontaneous nystagmus, positional nystagmus, gaze-induced nystagmus, smooth pursuit, random saccades, optokinetic stimulation, Dix-Hallpike testing, and caloric stimulation.

Audiogram: A basic hearing test. Generally speaking, an audiogram includes three parts: a record of the thresholds of hearing of an individual for various sound frequencies (pure tone audiometry), a record of the individual's ability to understand phonetically balanced words (speech audiometry), and a record of tympanic membrane compliance (tympanometry).

Otolith: Minute calciferous granules within the gelatinous membrane of the saccule and utricle. The otoliths, being heavier than the surrounding fluid, render the otolith organs sensitive to changes in position with respect to gravity.

Dix-Hallpike test: A maneuver that provokes the nystagmus and vertigo associated with benign paroxysmal positional vertigo.

Tinnitus: A noise in the ears, as ringing, buzzing, roaring, clicking, and so forth.

Canalith repositioning procedure: A therapeutic maneuver that moves misplaced otoliths from the posterior semicircular canal into the saccule.

Brandt-Daroff exercises: A therapeutic series of maneuvers that dissipate misplaced otoliths and that habituates the vertigo from these otoliths.

Clinical Approach

Dizziness and vertigo are not interchangeable. Dizziness is a common lay word that can be a catchphrase for any sensation in the head: lightheadedness, giddiness, imbalance, or spinning. Vertigo, however, is a very specific type of sensation. It is the sensation of spinning. This spinning can be perceived either as room-spinning or self-spinning. The perspective of spinning is not, in itself, particularly diagnostic. The sensation of spinning, as being different from other sensations of dizziness, is important.

The duration of vertigo is the next consideration. Very brief vertigo, that lasts only a second or two that is brought on by quick head movements, might indicate a vestibular lesion. These patients usually have a distant, antecedent history of more prolonged vertigo, as that of viral vestibular neuronitis. Vertigo that lasts 10 to 30 seconds and that recurs every time the patient assumes a particular position, such as rolling to one side while lying in bed usually indicates BPPV.

Vertigo that lasts for more than 1 day is indicative of an acute labyrinthine disorder. These can be further differentiated by those disorders which are associated with otitis media or cholesteatoma and those that are not. Lastly, vertigo that lasts 20 minutes to 24 hours is most commonly associated with Ménière disease.

Associated symptoms are important in differentiating factors in the history. These symptoms include aural pressure, tinnitus, and hearing loss. BPPV is not associated with any of these symptoms. Aural pressure describes the sensation of fullness or water in the ear. The physical examination will readily identify patients with serous or suppurative otitis media. Classically, aural pressure is a sign of Ménière disease.

Tinnitus is the perception of sound generated within the ear. Like dizziness, it has many different descriptions and manifestations. This discussion will be limited to tinnitus that occurs simultaneously with vertigo. Tinnitus, like hearing loss, is indicative of an inner ear cause of vertigo. Low-pitched, roaring tinnitus is usually associated with Ménière disease. High-pitched tinnitus is usually associated with high frequency sensorineural hearing loss.

Hearing loss is generally indicative of either a middle ear or inner ear disorder. An audiogram is the best way to measure hearing; however, a tuning fork examination is readily performed in the outpatient setting and can give useful information to the discerning physician: the **Weber test** and **Rinne test.** Uncomplicated otitis media produces a conductive hearing loss. Although it might be associated with a mild sensation of imbalance, it is usually not a cause of vertigo. Otitis media that has spread to involve the inner ear produces a suppurative labyrinthitis. This complication of otitis media produces a very severe, disabling vertigo, with nausea and vomiting, and sensorineural hearing loss. Cholesteatomas are benign tumors that occur within the middle ear, caused by in-growth of skin from the eardrum. Symptoms of cholesteatoma are conductive hearing loss and foul smelling otorrhea; the physical examination usually shows a whitish mass in the middle ear. Neglected cholesteatomas can grow to destroy the inner ear, cause facial paralysis, or erode the bone of the posterior cranial fossa and produce meningitis or brain abscess. For patients with middle ear disease, the physical examination is diagnostic and differentiates these forms of vertigo from those without middle ear disease.

Other symptoms that occur in association with vertigo or dizziness such as headache, difficulty speaking or swallowing, scintillations or other visual disturbances, or numbness or weakness of an extremity should point the clinician toward a central cause. Headache that occurs with symptoms of scintillations, nausea or vomiting, or numbness or weakness of an extremity, especially in the setting of a family history of migraine headaches, should direct the physician to a diagnosis of vestibular migraine.

Benign paroxysmal positional vertigo (BPPV) is perhaps one of the most common forms of vertigo. Its name is descriptive. It is called *benign* because it often is self-limited and lasts for a few days. It is called *paroxysmal* because the sensation comes on as a burst or spasm. This sensation can be very strong and disturbing to the patient. It is called *positional* since particular positions evoke the vertigo. Classically, lying down and rolling to one side will provoke this type of vertigo. Additionally, looking upward as one would while trying to reach for a top shelf can provoke this vertigo, giving rise to the synonym of *top shelf syndrome* (Table 37–1).

Clinical Evaluation

For most patients with vertigo, the physical examination is normal. The ears, cranial nerve function, and neurologic examination should be carefully assessed. Occasionally, when patients present very early in the disease course, nystagmus can be seen. Nystagmus can then be described by its principle movement direction: horizontal, vertical, rotatory, or direction changing. Vertical nystagmus and direction changing nystagmus are indicators of central pathology. Horizontal nystagmus is usually caused by an inner ear process. Typically the fast component is beating away from the affected ear. Lastly, rotatory nystagmus is also produced by an inner ear process, typically BPPV.

The important clinical finding in BPPV is a **latent geotropic, rotatory nystagmus** that **reverses** with an upright position and **fatigues** on repeat testing. These findings are produced with a Dix-Hallpike maneuver. This maneuver is begun with the patient sitting upright. He or she is asked to turn his or her head to one side and then to lie back with his or her head in that position. Having the patient recline quickly evokes a stronger response, and patients that are sensitized to this vertigo will often avoid or significantly retard lying back on the affected side. With the patient laying flat with the head to one side, the examiner looks for a downbeat (also called geotropic) rotatory nystagmus. This nystagmus has a latency period of between 1 to 5 seconds, but can take up to 30 seconds to appear. The nystagmus has a very characteristic crescendo-decrescendo onset that is very disorienting and disturbing to the patient. It is helpful for the clinician to provide reassurance to patient during this test that the dizziness will go away. Once the nystagmus has subsided, the patient is asked to return to a sitting position. Frequently, the nystagmus will return, although in this circumstance its direction will be opposite of that seen before. Once the nystagmus disappears, the test is repeated for the opposite side. Patients can have BPPV that affects both inner ears; however, the most common presentation is unilateral BPPV. The test can be performed with Frenzel lenses, which magnify the appearance of the eye movements and eliminate the possibility of visual fixation suppressing the nystagmus.

If a patient has a strong positive response during the initial Dix-Hallpike test, a repeat test will show a lessened or weakened nystagmus. This is the phenomenon of fatigability, and it is an important distinguisher of BPPV from other forms of positional nystagmus. Furthermore, nystagmus that lacks a latency period is probably not BPPV, and it is usually a sign of central pathology. Other clinical tests for vertigo include the head thrust test, head-shaking nystagmus, and the Fukuda marching test. They are usually diagnostic of a unilateral vestibular weakness, and they are not particularly helpful in diagnosing BPPV.

Table 37–1
DIFFERENTIAL DIAGNOSIS OF VERTIGO

DIAGNOSIS	DURATION OF VERTIGO ATTACKS	DURATION OF SYMPTOMS	ASSOCIATED SYMPTOMS	PRINCIPLE PHYSICAL FINDINGS	TREATMENT
BPPV	5 to 30 seconds	Repeated attacks over weeks, months, or even years	None	Latent, geotropic nystagmus with reversibility and fatigue on Dix-Hallpike testing	Canalith repositioning procedure, Brandt-Daroff exercises
Vestibular migraine	Seconds to minutes	Minutes to hours, recurrent attacks	Headache, scintillations, other neurologic symptoms (e.g., weakness or numbness of extremity, changes in speech, etc.)	Usually normal physical examination	Either suppressive or abortive therapy for migraine, refer to neurologist
Vestibular epilepsy	Seconds to minutes	Minutes, recurrent episodes	Loss of consciousness, other neurologic symptoms	Usually normal physical examination	Anti-epileptic therapy, refer to neurology
Vertebrobasilar insufficiency	Seconds to minutes	Repeated episodes or evolving symptoms over weeks	Changes in speech or swallowing, cerebellar symptoms, history consistent with atherosclerosis	Can be normal, might have cranial nerve findings, cerebellar signs, or carotid bruit	Anti-platelet therapy, management of risk factors

Ménière disease	20 minutes to 24 hours	Repeated episodes over weeks to months to years	Aural pressure, low pitch (roaring) tinnitus, low frequency hearing loss	Nystagmus during an attack, normal ear examination, might have hearing loss on audiogram, vestibular weakness on ENG	Low salt diet and diuretictherapy, might need vestibular suppressants, might vestibular ablative therapy or nerve section
Viral vestibular neuronitis	24 hours+	Several days, resolving over a few weeks as vestibular compensation occurs	Nausea and vomiting	Horizontal nystagmus when patient is seen early in course, otherwise normal examination, vestibular weakness on ENG	Supportive care, anti-emetics, possibly vestibular suppressants, might need vestibular rehabilitation therapy
Acute suppurative labyrinthitis	2–3 days	Several days, resolving over a few weeks as vestibular compensation occurs	Severely ill with nausea and vomiting, hearing loss, tinnitus, otorrhea	Otitis media or cholesteatoma, nystagmus early in presentation, possible facial paralysis from cholesteatoma	IV antibiotics and possibly surgery

(Continued)

Table 37–1

DIFFERENTIAL DIAGNOSIS OF VERTIGO (*Continued*)

DIAGNOSIS	DURATION OF VERTIGO ATTACKS	DURATION OF SYMPTOMS	ASSOCIATED SYMPTOMS	PRINCIPLE PHYSICAL FINDINGS	TREATMENT
Acute serous labyrinthitis	2–3 days	Several days, resolving over a few weeks as vestibular compensation occurs	Hearing loss, tinnitus, nausea and vomiting	History of past otologic surgery, nystagmus early in presentation	Supportive care with anti-emetics, possible vestibular suppressants, might need vestibular rehabilitation, use steroids if hearing loss is present
Herpes zoster oticus (Ramsay Hunt syndrome)	2–3 days	Acute illness lasts approximately 7–10 days, residual symptoms can be long lasting	Herpetic rash in ear, retro-auricular pain, hearing loss	Facial paralysis, hearing loss,	Antiviral medications, steroids, might need vestibular rehabilitation

BPPV, benign paroxysmal positional **vertigo;** ENG, **electronystagmogram.**

Testing

Laboratory testing for vertigo is directed by the history and physical findings. Patients that have signs of stroke or suspected cholesteatoma should be evaluated with imaging studies. However, most cases of vertigo do not produce changes that are seen on CT or MRI, and blood tests are not generally helpful. An ENG is the basic test of vestibular function. This test uses either electrodes placed around the eyes or infrared goggles to record eye movements. Patients are then given several different tasks or movements to perform. Finally cool or warm water is flooded into each ear canal to provoke a caloric response from the inner ear. During these tests, the rate of nystagmus is calculated and compared between the two sides or to standard norms. Although ENG does not disclose the cause of vertigo, it can be helpful in distinguishing peripheral from central causes or in determining which inner ear is involved.

Other tests of the vestibular and balance systems are the rotatory chair test and computerized dynamic posturography. Generally, the clinical utility of these tests have been limited by lack of third-party payment. However, both tests can be helpful when used in the right clinical situation.

Treatment

Since the early 1990s, BPPV has been treated with a canalith repositioning procedure. This procedure takes the patient through a series of head and body movements so that the canaliths are moved from the posterior semicircular canal back to the saccule. This procedure takes approximately 10 minutes to perform in the office setting and has a high rate of success. Many physicians have learned to perform this simple maneuver; additionally physical therapists that are trained in vestibular rehabilitation can perform this maneuver.

An alternative form of therapy is the habituating exercises described by Brandt and Daroff. During this exercise, the patient sits at the edge of the bed and moves his body laterally, so that he is lying on the affected side. After waiting for the vertigo to resolve, the patient then sits upright and moves laterally so that he is lying on the opposite side. This movement is repeated 10 times twice daily. The patient will generally be symptom free at the end of 2 weeks.

Although medications are widely prescribed for vertigo, dizziness, and nausea and vomiting, their usefulness in BPPV is very limited and should be avoided. The onset of vertigo is so abrupt and its duration is so short that these medications are not warranted. Patients that do not respond to standard treatment of BPPV should be referred to a specialist for further evaluation and treatment.

Comprehension Questions

[37.1] Which of the following tests is used to diagnose benign paroxysmal positional vertigo?

A. Weber test
B. Rinne test
C. Dix-Hallpike maneuver
D. Brandt-Daroff maneuver
E. Epley maneuver

[37.2] A 40-year-old woman has recurring episodes of disabling vertigo, lasting 30 minutes, and accompanied by roaring tinnitus, aural pressure and low frequency hearing loss. Her physical examination is normal. What is the most likely diagnosis?

A. Benign paroxysmal positional vertigo
B. Acute suppurative labyrinthitis
C. Acute serous labyrinthitis
D. Ménière disease
E. Vertebrobasilar insufficiency

[37.3] A 45-year-old woman complains of recurring episodes of vertigo that began after she bumped her head rather forcefully 2 weeks ago. Her spells last 10 to 15 seconds and occur whenever she goes to bed or wakes up. She denies any hearing loss or tinnitus. Her physical examination is normal except for a latent, rotatory nystagmus when she is lying with the right ear down. What is the most likely diagnosis?

A. Acute serous labyrinthitis
B. Benign paroxysmal positional vertigo
C. Vestibular migraine
D. Ménière disease
E. Viral vestibular neuronitis

Answers

[37.1] **C.** The Dix-Hallpike maneuver is used to diagnose BPPV. It consists, of positioning the patient from a sitting position to that of lying down with one ear down. The important findings of this test are a latent, geotropic, rotatory nystagmus. Frequently a reverse of the nystagmus is found on return to a sitting position. The Weber and Rinne test are tuning fork tests for hearing assessment. The Epley maneuver and Brandt-Daroff exercises are used in the treatment of BPPV.

[37.2] **D.** The symptoms described are the classic findings in Ménière disease. BPPV is characterized by rotatory nystagmus and has no associated hearing loss or tinnitus. Acute serous labyrinthitis and acute suppurative labyrinthitis produce vertigo that usually lasts for more than one day. Vertebrobasilar insufficiency is generally associated with other cranial nerve or central nervous system symptoms in the setting of risk factors for atherosclerosis.

[37.3] **B.** The symptoms and physical findings are those of BPPV. Acute serous labyrinthitis and viral vestibular neuronitis have vertigo that lasts for more than one day. In vestibular migraine vertigo is associated with headache, especially when other neurologic symptoms and a family history suggestive of migraine. Ménière disease has vertigo that lasts at least 20 minutes and is usually associated with hearing loss, roaring tinnitus, and aural pressure.

CLINICAL PEARLS

❖ Symptoms of BPPV can occur with ingestion of aspirin or phenytoin (Dilantin), or alcohol intoxication.

❖ Onset of vertigo should be evaluated immediately, if the following symptoms occur: headache or ear pain, fever, stiff neck, sensitivity of eyes to light, ringing or rushing noises in the ear, speech difficulties, weakness or numbness on one side of the body or face, hearing loss, and fainting.

❖ Rarely is BPPV a problem that won't go away. If it continues, a specialist such as an otolaryngologist, head and neck surgeon, or a neurologist needs to be involved.

REFERENCES

Dorland's Illustrated Medical Dictionary, 27th ed. Philadelphia, PA: WB Saunders; 1988.

Epley JM. The canalith repositioning procedure: for treatment of benign paroxysmal positional vertigo. Otolaryngol Head Neck Surg 1992 Sep;107(3):399–404.

Furman JM, Cass SP. Benign paroxysmal positional vertigo. N Engl J Med 1999 Nov 18;341(21):1590–1596.

Hilton M, Pinder D. The Epley (canalith repositioning) maneuvre for benign paroxysmal positional vertigo. Cochrane Database Syst Rev 2004;(2):CD003162.

Semont A, Freyss G, Vitte E. [Benign paroxysmal positional vertigo and provocative maneuvers] Ann Otolaryngol Chir Cervicofac 1989;106(7):473–476.

Soto Varela A, Bartual Magro J, Santos Perez S, et al. Benign paroxysmal vertigo: a comparative prospective study of the efficacy of Brandt and Daroff exercises, Semont and Epley maneuver. Rev Laryngol Otol Rhinol (Bord) 2001;122(3): 179–183.

A 64-year-man is referred to a neurologist by his primary care physician for a 3-year history of progressive weakness in his lower extremities resulting in frequent falls, difficulty standing from a chair, and painful burning in his feet and finger tips. The patient has a past medical history of high blood pressure. His physical examination is significant for weakness in his lower extremities, specifically of the hip flexors, and ankle/foot muscles. The patient also has mild weakness of his finger extensors. The sensory examination is significant for loss of sensation in his extremities, worse in the toes and fingers and extending above the knee and at the wrist. The deep tendon reflexes are absent in the upper and lower extremities. The rest of the neurologic examination is normal. His extensive laboratory studies are normal, including a normal blood glucose and a normal glycosylated hemoglobin level. MRI of his brain is normal, and MRI of his spine shows minimal arthritis, but no cord or nerve compression. Electrodiagnostic study of his muscle (electromyography) and nerve (nerve conduction study) confirm a sensory and motor polyneuropathy involving both his lower extremities and upper extremities.

◆ **What is the most likely diagnosis?**

◆ **What is the next diagnostic step?**

◆ **What is the next step in therapy?**

ANSWERS TO CASE 38: Chronic Inflammatory Demyelinating Polyneuropathy

Summary: This 64-year-old hypertensive gentleman with a slowly progressive condition that causes skeletal muscle weakness and sensory loss of his extremities. His examination reveals absent reflexes, proximal (hips) and distal (fingers, ankle/feet) weakness, and a stocking-and-glove distribution of sensory loss in his upper and lower extremities. His studies confirm that his symptoms are caused by a neuropathy involving both of his arms and legs. Thus, this patient has a symmetric, bilateral sensory and motor polyneuropathy.

 Most likely diagnosis: Chronic inflammatory demyelinating polyneuropathy

 Next diagnostic step: Analysis of the cerebrospinal fluid

 Next step in therapy: Immunosuppressive therapy such as corticosteroids or intravenous immunoglobulins

Analysis

Objectives

1. Know diagnostic approach to polyneuropathy including laboratory and pathologic studies and electrodiagnostic tests.
2. Be familiar with the common etiologies of chronic polyneuropathy.
3. Be familiar with the management of chronic demyelinating polyneuropathy.

Considerations

This patient likely has a chronic polyneuropathy. The term **polyneuropathy** describes nerve dysfunction (neuropathy) involving multiple nerves (>3–4) of the legs and arms. He presents with a slowly progressive symmetrical weakness and sensory abnormalities of the hands and legs. This patient's examination is consistent with a **peripheral nervous system process,** as reflected by weakness that is flaccid or associated with decreased **or absent reflexes.** The sensory deficits point toward peripheral nerve involvement, rather than that of motor neuron cells, nerve-muscle junction, or solely muscle since disorders of these structures result in pure motor involvement. Other conditions that can cause a peripheral neuropathy include toxins such as lead, arsenic, thallium, chemotherapy drugs, and certain antiretroviral therapy; metabolic conditions classically diabetes mellitus, with an estimated 50% of diabetics having some form of neuropathy, although many are asymptomatic. Diabetic polyneuropathy is a diagnosis of exclusion, and usually involve people with diabetes mellitus for at least 25 years.

Chronic polyneuropathies without an underlying etiology are considered primary or idiopathic polyneuropathies, although these can be associated with a number of conditions, such as malignancy and HIV. Chronic acquired inflammatory demyelinating polyneuropathy is a neurological disorder characterized by progressive weakness and impaired sensory function in the legs and arms caused by damage to the myelin sheath (the fatty covering that wraps around and protects nerve fibers) and is one of the few peripheral neuropathies amenable to treatment. In this case, the patient's presentation is consistent with a chronic polyneuropathy, likely a primarily acquired disorder suggestive of chronic inflammatory demyelinating polyneuropathy. Electromyograph (EMG) and nerve conduction studies would help confirm the diagnosis.

APPROACH TO CHRONIC INFLAMMATORY DEMYELINATING POLYNEUROPATHY

Definitions

Myelin: An electrically insulating phospholipid layer that surrounds the axons of many neurons. It is an outgrowth of Schwann cells, a glial cell that supplies the myelin for peripheral neurons whereas oligodendrocytes supply it to those of the central nervous system.

Axon: Nerve fiber projection of a motor or sensory neuron that conducts electrical impulses away from the neuron cell body or soma.

Clinical Approach

Clinical Features and Epidemiology

The prevalence of chronic inflammatory demyelinating polyneuropathy (CIDP) is approximately 1.24 to 1.9 per 100,000. The estimated annual incidence is 0.15 per 100,000 population. However, the true incidence of CIDP is likely underestimated because of stringent diagnostic criteria and clinical and pathological variability of the disorder.

In neuromuscular disease referral centers, however, CIDP represents approximately 20% of undiagnosed neuropathies and accounts for approximately 10% of all patients referred.

CIDP can occur at any age including childhood in 10% of cases. However, the mean age of onset is approximately 47.6 years (median, 53.5 years). Males are more affected than females by 2:1.

Chronic inflammatory demyelinating polyneuropathy (CIDP) is an acquired peripheral neuropathy with an extremely variable clinical presentation and course. At symptom onset, patients usually present with a generalized pattern of **numbness and weakness** in **upper and lower extremities** and spontaneous pain that develops **gradually** over several weeks. Some patients present with a progressive sensory ataxia; in other patients motor deficits predominate. Proximal and distal limbs are commonly affected in a roughly **symmetrical** pattern. Yet occasionally, the demyelinating neuropathy is focal, leading to focal or multifocal motor dysfunction. Motor deficits occur in 83–94%, sensory deficit in 72–89%, loss of tendon reflexes in 86–94%, and facial palsy in 4–15% of patients. Symptoms typically develop gradually in 84%, but can occur more acutely in 16% of patients who reach maximal disability within 4 weeks. Often these rapidly progressing patients are initially diagnosed with Guillain-Barré syndrome or acute inflammatory demyelinating polyneuropathy (see Case 39), but the diagnosis is usually changed to CIDP or CIDP-variant when symptoms persist or progress beyond 8 weeks. A variable proportion of cases follow a relapsing course, with many of these patients, often younger, developing a secondarily progressive course, similar to that observed in multiple sclerosis patients.

Etiology and Pathogenesis

Chronic inflammatory demyelinating polyneuropathy is presumably immunological in origin. It is characterized morphologically by longstanding multifocal demyelination that predominantly affects spinal roots, major plexuses, and proximal nerve trunks and is associated with a mild to moderate immune inflammation. Although no genetic susceptibility genes or factors have been identified, there are certain predisposing factors reportedly linked to the disease, including a history of vaccination or infection within 6 weeks of symptom onset, pregnancy or postpartum period, and surgery.

Pathologically, lesions consist of patchy regions of demyelination and edema with variable inflammatory infiltrates of macrophages and T cells, which are diagnostic of CIDP. Both cell-mediated mechanisms and antibody-mediated responses to major glycolipid or myelin protein antigens have been implicated. CD 4+ and CD 8T cells can be demonstrated in nerve biopsy specimens, but macrophages constitute the major cell component of the inflammatory infiltrate.

Diagnosis

CIDP should be considered in patients with a progressive symmetrical or asymmetrical polyneuropathy that is relapsing and remitting or progresses for more than 2 months. Sensory symptoms, proximal weakness, areflexia without wasting, or preferential loss of vibration or joint position sense are especially suggestive. **The major diagnostic tests for chronic inflammatory demyelinating polyneuropathy are electrophysiologic studies (EMG and nerve conduction studies [NCV]), cerebrospinal fluid (CSF) examination, and nerve biopsy.**

Increased CSF protein content in association with less than 10 cells/mm^3, **cytoalbuminologic dissociation**, is also a feature of CIDP. EMG is useful to differentiate other causes of muscle weakness, such as myopathy, axonal neuropathies, and disorders of nerve muscle transmission. Nerve conduction studies will often show a reduction or block in nerve conduction velocities, which is consistent with demyelination. These studies, however, may be nonspecific.

In many instances, the electrophysiologic tests for the diagnosis of a demyelinating neuropathy will provide mixed results because of the accompanying secondary nerve axon degeneration that can occur with demyelination. A nerve biopsy should be considered in patients when a clinical suspicion of an inflammatory demyelinating neuropathy remains even if they fail to meet the proposed criteria for CIDP. The nerve biopsy may show only nonspecific lesions when the demyelination and inflammation are proximal to the site of the biopsy (sampling error). MRI can be supportive in difficult diagnostic cases and can show hypertrophy and contrast enhancement of nerve roots and nerve plexi and is helpful in ruling out infiltrative processes or spinal disease.

Laboratory studies should also be performed to rule out other causes or associated conditions including a fasting glucose or glucose tolerance test to rule out diabetes or prediabetic state, thyroid dysfunction, vitamin deficiencies (B_{12}, folate), rheumatologic disorders, leukemias or paraproteinemias, and infection (HIV).

Although this patient does not have diabetes mellitus, many diabetics will develop a chronic progressive symmetric polyneuropathy. However, these patients usually develop a predominantly motor and ataxic polyneuropathy, and the nerve conduction studies usually show more severe axonal loss.

Treatment and Management

Corticosteroids, intravenous immunoglobulins, plasma exchanges, and immunosuppressive drugs are the main treatments used in this condition. Nearly all patients with CIDP will show an initial response to immunomodulatory therapy. However, evaluation of response to treatment is hampered by the lack of objective measures, poor correlation with electrophysiological data, variable incidence of axonal degeneration, which is unlikely to respond quickly to treatments and the variability of the disease course.

Patients with very mild symptoms which do not or only slightly interfere with activities of daily living may be monitored without treatment. **Urgent treatment with corticosteroids or** intravenous immunoglobulin **(IVIg)** should be considered for patients with moderate or severe disability, for example, when hospitalization is required or ambulation is severely impaired. Contraindications to corticosteroids will influence the choice toward IVIg and vice versa. For pure motor CIDP IVIg treatment should be first choice. If corticosteroids are used, patients should be monitored closely for adverse events related to steroid therapy. Occupation and physical therapy are often helpful in maintaining muscle conditioning and safe mobility.

Comprehension Questions

[38.1] Which of the following test results is diagnostic of definite CIDP?

    A. Cytoalbuminologic dissociation
    B. Decreased nerve conduction velocities
    C. Hypertrophy of nerve roots
    D. Segmental demyelination of nerve axons

[38.2] Which patient will often present with relapsing CIDP?

    A. Older patients
    B. Presence of diabetes
    C. HIV-infected patients
    D. Younger patients

[38.3] Which of the following therapies is effective in treating CIDP?

    A. Corticosteroids, physical therapy, radiation therapy
    B. Corticosteroids, physical therapy, immune globulins
    C. Corticosteroids, plasma exchange, surgery
    D. Corticosteroids, immune globulins, nerve growth factor

Answers

[38.1] **D.** Segmental demyelination of nerve axons is diagnostic of CIDP.

[38.2] **D.** Younger patients are more prone to a relapsing course.

[38.3] **B.** Corticosteroids, physical therapy, and immunoglobulins are effective therapy in CIDP.

CLINICAL PEARLS

❖ **Chronic inflammatory demyelinating polyneuropathy (CIDP)** is the second most frequently diagnosed neuropathy in patients 70–79 years of age.

❖ Clinical diversity in presentation and course are the most remarkable features of CIDP.

❖ Cranial nerves can be involved, particularly cranial nerve VII resulting in diplopia.

❖ Papilledema with pseudotumor cerebri syndrome are rarely observed in patients with CIDP and is caused by high CSF protein levels (usually >1000 mg/mL).

REFERENCES

European Federation of Neurological Societies; Peripheral Nerve Society. Guideline on management of paraproteinaemic demyelinating neuropathies: report of a joint task force of the European Federation of Neurological Societies and the Peripheral Nerve Society. Eur J Neurol 2006 Aug;13(8):809–818.

Neuromuscular Disease Center. Home page. Available at : http://www.neuro.wustl. edu/neuromuscular/. Said G. Chronic inflammatory demyelinating polyneuropathy. Neuromuscul Disord 2006 May;16(5):293–303.

A 25-year-old female is brought into the emergency room (ER) after tripping during a volleyball match. Her teammate notes that she had been stumbling and was starting to have more difficulty with her serve. On arrival, she can no longer raise her legs and labors to adjust herself in bed. She has also begun to complain of shortness of breath. She denies fever but states that 3 weeks ago the entire team suffered from abdominal cramps and diarrhea after a championship cookout. The patient denies previous health problems. On examination, she appears weak and slightly dyspneic. Her temperature is 36.6°C (98°F); heart rate, 50 beats/min; respiration rate, 26 breaths/min; and blood pressure, 90/60 mmHg. Her pupils are sluggish, and she constantly clears her throat. She can only keep her arms up against gravity for 10 seconds, and her hands are limp. She has slight movement of her legs with decreased sensation of pain and fine touch to her knees. Her reflexes are absent. She has no skin lesions. Her heart and lung examinations are unremarkable except for bradycardia and poor inspiratory effort. The abdominal examination reveals normoactive bowel sounds and no masses. Her complete blood count is unremarkable. The pregnancy test is negative. MRI of the brain and spine are normal.

 What is the most likely diagnosis?

 What is the next diagnostic step?

 What is the next step in therapy?

ANSWERS TO CASE 39: Guillain-Barré Syndrome

Summary: A 25-year-old healthy female presents to the ER with rapid progression of ascending weakness with diaphragmatic involvement. She has a history of gastroenteritis 5 weeks before presentation. She is bradycardic, tachypneic, and hypotensive. The neurologic examination is significant for areflexia, paralysis of her legs with sensory deficits, severe weakness of her arms, and some difficulty swallowing and breathing. The pregnancy test is negative.

◆ **Most likely diagnosis:** Guillain-Barré syndrome or acute inflammatory demyelinating polyneuropathy (AIDP)

◆ **Next diagnostic step:** Lumbar puncture for elevated protein level with few cells (albuminocytologic dissociation)

◆ **Next step in therapy:** Forced vital capacity with prophylactic intubation and mechanical ventilation for forced vital capacity (FVC) less than 15–20 mL/kg

Analysis

Objectives

1. Know a diagnostic approach to Guillain-Barre syndrome including historical clues and examination findings, and understand the differential diagnosis.
2. Understand that addressing respiratory failure should be the first priority in treating acute weakness caused by Guillain-Barré syndrome.
3. Be familiar with a rational workup for Guillain-Barré syndrome, and know the subtypes including the Miller Fisher variant.

Considerations

This 25-year-old woman developed acute symmetric ascending paralysis with progressive involvement of diaphragmatic muscles. Her most immediate problem is impending respiratory failure. The **first priority** should be to **determine the progression of respiratory insufficiency,** usually by serially measuring FVC. The negative inspiratory force should also be followed. Oxygen desaturation occurs much too late to be a safe indicator. An FVC less than 15–20 mL/kg or maximum inspiratory pressure less than 30 cm H_2O usually signals imminent need for intubation and mechanical ventilation. After determining the need for intubation, the next priority is to determine the etiology of the weakness. **Guillain-Barré syndrome is the most common cause of acute flaccid paralysis in the United States,** occurring in 1–3 out of every 100,000 people with a bimodal distribution affecting patients 15–35 years of age and 50–75 years of age. This patient has the classic history of a bacterial or viral gastrointestinal illness 2–4 weeks prior to onset of paresthesia and weakness. She had been exposed to poorly cooked meat, which predisposes her to *Campylobacter jejuni.* Forty percent of Guillain-Barré patients have positive *C. jejuni* serum antibodies and/or stool cultures. Areflexia is a hallmark examination finding, particularly in conjunction with proximal lower extremity weakness with distal sensory changes and ascending progression. Diaphragmatic and cranial nerve muscles can be affected as well, with up to one-third of patients requiring intubation, as well as autonomic involvement causing the bradycardia and hypotension.

APPROACH TO ACUTE WEAKNESS

Definitions

Acute weakness: Ascends from legs to arms and cranial nerves over hours to days.

Inflammatory: Autoimmune humoral and cell-mediated response to recent infection capable of molecular mimicry to stimulate production of antiganglioside antibodies against surface molecules of peripheral nerves.

Demyelinating: Immune-mediated damage to myelin surrounding the peripheral nerves, spinal roots, and cranial nerves resulting in clinical weakness and numbness, and electromyographic evidence of profoundly delayed or absent nerve conduction velocities.

Polyneuropathy: Symmetric damage to peripheral nerves in multiple extremities.

Flaccid: Lower motor neuron weakness with hypo- or areflexia, hypotonia, and, in the case of chronic disease, muscle atrophy.

Clinical Approach

Acute motor weakness can be associated with conditions affecting all levels of the nervous system. However, the pattern of weakness, presence of other signs (sensory loss, incoordination, altered mental status) and degree of hypo- or hyperreflexia helps to distinguish the anatomic site of disease.

Disorders of the brain that cause acute weakness include acute stroke, space occupying lesion, or an inflammatory or infectious cause. Often these conditions affect multiple pathways resulting in not only motor weakness, but sensory changes, speech changes, and altered mental status. In this case, the patient presented with a rapidly ascending, bilateral weakness and respiratory weakness, in the absence of speech changes. Her reflexes were absent, and her level of consciousness is intact. Therefore, it is unlikely that her condition is caused by disease of the brain. Further CNS disease often results in unilateral involvement in association with increased reflexes. Further, those conditions that affect both sides of the brain and cause bilateral weakness, are often diffuse and affect speech and mentation. The exception to this is spinal cord disease, which can result in symmetric weakness and sensory loss that can ascend from the legs, depending on the condition. Therefore, it is often worthwhile to image the spinal cord in such clinical presentations. In this case, the patient's spinal cord was normal. Therefore, the presentation is most consistent with a condition of the peripheral nervous system.

The peripheral nervous system (PNS) is made up of the nerve root, peripheral nerve, nerve-muscle junction, and muscle. Myopathies of various etiologies often present with a subacute or chronic course associated with proximal muscle weakness, which typically does not ascend. Although muscle diseases such as inflammatory myopathies, muscular dystrophies, and metabolic myopathies can be associated with respiratory impairment, the sensory and autonomic systems are not affected.

Nerve-muscle junctional disorders such as myasthenia gravis can present with acute and subacute motor weakness that fatigues with repetitive activity. However, the examination in this case did not reveal impairment or fatigue of the neuromuscular junction.

In this case, the acute onset of a flaccid ascending, symmetric weakness and presence of autonomic dysfunction is most consistent with an acute polyneuropathy. The etiologies of acute or subacute polyneuropathy is not extensive. In an otherwise healthy young girl, the presentation is most consistent with acute inflammatory demyelinating polyneuropathy (AIDP) or Guillain-Barré syndrome.

Guillain-Barré syndrome can be associated with *C. jejuni* as well as other bacterial etiologies including *Haemophilus influenzae, Mycoplasma pneumoniae,* and *Borrelia burgdorferi,* and viral etiologies such as HIV, Cytomegalovirus (CMV), and Epstein-Barr virus (EBV). Postvaccination disease, especially influenza, has been reported, as well as rare cases associated with systemic lupus erythematosus, sarcoidosis, lymphoma, postpregnancy, and certain medications. There are five major subtypes of Guillain-Barré syndrome, the most common by far being AIDP. The Miller-Fisher variant presents with the textbook triad of areflexia, ataxia (out of proportion to sensory deficits), and ophthalmoplegia, predominant cranial nerve weakness rather than extremities, and positive anti-GQ1b (ganglioside) antibodies. Acute motor-axonal neuropathy (AMAN) is purely motor and affects mostly children, with greater than 70% being seropositive for *C. jejuni*. It usually carries a better prognosis for recovery. Acute motor-sensory axonal neuropathy (AMSAN) affects more adults, with significant muscle atrophy and poor recovery. Acute panautonomic neuropathy is the rarest subtype with mortality from cardiovascular involvement and dysrhythmias. The differential diagnosis for acute flaccid paralysis with gastrointestinal symptoms includes two very important etiologies that carry high morbidity but, if identified and treated quickly, can be reversed: botulism and tick paralysis. Botulism is caused by the *Clostridium botulinum* neurotoxin, the most lethal toxin known to man, and is frequently food-borne but can also present with intravenous drug use, surgery, and wounds. The difference is that patients present with a descending paralysis, beginning with the Dozen Ds of cranial nerve progression—dry mouth, double vision, pupil dilation, droopy eyelids, facial droop, diminished gag reflex, dysphagia, dysarthria, dysphonia, difficulty lifting head, descending paralysis, and diaphragmatic paralysis. Rapid administration of botulism antitoxin halts worsening, although mechanical ventilation can still be required. Tick paralysis produces a rapidly ascending paralysis with areflexia, ataxia, and respiratory insufficiency much like Guillain-Barré syndrome, particularly in children with a history of outdoor exposure. Removal of the discovered female tick can be curative by elimination of the source of the neurotoxin.

Clinical Presentation

The mean interval from onset of Guillain-Barré syndrome to the most severe degree of impairment is 12 days, with 98% of patients reaching the end point of clinical worsening (nadir) by 4 weeks. The mean time to improvement starts at 28 days, and clinical recovery usually occurs by 200 days. Eighty-five percent of patients recover completely, although up to 15% have permanent deficits. Three to eight percent of patients die in spite of intensive care management. A major cause of mortality in elderly victims is arrhythmias.

The history should be meticulous to identify corroborating symptomatology and triggers as discussed above, and to rule out other causes of acute flaccid paralysis. The physical examination should focus on the vital signs, reflexes, and extent of weakness in the extremities, diaphragm, and cranial nerves. Fever and mental status changes are unusual, and signal hypoxic respiratory failure or a different etiology. The principal laboratory test is the lumbar puncture showing rising protein levels up to 400 mg/L with no associated increase in cell count (*albuminocytologic dissociation*), although protein elevation may not be seen until 1–2 weeks after onset, and 10% remain normal. Antibodies and stool culture for *C. jejuni* are frequently checked. Other helpful tests include sedimentation rate, antiganglioside antibodies, anti-GQ1b antibodies for Miller Fisher presentations, and pregnancy test. Presence of anti-GM1 antibodies signals a poorer prognosis. Nerve conduction studies show early changes indicative of nerve root demyelination. MRI of the brain and spine can show anterior nerve root enhancement, which is more specific for Guillain-Barré syndrome, but should be obtained for difficult cases to rule out secondary causes, such as malignancy, vasculitic, or viral infection, and spinal cord pathology. Measurement of respiratory strength (FVC) is crucial for cases with respiratory involvement as above. Electrocardiograph (ECG) should be performed to screen for atrioventricular block, ST segment changes, and arrhythmias.

The patient should be admitted for further monitoring and treatment. If the etiology is still unclear and the patient continues to deteriorate, consultation with a neurologist is indicated.

Treatment

Intubation and mechanical ventilation should be considered for FVC less than 15 mL/kg with intensive care monitoring for arrhythmias and blood pressure instability. Because of the immune-mediated pathogenesis of the disease, the only proven therapies are IV immune globulin therapy (5 days) and plasma exchange (10 days), both of which can hasten recovery by 50% if initiated early in the course of the disease. There is no data to support the use of steroids. Complications of immobility, hospitalization, and respiratory insufficiency should be avoided by implementing prophylactic measures for deep venous thrombosis, decubitus ulcers, gastritis, and aspiration. Recurrence is rare but can occur in up to 5% of cases.

Comprehension Questions

Match the following etiologies (A–E) to the clinical situation [39.1] to [39.4]:

    A. Acute inflammatory demyelinating polyneuropathy
    B. Acute stroke
    C. Myasthenia gravis
    D. Inflammatory myopathy
    E. Tick paralysis
    F. Transverse cord myelitis

[39.1] A 19-year-old man, who works at a hamburger stand, develops diarrhea, and 2 weeks later experiences gait difficulties and foot tingling.

[39.2] An 18-year-old woman comes back from a camping trip complaining of blurry vision, facial weakness, and difficulty swallowing followed by arm then leg weakness.

[39.3] A 62-year-old man with hypertension and diabetes presents with acute right face, arm, leg weakness, slurred speech, and right-sided hyperreflexia.

[39.4] A 34-year-old woman presents with fatigable muscle weakness with climbing stairs or blow drying her hair. This is associated with some shortness of breath, which improves with rest.

Answers

[39.1] **A.** AIDP is the most common presentation of Guillain-Barré syndrome, with up to 40% of patients seropositive for *C. jejuni*, which is found in poorly cooked meats.

[39.2] **E.** Tick paralysis presents with ascending paralysis and resolves with removal of the tick.

[39.3] **B.** Unilateral face, arm, leg weakness and dysarthria in a patient with risk factors for vascular disease is consistent with an acute cerebrovascular event.

[39.4] **C.** Myasthenia gravis is an acquired neuromuscular junction disorder caused by antibody-mediated impairment of the skeletal muscle acetylcholine receptor.

CLINICAL PEARLS

❖ The majority of Guillain-Barré cases are associated with a history of preceding *C. jejuni* or other flu-like or gastrointestinal syndrome.

❖ Most Guillain-Barré patients experience proximal lower extremity weakness with ascending paralysis within hours to days.

❖ One should be wary that the examination can worsen rapidly from one visit to the next with the possibility of respiratory failure.

❖ Significant autonomic instability can accompany Guillain-Barré symptoms and require intensive care monitoring.

❖ IV immunoglobulin and plasma exchange are the two therapeutic options that have been shown to improve recovery.

REFERENCES

Hughes RA, Cornblath DR. Guillain-Barré syndrome. Lancet 2005 Nov 5;366(9497):1653–1666.

Miller A. Guillain-Barré syndrome. Available at: http://www.emedicine.com/EMERG/topic222.htm.

A 31-year-old woman presents with a 3-month history of muscle soreness, cramps, and muscle fatigue with climbing stairs and carrying objects. The patient has recently noted a rash on her cheeks, necks, chest, and back and swelling around her eyes. Her review of symptoms is significant for recent sensitivity of her fingers to cold temperatures, difficulty swallowing certain foods and pills, and some shortness of breath with exertion. The physical examination is significant for an erythematous rash across her cheeks, neck, chest, and back and mild lid edema. The cardiac exam is significant for occasional skipped beats. The neurologic examination shows proximal muscle weakness of the patient's deltoids, biceps, hip flexors, and knee flexors. The sensory and coordination examination is normal. Laboratory studies are normal except for elevated serum creatine kinase of 770 (normal 50–200). Electromyography and nerve conduction studies reveal an irritative myopathy and normal nerve conductions.

◆ **What is the most likely diagnosis?**

◆ **What is the next diagnostic step?**

◆ **What is the next step in therapy?**

ANSWERS TO CASE 40: Dermatomyositis

Summary: A young woman complains of subacute onset of proximal muscle weakness and myalgias, skin rash, and a clinical history of Raynaud phenomena, dysphagia, and cardiac arrhythmia. The diagnostic studies reveal an irritative and damaging myopathy that is likely inflammatory in etiology.

◆ **Most likely diagnosis:** Dermatomyositis

◆ **Next diagnostic step:** Skeletal muscle biopsy

◆ **Next step in therapy:** Immunomodulatory therapy; cardiac and respiratory evaluation

Analysis

Objectives

1. Describe the most common types of inflammatory myopathies.
2. Be familiar with the diagnostic workup of inflammatory myopathies.
3. Be familiar with the treatment and management of dermatomyositis.

Clinical Considerations

The patient presented in this case has a subacute onset of proximal muscle pain and weakness, some swallowing (dysphagia) difficulties, and rash. This clinical presentation is consistent with dermatomyositis. The two most common inflammatory myopathies are dermatomyositis and polymyositis. Both diseases share the common symptom of proximal muscle weakness. **Dermatomyositis differs from polymyositis by its immunopathogenesis but also by the involvement of skin, with rash, discoloration, and tissue calcification.** Inclusion body myositis (IBM) is another inflammatory myopathy that shares some features with polymyositis and dermatomyositis. However, IBM occurs in older patients, usually >50 years of age, and affects men more than women. Inclusion body myositis tends to present with a more gradual onset of weakness, which can date back several years by the time of diagnosis. It generally follows a more indolent course and is more refractory to therapy.

APPROACH TO DERMATOMYOSITIS

Definitions

Heliotrope rash: Bluish-purple discolorations on the face, lids, neck, shoulders, upper chest, elbows, knees, knuckles, and back of patients with dermatomyositis.

Gottron nodules: Flat-topped raised nonpruritic lesions found over the dorsum of the metacarpophalangeal, proximal interphalangeal, and distal interphalangeal joints.

Anti-Jo-1 antibody: Antibody that recognizes a cytoplasmic histidyl transfer RNA synthetase.

Creatine kinase (CK): An enzyme found primarily in the heart and **skeletal muscles**, and to a lesser extent in the brain. Significant injury to any of these structures will lead to a measurable increase in CK levels.

Raynaud phenomenon: A condition resulting from poor circulation in the extremities (i.e., fingers and toes). In a person with Raynaud phenomenon, when his or her skin is exposed to cold or the person becomes emotionally upset, the blood vessels under the skin spasm, and the blood flow slows. This is called vasospasm. These areas can become cyanotic and cold.

Clinical Approach

Polymyositis and dermatomyositis are frequently considered together because they have similar clinical, laboratory, and pathologic features and because they progress at the same tempo. Although inclusion body myositis shares some features with polymyositis and dermatomyositis, it generally follows a more indolent course and is more refractory to therapy.

Epidemiology and Clinical Features

Dermatomyositis is more rare than polymyositis, affecting 10 people out of every 1 million. Although there is a juvenile form of this disease that begins between the ages of 5 and 15 years, it most commonly begins between the ages of 40 and 60 years. Dermatomyositis has a subacute (somewhat short and relatively severe) onset, usually worsening over a period of days or weeks, although it might also last for months.

The distinguishing characteristic of dermatomyositis is a rash accompanying, or more often, preceding muscle weakness. The rash is described as patchy, bluish-purple discolorations on the face, neck, shoulders, upper chest, elbows, knees, knuckles, and back. Some patients might also develop hardened bumps of calcium deposits under the skin. Trouble with swallowing (dysphagia) might also occur. In approximately one-fourth of adult cases, muscles ache and are tender to the touch. In the juvenile form, these myalgias can be seen in as many as 50 percent.

Polymyositis also causes varying degrees of decreased muscle function. The disease has a more gradual onset compared to dermatomyositis and generally begins in the second decade of life. Polymyositis rarely affects people younger than18 years of age. Like dermatomyositis, difficulty with swallowing occurs and is more common with polymyositis, which can affect nutrition as well increase the risk of aspiration pneumonia. Approximately one-third of patients with polymyositis or dermatomyositis experience muscle tenderness and cramps.

The chief clinical feature of polymyositis and dermatomyositis is progressive, painless symmetrical proximal muscle weakness, with symptoms possibly dating back to 3 to 6 months by the time of the diagnosis. Upper-extremity muscle weakness manifests as difficulty in performing activities that require holding the arms up, such as hair washing, shaving, or reaching into overhead cupboards. Neck muscle weakness may lead to difficulty raising the head from a pillow or even holding it up while standing. Involvement of pharyngeal muscles may result in hoarseness, dysphonia, dysphagia, and nasal regurgitation after swallowing. Lower-extremity proximal muscle weakness manifests as difficulty climbing stairs and rising from a seated or squatting position. Patients will often seek chairs with armrests to push off from or grab the sink or towel bar to rise from the toilet.

Other Clinical Features

Weakness is the major complaint, but proximal myalgias and constitutional symptoms such as fever, fatigue, and weight loss can occur.

Interstitial pneumonitis occurs in approximately 10% of patients with polymyositis, usually developing gradually over the course of the illness. Myocardial involvement in polymyositis and dermatomyositis is well described. The reported frequency of congestive heart failure (with or without cardiomegaly) ranges from fewer than 5% of patients to 27–45%. Electrocardiographic abnormalities are more common, with left anterior fascicular block and right bundle-branch block representing the most frequent conduction defects.

Both polymyositis and dermatomyositis were associated with an increased risk of malignancy, with a threefold risk demonstrated in patients with dermatomyositis and a 1.4-fold risk for patients with polymyositis. The types of malignancy generally reflected those expected for age and sex although ovarian cancer was overrepresented in women with dermatomyositis, and both groups of patients displayed a greater-than- expected occurrence of non-Hodgkin lymphoma.

Cutaneous Features of Dermatomyositis

In dermatomyositis, patients can have an erythematous, often pruritic rash over the face, including the cheeks, nasolabial folds, chin, and forehead. Heliotrope (purplish) discoloration over the upper eyelids with periorbital edema is characteristic (Fig. 40–1), as is the *shawl sign*, which describes the pattern of an erythematous rash in V distribution on the chest and across the shoulders. **Gottron papules**—flat-topped raised nonpruritic lesions found over the dorsum of the metacarpophalangeal, proximal interphalangeal, and

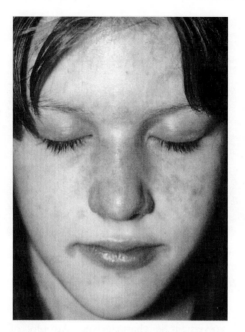

Figure 40–1. Heliotrope rash. *(With permission from Kasper DL, Braunwal E, Fauci A, et al. Harrison's principles of internal medicine, 16th ed. New York: McGraw-Hill; 2004: Fig. 49–3.)*

distal interphalangeal joints—are virtually pathognomonic for dermatomyositis (Fig. 40–2). Often pinkish to violaceous, sometimes with a slight scale, they are distinguished from cutaneous lupus in that lupus has a predilection for the dorsum of the fingers between the joints.

Calcinosis Cutis

Children with dermatomyositis are also particularly prone to calcinosis cutis, which is the development of dystrophic calcification in the soft tissues and muscles, leading to skin ulceration, secondary infection, and joint contracture. Calcinosis cutis occurs in up to 40% of children with dermatomyositis and less commonly in adults; there is no proven therapy to prevent this complication.

Inclusion Body Myositis

Inclusion body myositis tends to present with a more gradual onset of weakness, which can date back several years by the time of diagnosis. Although the muscle weakness is proximal, distal muscle groups can also be affected, and

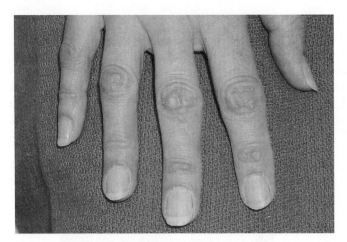

Figure 40–2. Gottron papules. *(With permission from Kasper DL, Braunwal E, Fauci A, et al. Harrison's principles of internal medicine, 16th ed. New York: McGraw-Hill; 2004: Fig. 49–4.)*

asymmetry of involvement is characteristic. Atrophy of the deltoids and quadriceps is often present, and weakness of forearm muscles (especially finger flexors) and ankle dorsiflexors is typical. Peripheral neuropathy with loss of deep tendon reflexes can be present in some patients.

Diagnosis

Because both polymyositis and dermatomyositis are relatively rare, there is not a clearly defined approach to diagnosing these conditions. The diagnosis is further complicated by the similarity of these diseases to other, more common diseases and disorders. Both polymyositis and dermatomyositis are often diagnosed by ruling out other conditions.

Laboratory studies include a creatine kinase serum level. The laboratory hallmark of polymyositis and dermatomyositis, although not specific to either of these, is a dramatic elevation of the serum creatine kinase, often in the range of 1,000 to 10,000 mg/dL. Although early in the disease process milder elevations can be seen. In inclusion body myositis, creatine kinase elevations tend to be less striking, often increasing only to the 600 to 800 mg/dL range; 20% to 30% of patients with inclusion body myositis can have a normal creatine kinase at presentation. With initiation of effective treatment, creatine kinase levels decrease rapidly, and periodic measurements are used to follow up disease activity over the course of the long term. **Caution is advised** when interpreting creatine kinase elevations, as levels can remain mildly elevated with clinically quiescent disease. Therefore, the degree of elevation does not necessarily correlate with the degree of muscle weakness, although disease exacerbation is often associated with increased levels. Elevated serum levels of aldolase, lactate dehydrogenase (LDH), aspartate aminotransferase (AST), and alanine aminotransferase (ALT) are less sensitive and specific for active myositis.

Autoantibodies can be present in polymyositis and dermatomyositis, but they are generally absent in inclusion body myositis. Autoantibodies present in polymyositis and dermatomyositis include the myositis specific autoantibodies anti-Jo-1, seen in 20% of patients, and the less commonly encountered anti-PL-7, anti-PL-12, anti-OJ, and anti-EJ. These antibodies recognize cytoplasmic transfer RNA synthetases (for transfer RNA synthetase), and they are markers of the subset of polymyositis and dermatomyositis patients described as having antisynthetase syndrome, which is characterized by fever, inflammatory arthritis, Raynaud phenomenon, and interstitial lung disease and is associated with a reduction in survival compared with uncomplicated polymyositis and dermatomyositis.

The evaluation of the patient with suspected myositis should include **electromyography and nerve conduction studies** that will show changes in muscle activity at rest and with contraction suggestive of an *irritative* or inflammatory myopathy. A **muscle biopsy** specimen demonstrating typical histologic features in the absence of markers of metabolic myopathy, infection, or drug effect establishes the diagnosis of polymyositis. Muscle biopsy may not be necessary in a patient presenting with proximal muscle weakness, creatine kinase elevation, and the classic cutaneous manifestations of dermatomyositis. When biopsy is performed, however, care must be taken not to select a muscle that is so weak or atrophic that the biopsy reveals endstage disease. The common pathophysiologic features of polymyositis, dermatomyositis, and inclusion body myositis are chronic inflammation, an attempt at healing by fibrosis, and a net loss of myofibrils. The inflammatory infiltrate is composed mainly of lymphocytes. In polymyositis and inclusion body myositis, the lymphocytes are found predominantly within the fascicles, made up of CD8+ T lymphocytes. In dermatomyositis, the cells are found predominantly in the perivascular and perifascicular regions, mostly macrophages and CD4+ lymphocytes. Perifascicular atrophy is diagnostic of dermatomyositis regardless of the presence of inflammatory cells.

For inclusion body myositis, the muscle cells exhibit a variety of abnormal inclusions, including eosinophilic cytoplasmic inclusions, vacuoles rimmed with basophilic granules, and foci that stain positively with Congo red, consistent with amyloid deposits. On electron microscopy, inclusion body myositis is characterized by the presence of cytoplasmic helical filaments (tonofilaments), which contain beta-amyloid protein and a number of other proteins implicated in neurodegeneration.

Often the clinical presentation is straightforward and can help distinguish between the most common types (polymyositis [PM], dermatomyositis [DM], IBM, see Table 40–1). However, other conditions can present with myalgia, weakness, or serum creatine kinase elevation or any combination of these features and need to be ruled out. Often these conditions may or may not be associated with an infiltrate of inflammatory cells on muscle biopsy. Many drugs

Table 40–1

IDIOPATHIC INFLAMMATORY MYOPATHIES: CLINICAL
& LABORATORY FEATURES

	IBM	PM	DM
Age of onset	>50 years	Adult	All ages
Gender	Males	Females	Females
Family history	Rare	No	No
Malignancy associated	No	Slight	Yes
Rash	No	No	Yes
CK level	< 10 × normal	50 × normal	50 × normal
Therapeutic response	Poor	Variable	Good
Biopsy finding	Vacuoles, amyloid deposits	Inflammatory complement deposits	Inflammation

CK, creatine kinase; DM, dermatomyositis; IBM, inclusion body myositis; PM, polymyositis.

and toxins can induce a metabolic myopathy with weakness, serum creatine kinase elevation, and myalgia, such as statins (cholesterol lowering medications). Penicillamine and zidovudine are associated with inflammatory infiltrates. Infection, endocrinopathy, metabolic myopathy, fibromyalgia, polymyalgia rheumatica, sarcoid, and paraneoplastic phenomena, and some genetically acquired muscular dystrophies also require consideration. Therefore, a thorough history including family, past medical, medication use, and exposures should be obtained.

Treatment and Management

Currently, there is no cure for inflammatory myopathies. However, there are several approaches to treatment. Several **immunosuppressant medicines** have been shown to be quite effective in treating dermatomyositis and polymyositis. The mainstay of therapy is oral prednisone given initially at a dose of 1 mg/kg in the morning. Tapering the dose can be attempted after 4 to 6 weeks, with very gradual tapering. In patients whose disease responds only partially to corticosteroids, or who are unable to tolerate chronic or high doses, other agents such as methotrexate or azathioprine may be used. Use of either agent requires an understanding of its toxicity profile and careful monitoring for adverse effects. Intravenous immunoglobulin infusion on a monthly basis can be helpful in some patients with refractory dermatomyositis. Inclusion body myositis is considered to be refractory to any medical therapy, although a few case series have reported stabilization and even improvement in patients treated with prednisone alone or in combination with azathioprine or methotrexate. Intravenous immunoglobulin therapy has some reported benefit in patients with dysphagia, or swallowing difficulties.

Screening

Patients also require evaluation of pulmonary and cardiac function with chest x-ray, formal pulmonary function testing, electrocardiogram (ECG), and referrals to cardiology and pulmonology. **Dermatomyositis and polymyositis are often associated with underlying malignancy.** If malignancy is suspected, a thorough primary screening is indicated including relevant radiography, gynecologic evaluation, colonoscopy, and breast mammography. Even if an initial evaluation for malignancy at the time of presentation of myositis is unrevealing, **the clinician should remain alert to signs and symptoms of new malignancy in the first several years of follow-up.**

Physical Therapy

Physical therapy is important in helping patients manage the muscle weakness associated with inflammatory myopathies. A physical therapist will assist a patient in designing an appropriate exercise program, as well as help the patient make progress throughout the program. Some patients might require assistive devices such as a walker, and a physical therapist will assist in determining the most suitable device.

Speech Therapy

Some patients who have swallowing problems need the assistance of a speech therapist. A speech therapist can recommend exercises that might improve swallowing, as well as provide general tips and guidance for overcoming swallowing difficulties. As with many other conditions, education about inflammatory myopathies and local support groups can be the greatest tools for managing the disorder and preventing complications.

Comprehension Questions

[40.1] Which of the following is not a dermatologic manifestation of dermatomyositis?

A. Calcinosis cutis
B. Malar rash
C. Gottron papules
D. Heliotrope rash

[40.2] Which of the following statements is true of IBM?

A. IBM differs from polymyositis only in regards to response to immune therapy.
B. IBM is the most common acquired myopathy in patients older than 50 years of age.
C. Inflammation must be present on muscle biopsy in order to confirm a diagnosis of IBM.
D. The presence of *rimmed vacuoles* on the muscle biopsy of IBM patients is caused by effects of chronic immune suppressant therapy.

[40.3] Which of the following conditions are associated with polymyositis and dermatomyositis?

A. Interstitial lung disease, psoriasis, dysphagia
B. Interstitial lung disease, heart failure, malignancy
C. Malignancy, cardiac arrhythmias, meningitis
D. Malignancy, interstitial lung disease, meningitis

Answers

[40.1] **B.** Malar rash, also called *butterfly rash*, involves both cheeks and extends across the bridge of the nose and is often seen in patients with systemic lupus erythematosus.

[40.2] **B.** It is the most common acquired muscle disease occurring in persons older than 50 years of age, with a prevalence estimated at 4–9:1,000,000. It affects men more frequently than women, greater than 2:1

[40.3] **B.** Dermatomyositis and polymyositis are associated with a greater risk of malignancy, although to varying degrees, and a 10% incidence of lung and cardiac involvement.

CLINICAL PEARLS

❖ IBM is not a variant of polymyositis, but it is the most common acquired muscle disease occurring in persons older than 50 years of age.

❖ There are abnormal accumulations of proteins commonly seen in neurodegenerative disorders (Alzheimer disease, Parkinson disease, etc.) in muscle fibers of inclusion body myositis patients.

❖ Most patients with PM have some distal weakness, although it is usually not as severe as the proximal weakness.

❖ The most common reason for a misdiagnosis of an inflammatory myopathy is erroneous pathologic interpretation of the biopsy.

REFERENCES

Kissel JT. Misunderstandings, misperceptions, and mistakes in the management of the inflammatory myopathies. Semin Neurol 2002 Mar;22(1):41–51.

Neuromuscular Disease Center. Home page. Available at: http://www.neuro.wustl.edu/neuromuscular/.

Rendt K. Inflammatory myopathies: narrowing the differential diagnosis. Cleve Clin J Med 2001 Jun;68(6):505, 509–514, 517–519.

A 64-year-old male comes to a neurologist with an 11-month history of progressive weakness. He first noticed weakness of his right hand with difficulty holding onto things. This progressed to right shoulder and upper arm weakness, with difficulty raising his arm above his head or carrying things. The patient's only health problems are high blood pressure and arthritis in his knees. On examination, the patient is otherwise well developed and cognitively intact. General examination reveals muscle atrophy and wasting of the intrinsic and small muscles of his right hand, right triceps, and muscles of his right shoulder. There is visible muscle twitching of both arm muscles and paraspinal muscles of his back. The neurologic examination reveals significant weakness of the right upper extremity and some moderate weakness of his left deltoid and biceps, and right hip flexors. His reflexes are increased in both legs and left arm. His sensory and cerebellar examinations are normal. MRI of the brain and spine are normal. Laboratory studies are normal. Electrodiagnostic studies (EMG/NCV) reveal diffuse muscle denervation in his arms, legs, and paraspinal muscles. There is no evidence of neuropathy or myopathy.

◆ **What is the most likely diagnosis?**

◆ **What is the next diagnostic step?**

◆ **What is the next step in therapy?**

ANSWERS TO CASE 41: Amyotrophic Lateral Sclerosis

Summary: A 64-year-old relatively healthy man presents with progressive skeletal muscle weakness of both upper extremities and lower extremity. His examination and diagnostic workup reveals pure motor weakness, without sensory and cerebellar involvement or spinal cord and brain abnormalities.

 Most likely diagnosis: Motor neuron disease—amyotrophic lateral sclerosis

 Next diagnostic step: Electromyography of skeletal muscle and nerve conduction study of peripheral nerve and nerve roots

◆ **Next step in therapy:** Supportive management of mobility and monitoring of respiratory and swallowing function

Analysis

Objectives

1. Describe the diagnostic approach to motor neuron disease/amyotrophic lateral sclerosis including neuroimaging, laboratory and pathologic studies, and electrodiagnostic tests.
2. Understand that amyotrophic lateral sclerosis is a diagnosis based on the exclusion of other pure or predominantly motor syndromes.
3. Be familiar with the management of amyotrophic lateral sclerosis.

Clinical Considerations

This 64-year-old man complains of progressive skeletal muscle weakness of his right upper extremity associated with muscle wasting (atrophy). The examination is also significant for weakness in the left upper extremity and lower extremity as well. There is no loss of sensation by history or examination, thus this is a pure skeletal muscle (motor) process. The possible site(s) of pathology or disease for a pure motor process includes the area for voluntary motor control (the motor cortex), the neurons, which control voluntary motor movement (motor neurons); the individual motor roots originating from the cord, the motor nerves, which are made up of more than one motor root; or the muscle. These sites can be grouped into upper motor pathways and lower motor pathways.

Upper motor pathways include the upper motor neuron located in the motor cortex of the brain. Myelinated nerve fibers (corticospinal tract) originate from these neurons and travel to synapse on lower motor neurons located in the brainstem and spinal cord. It is at the level of the lower motor neuron that the lower motor neuron pathway originates. From the lower motor neuron, the motor nerve root originates and in combination with other nerve roots becomes a nerve, which synapses with the skeletal muscle and thus controls skeletal muscle movement of the face and body. Diseases that affect motor pathways can often be distinguished based on whether the upper or lower motor pathways are purely or predominantly effected. Patients with upper motor pathway disease will present with spastic muscle weakness associated with increased reflexes, whereas those with lower motor pathway disease will present with flaccid skeletal muscle weakness associated with muscle atrophy and decreased or absent reflexes. The latter presentation is caused by loss of direct innervation of the muscle and can also be accompanied with muscle twitching (fasciculations) and/or muscle cramping.

Diagnoses to consider when the presentation is predominantly a lower motor pathway syndrome include processes that affect lower motor neurons, motor roots, nerves, or muscle, including spinal cord and root compression, motor neuropathies (Guillain-Barré syndrome), and myopathies (polymyositis). Diagnoses to consider when the presentation is predominantly an upper motor pathway syndrome include processes that affect upper motor neurons, motor cortex, and associated pathways, such as stroke, tumors, and demyelinating disease, such as multiple sclerosis. Of note, spinal cord compression can cause signs and symptoms of both upper and lower motor syndromes when compression involves descending motor pathways and contiguous motor nerve roots at that level of the cord.

In this case, the man presents with signs and symptoms of both upper and lower motor dysfunction. Neuroimaging of his brain and spinal cord rules out a brain, cord, or root process. Electrodiagnostic studies of his muscles and nerves rule out a neuropathy or myopathy. Thus, his presentation is consistent with a motor neuron process affecting both upper and lower motor neurons, such as amyotrophic lateral sclerosis.

APPROACH TO PURE MOTOR WEAKNESS

Definitions

Upper motor neuron disease: Pathologic process resulting in skeletal muscle weakness, spasticity, and increased reflexes with normal sensation

Lower motor neuron disease: Pathologic process resulting in skeletal muscle weakness, flaccidity, decreased or absent reflexes, muscle atrophy, and fasciculations with normal sensation

Myelopathy: Pathologic process that is extrinsic or intrinsic to the spinal cord, which can result in muscle weakness, spasticity, and sensory abnormalities at and below the level of the cord pathology

Radiculopathy: Pathologic process affecting the motor and/or sensory nerve roots, which originate from or enter to the spinal cord; usually caused by compression or narrowing of nerve root foramen (nerve/root canal) associated with degenerative spine or disc disease (spondylosis or spondylolisthesis)

Clinical Approach

Clinical Features and Epidemiology

Amyotrophic lateral sclerosis (**ALS**) **is caused by the degeneration of both upper (corticospinal) and lower (spinal) motor neurons**, resulting in **skeletal muscle atrophy and weakness**, and culminating in **respiratory insufficiency**. Onset is usually insidious over months with limb onset occurring in 56–75% of patients. Involvement of speech (dysarthria) and/or swallowing (dysphagia) is defined as bulbar dysfunction and occurs as the primary symptom in 25–44% of patients. Bulbar dysfunction is uncommon when ALS presents in the third and fourth decade, and represents more than 50% of patients when ALS presents in the sixth and seventh decades, especially in women.

The incidence (number of new cases per 100,000 per year) and prevalence (the number of existing cases per 100,000 per year) are 1–2 cases and 4–6, respectively. There is an overall male predominance of 1.5 to 1 in sporadic cases, with a ratio of 3–4 to 1 when ALS presents in the third and fourth decades, and 1 to 1 when ALS presents in the sixth and seventh decades. The time interval between first symptom and diagnosis ranges from 9 to 20 months, with an average time interval of 13 months. The overall survival is 3–5 years for over 50% of patients, although this can vary between 1–20 years. Age of onset is clearly a prognostic factor for survival. Improved survival is also associated with limb onset and slow rate of progression, whereas a poorer prognosis is associated with bulbar (speech and swallowing dysfunction) onset and a faster rate of progression.

Etiology and Pathogenesis

The etiology of ALS is unknown, but 10% of cases are transmitted as a dominant or recessive trait, whereas 90% of cases are sporadic. Of the familial cases, 25% are caused by mutations of the copper-zinc (Cu/Zn) superoxide dismutase gene (SOD1) located on chromosome 21. More than 100 mutations of the SOD1 gene have been linked to familial ALS. For many of these mutations, enzyme activity is actually normal or elevated. Therefore, the mutation of SOD1 gene causes disease by a gain of a toxic, injurious property rather than a loss of enzyme function. Several disease processes (pathogenic mechanisms) are implicated in motor neuron degeneration, including overactivation of excitatory neural synapses (excitotoxicity), immune activation and inflammation, mitochondrial dysfunction or altered energy metabolism, impaired clearing of aggregated proteins, and premature cell death (apoptosis). Although disturbances in each of these pathways can contribute to amplification or even initiation of motor neuron injury, the temporal relationship of these pathways and their primacy in dictating disease onset and progression is unclear.

Diagnosis

No one test can provide a definitive diagnosis of ALS, although the **presence of upper and lower motor neuron signs in a single limb** is strongly suggestive of the disorder. The diagnosis of ALS is primarily based on the symptoms and signs the physician observes in the patient and a series of tests to rule out other diseases. A full medical history and neurologic examination at regular intervals can assess whether symptoms such as muscle weakness, atrophy of muscles, hyperreflexia, and spasticity are getting progressively worse.

Because symptoms of ALS can be similar to those of a wide variety of other, more treatable diseases or disorders, appropriate tests must be conducted to exclude the possibility of other conditions. These tests include *electromyograph* (EMG), *nerve conduction velocity* (NCV), MRI, which can diagnose conditions such as a spinal cord tumor, a herniated disk in the neck, fluid-filled spaces within the cord (syringomyelia), or cervical spine degenerative diseases (spondylosis or spondylolisthesis).

Based on the patient's symptoms and findings from the examination and from these tests, the physician can order tests on blood and urine samples to eliminate the possibility of other diseases as well as routine laboratory tests. In some cases, for example, if a physician suspects that the patient has a myopathy rather than ALS, a muscle biopsy can be performed. Infectious diseases such as HIV, human T-cell leukemia virus (HTLV), and Lyme disease caused by *Borrelia burgdorferi* infection can in some cases cause ALS-like symptoms. Neurologic disorders such as multiple sclerosis, postpolio syndrome, multifocal motor neuropathy, and spinal muscular atrophy (lower motor neuron disease) also can mimic certain facets of the disease and should be considered by physicians attempting to make a diagnosis.

Due to the prognosis of this diagnosis and the variety of diseases or disorders that can resemble ALS in the early stages of the disease, patients may wish to obtain a second neurologic opinion. Based on El Escorial diagnostic criteria determined by World Federation of Neurology Research Group on Motor Neuron Diseases, a definite diagnosis of ALS requires the presence of both upper and lower motor neuron signs in at least three separate regions, including upper and/or lower extremities, tongue/speech, and paraspinal muscles using clinical, laboratory, radiographic, and pathologic results.

Treatment and Management

No cure has yet been found for ALS. However, the FDA has approved the first drug treatment for the disease—riluzole (Rilutek). Riluzole is believed to reduce damage to motor neurons by decreasing the release of glutamate, a neurotransmitter involved in excitotoxicity; one of the disease mechanism implicated in ALS. Clinical trials with ALS patients showed that riluzole prolongs survival by several months, mainly in those with difficulty swallowing. The drug also extends the time before a patient needs ventilation support. Riluzole does not reverse the damage already done to motor neurons, and patients taking the drug must be monitored for liver damage and other possible side effects. However, this drug offers hope that the progression of ALS may one day be slowed by new medications or combinations of drugs.

Other treatments for ALS are designed to relieve symptoms and improve the quality of life for patients. This supportive care is best provided by multidisciplinary teams of healthcare professionals such as physicians; pharmacists; physical, occupational, and speech therapists; nutritionists; social workers; and home care and hospice nurses. Working with patients and caregivers, these teams can design an individualized plan of medical and physical therapy and provide special equipment aimed at keeping patients as mobile and comfortable as possible.

Physicians can prescribe medications to help reduce fatigue, ease muscle cramps, control spasticity, and reduce excess saliva and phlegm. Drugs also are available to help patients with pain, depression, sleep disturbances, and constipation. Physical therapy and special equipment can improve and maintain the patient's independence and safety throughout the course of the disease. Low-impact aerobic exercise such as walking, swimming, and stationary bicycling can strengthen unaffected muscles, improve cardiovascular health, and help patients fight fatigue and depression. Range of motion and stretching exercises can help prevent painful spasticity and shortening (contracture) of muscles. Physical therapists can recommend exercises that provide these benefits without overworking muscles. Occupational therapists can suggest devices such as ramps, braces, walkers, and wheelchairs that help patients conserve energy and remain mobile.

ALS patients who have difficulty speaking can benefit from working with a speech therapist. These health professionals can teach patients adaptive strategies such as techniques to help them speak louder and more clearly. As ALS progresses, speech therapists can help patients develop ways for responding to yes-or-no questions with their eyes or by other nonverbal means and can recommend aids such as speech synthesizers and computer-based communication systems. These methods and devices help patients communicate when they can no longer speak or produce vocal sounds.

Patients and caregivers can learn from speech therapists and nutritionists how to plan and prepare numerous small meals throughout the day that provide enough calories, fiber, and fluid and how to avoid foods that are difficult to swallow. Patients may begin using suction devices to remove excess fluids or saliva and prevent choking. When patients can no longer get enough nourishment from eating, doctors may advise inserting a feeding tube into the stomach. The use of a feeding tube also reduces the risk of choking and pneumonia that can result from inhaling liquids into the lungs. The tube is not painful and does not prevent patients from eating food orally if they wish.

When the muscles that assist in breathing weaken, use of noninvasive ventilatory assistance (*intermittent positive-pressure ventilation* [IPPV] or *bilevel positive airway pressure* [BIPAP]) can be used to aid breathing during sleep. Such devices artificially inflate the patient's lungs from various external sources that are applied directly to the face or body. When muscles are no longer able to maintain oxygen and carbon dioxide levels, patients can consider more invasive and permanent forms of mechanical ventilation (respirators) in which a machine inflates and deflates the lungs. This requires a tracheostomy, in which the breathing tube is inserted directly in the patient's trachea. Patients and their families should consider several factors when deciding whether and when to use one of these options. Ventilation devices differ in their effect on the patient's quality of life and in cost. Although ventilation support can ease problems with breathing and prolong survival, it does not affect the progression of ALS. Patients need to be fully informed about these considerations and the long-term effects of life without movement before they make decisions about ventilation support.

Social workers and home care and hospice nurses help patients, families, and caregivers with the medical, emotional, and financial challenges of coping with ALS, particularly during the final stages of the disease. Social workers provide support such as assistance in obtaining financial aid, arranging durable power of attorney, preparing a living will, and finding support groups for patients and caregivers. Respiratory therapists can help caregivers with tasks such as operating and maintaining respirators, and home care nurses are available not only to provide medical care but also to teach caregivers about giving tube feedings and moving patients to avoid painful skin problems and contractures. Home hospice nurses work in consultation with physicians to ensure proper medication, pain control, and other care affecting the quality of life of patients who wish to remain at home. The home hospice team can also counsel patients and caregivers about end-of-life issues.

Comprehension Questions

[41.1] Which of the following diagnostic studies is critical to diagnosing ALS?

    A. Cerebrospinal fluid (CSF) analysis
    B. Electroencephalograph (EEG)
    C. EMG/NCV
    D. Genetic testing

[41.2] What percentage of ALS cases are familial?

    A. 10%
    B. 25%
    C. 50%
    D. 100%

[41.3] Which of the following clinical features is associated with ALS?

    A. Sensory loss on face

    B. Resting tremor of the hands

    C. Slurred speech

    D. Loss of position sense of the toes

Answers

[41.1] **C.** Although several diagnostic studies help to support a diagnosis of ALS, the EMG/NCV is critical to determine the pattern of involvement along with the physical examination.

[41.2] **A.** Ten percent of all ALS cases show an autosomal dominant inheritance pattern.

[41.3] **C.** ALS is motor neuron disorder and is not associated with sensory symptoms.

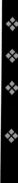

CLINICAL PEARLS

❖ ALS is a progressive neurodegenerative disease, which is sporadic in 90–95% of cases.

❖ Cervical myelopathy is a common mimic of ALS and must be ruled out by appropriate imaging studies.

❖ ALS is a diagnosis of exclusion and requires evaluation for metabolic, structural, and infectious or inflammatory disorders that can produce an ALS-like presentation.

❖ Riluzole is the only FDA approved drug for ALS and has been shown to prolong survival by 10% as defined by a delay in initiating invasive ventilatory support by 3 months.

REFERENCES

National Institute of Neurological Disorders and Stroke. Amyotrophic lateral sclerosis fact sheet. Available at: http://www.ninds.nih.gov/disorders/amyotrophiclateralsclerosis/detail_amyotrophiclateralsclerosis.htm.

Rocha JA, Reis C, Simoes F, et al. Diagnostic investigation and multidisciplinary management in motor neuron disease. J Neurol 2005 Dec;252(12):1435–1447.

Simpson EP, Yen AA, Appel SH. Oxidative stress: a common denominator in the pathogenesis of amyotrophic lateral sclerosis. Curr Opin Rheumatol 2003 Nov;15(6):730–736.

Traynor BJ, Codd MB, Corr B, et al. Clinical features of amyotrophic lateral sclerosis according to the El Escorial and Airlie House diagnostic criteria: a population-based study. Arch Neurol 2000 Aug;57(8):1171–1176.

University of Bristol Department of Anatomy. Upper motor neuron pathways: a tutorial. Available at: http://d-mis-web.ana.bris.ac.uk/calnet/UMN/page2.htm.

A 45-year-old right-handed office secretary presents with a 5-month complaint of numbness and pain of her right index and middle fingers, which is worse with driving or typing on her keyboard at work. The symptoms often awake the patient from sleep. She has also recently noticed decreased grip strength associated with frequent dropping of heavy objects. Her medical history is only significant for a diagnosis with hypothyroidism 7 months prior. Her neurologic and physical examinations are significant for numbness to pinprick sensation along the right side of her palm, thumb, index and middle fingers of her right hand. There is only mild weakness of finger flexion limited to these digits. Symptoms are worsened with tapping on the ventral or palm side of her wrist. The rest of her examination, including muscle and sensory testing are normal. Her deep tendon reflexes are normal, throughout. There are no musculoskeletal or joint abnormalities observed.

◆ **What is most likely diagnosis?**

◆ **What is the next diagnostic step?**

◆ **What is the next step in therapy?**

ANSWERS TO CASE 42: Median Nerve Mononeuropathy

A 45-year-old right handed office secretary with hypothyroidism presents with a 5-month complaint of numbness and pain of her right index and middle fingers, worsened with activity of the fingers. The symptoms often awaken the patient from sleep. There are both motor and sensory deficits of the median nerve distribution. There is the positive Tinel sign. The rest of her examination, including muscle and sensory testing are normal. Her deep tendon reflexes are normal, throughout.

◆ **Most likely diagnosis:** Right median nerve mononeuropathy (carpal tunnel syndrome [CTS])

◆ **Next diagnostic step:** Electromyography and nerve conduction studies

◆ **Next step in therapy:** Wrist splints, analgesics, rehabilitation, surgical evaluation

Analysis

Objectives

1. Know the signs and symptoms of median mononeuropathy.
2. Be familiar with the differential diagnosis of focal weakness and sensory deficits.
3. Be familiar with the treatment and management of median nerve mononeuropathy.

Considerations

The patient presents with signs and symptoms of focal right hand numbness, pain, and weakness. Her examination reveals sensory deficit affecting the lateral aspect of the hand and fingers. Symptoms are worsened or reproduced with tapping or pressure on the anterior or palm side of her wrist. Her examination is otherwise normal. Her clinical history is also significant for working as a secretary with associated worsening of symptoms with typing, in addition to driving and while sleeping. Based upon this presentation, the *site of lesion* is likely located at the wrist. The distribution of her sensory and motor impairment to the lateral aspect (thumb side) of her palm and to digits 2–4 of her hand fits the distribution of the median nerve, which is *fed* or innervated by cervical roots 5–7 originating from the cervical spinal cord on the same side. This presentation is consistent with a right median mononeuropathy or CTS originating from the wrist, although nerve root(s) compression of these nerve roots at the level of the cervical spine or involvement of the plexus of nerves of the arm, should not be ruled out.

APPROACH TO CARPAL TUNNEL SYNDROME

Definitions

Carpal tunnel: A narrow, rigid passageway of ligament and bones at the base of the hand through which the median nerve travels.

Tinel sign: Reproduction of numbness, tingling, or pain with tapping or pressing on the median nerve at the level of the patient's wrist.

Phalen sign: Test involves having the patient hold his or her forearms upright by pointing the fingers down and pressing the backs of the hands together. The presence of CTS is suggested if one or more symptoms, such as tingling or increasing numbness, is felt in the fingers within 1 minute

Cervical radiculopathy: Results from mechanical nerve root compression or intense inflammation of nerve root (s) (i.e., radiculitis), resulting in an acute shooting pain and /or weakness in the distribution of that nerve root

Brachial plexopathy: Bundle of nerves that lies between the neck and the axilla with the distal portion lying behind the clavicle and the pectoral muscles. It is formed from the C5, C6, C7, C8, and T1 nerve roots and is best understood by dividing it into three parts; trunks, divisions, and cords.

Clinical Approach

Epidemiology and Clinical Features

CTS occurs when the median nerve, which runs from the forearm into the hand, becomes pressed or squeezed at the wrist. The median nerve controls sensations to the palm side of the thumb (I), index finger (II), middle finer (III), and lateral (thumb side) of the ring finger (IV) as well as impulses to some small muscles in the hand that allow the fingers and thumb to move. The carpal tunnel is a narrow, rigid passageway of ligament and bones at the base of the hand, which houses the median nerve and tendons. Sometimes, thickening from irritated tendons or other swelling narrows the tunnel and causes the median nerve to be compressed. The result can be pain, weakness, or numbness in the hand and wrist, radiating up the arm. Although painful sensations can indicate other conditions, CTS is the most common and widely known of the entrapment neuropathies in which the body's peripheral nerves are compressed or traumatized.

Symptoms usually start gradually, with frequent burning, tingling, or itching numbness in the palm of the hand and the fingers, especially the thumb and the index and middle fingers. Some carpal tunnel sufferers say their fingers feel useless and swollen, even though little or no swelling is apparent. The symptoms often first appear in one or both hands during the night, because many people sleep with flexed wrists. A person with CTS can wake up feeling the need to "shake out" the hand or wrist. As symptoms worsen, people might feel tingling during the day. Decreased grip strength may make it difficult to form a fist, grasp small objects, or perform other manual tasks. In chronic and/or untreated cases, the muscles at the base of the thumb can waste away.

Not infrequently, patients report symptoms in the whole hand. Many patients with CTS also complain of a tight or swollen feeling in the hands and/or temperature changes (e.g., hands being cold/hot all the time). Many patients also report sensitivity to changes in temperature (particularly cold) and a difference in skin color. In rare cases, there are complaints of changes in sweating. In all likelihood, these symptoms are caused by autonomic nerve fiber involvement (the median nerve carries most autonomic fibers to the whole hand).

CTS is often the result of a combination of factors that increase pressure on the median nerve and tendons in the carpal tunnel, rather than a problem with the nerve itself. Most likely the disorder is caused by a congenital predisposition—the carpal tunnel is simply smaller in some people than in others. Other contributing factors include trauma or injury to the wrist that cause swelling, such as sprain or fracture; overactivity of the pituitary gland (e.g., acromegaly); hypothyroidism; diabetes, rheumatoid arthritis; mechanical problems in the wrist joint; work stress; repeated use of vibrating hand tools; fluid retention during pregnancy or menopause; or the development of a cyst or tumor in the canal. Some rare diseases can cause deposition of abnormal substances in and around the carpal tunnel, leading to nerve irritation. These diseases include **amyloidosis, sarcoidosis, multiple myeloma,** and **leukemia.** In some cases no cause can be identified.

There is little clinical data to prove whether repetitive and forceful movements of the hand and wrist during work or leisure activities can cause CTS. Repeated motions performed in the course of normal work or other daily activities can result in repetitive motion disorders such as bursitis and tendonitis. Writer's cramp—a condition in which a lack of fine motor skill coordination and ache and pressure in the fingers, wrist, or forearm is brought on by repetitive activity—is not a symptom of CTS.

Women are three times more likely than men to develop CTS, perhaps because the carpal tunnel itself can be smaller in women than in men. The dominant hand is usually affected first and produces the most severe pain. CTS usually occurs only in adults.

In the United States, the incidence is 1–3 cases per 1000 subjects per year; prevalence is approximately 50 cases per 1000 subjects in the general population. Incidence can increase as high as 150 cases per 1000 subjects per year, with prevalence rates greater than 500 cases per 1000 subjects in certain high-risk groups. Whites are probably at highest risk. The syndrome appears to be very rare in other non-white racial groups. The peak age of development of CTS is from 45–60 years of age. Only 10% of CTS patients are younger than 31 years of age.

Diagnosis

Early diagnosis and treatment are important to avoid permanent damage to the median nerve. A physical examination of the hands, arms, shoulders, and neck can help determine if the patient's complaints are related to daily activities or to an underlying disorder, and can rule out other painful conditions that mimic CTS.

Carpal tunnel mimic syndromes include cervical radiculopathies or brachial plexopathies that can affect more than one nerve root or peripheral nerve.

Cervical radiculopathy results from mechanical nerve root compression or intense inflammation of nerve root (s) (i.e., radiculitis), resulting in an acute shooting pain in the distribution of that nerve root. The cervical region accounts for 5–36% of all radiculopathies encountered. Incidence of cervical radiculopathies by nerve root level is as follows: C7 (70%), C6 (19–25%), C8 (4–10%), and C5 (2%). However, the distribution of numbness, pain, or weakness will often follow the distribution of the nerve roots(s). As nerve roots contribute to more than one nerve, radiculopathies often affect muscles and dermatomal patterns innervated by more than one peripheral nerve. This is often a clue to distinguishing between a mononeuropathy versus a radiculopathy. This likewise applies to conditions affecting the brachial plexus which often involves more than one nerve. Although the median nerve is innervated by cervical roots C5–7, these same roots also provide innervation to other peripheral nerves of the shoulder and arm. The median nerve provides motor and sensory innervation to the lateral, flexor compartment of the forearm and hand (Fig. 42–1).

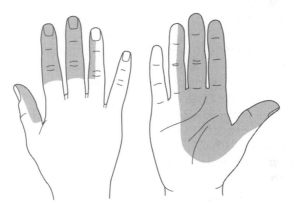

A. Sensory distribution of the median nerve

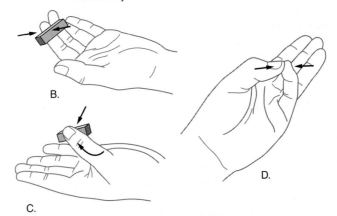

B.

C.

D.

Figure 42–1. Sensory distribution for the median nerve.

Clinically, the wrist is examined for tenderness, swelling, warmth, and discoloration. Each finger should be tested for sensation, and the muscles at the base of the hand should be examined for strength and signs of atrophy. Routine laboratory tests and x-rays can reveal diabetes, arthritis, and fractures.

Physicians can use specific tests to try to reproduce the symptoms of CTS. In the Tinel test, the doctor taps on or presses on the median nerve in the patient's wrist. The test is positive when tingling in the fingers or a resultant shock-like sensation occurs. The Phalen, or wrist-flexion, test involves having the patient hold his or her forearms upright by pointing the fingers down and pressing the backs of the hands together. The presence of CTS is suggested if one or more symptoms, such as tingling or increasing numbness is felt in the fingers within 1 minute. Doctors may also ask patients to reproduce a movement that brings on symptoms.

Often it is necessary to confirm the diagnosis by use of electrodiagnostic tests, electromyography/nerve conduction studies (EMG/NCV). In a nerve conduction study, electrodes are placed on the hand and wrist. Small electric shocks are applied and the speed with which nerves transmit impulses is measured. In electromyography, a fine needle is inserted into a muscle; electrical activity viewed on a screen can determine the severity of damage to the median nerve. Ultrasound imaging can show impaired movement of the median nerve. MRI can show the anatomy of the wrist but to date has not been especially useful in diagnosing CTS. Blood tests can be performed to identify medical conditions associated with CTS. These tests include thyroid hormone levels, complete blood counts, and blood sugar and protein analysis. X-ray tests of the wrist and hand might also be helpful.

Treatment

Treatments for CTS should begin as early as possible, under a doctor's direction. Underlying causes such as diabetes or arthritis should be treated first. Initial treatment generally involves resting the affected hand and wrist for at least 2 weeks, avoiding activities that can worsen symptoms, and immobilizing the wrist in a splint to avoid further damage from twisting or bending. If there is inflammation, applying cool packs can help reduce swelling.

Nonsurgical Treatments

In special circumstances, various drugs can ease the pain and swelling associated with CTS. Nonsteroidal antiinflammatory drugs, such as aspirin, ibuprofen, and other nonprescription pain relievers, can ease symptoms that have been present for a short time or have been caused by strenuous activity. Orally administered diuretics ("water pills") can decrease swelling. Corticosteroids (such as prednisone) or the drug lidocaine can be injected directly into the wrist or taken by mouth (in the case of prednisone) to relieve pressure on the median nerve and provide immediate, temporary relief to persons with mild or intermittent symptoms. Vitamin B_6 (pyridoxine) supplements have been shown to ease the symptoms of CTS.

Stretching and strengthening exercises can be helpful in people whose symptoms have abated. These exercises may be supervised by a physical therapist, who is trained to use exercises to treat physical impairments, or an occupational therapist, who is trained in evaluating people with physical impairments and helping them build skills to improve their health and well-being. Acupuncture and chiropractic care have benefited some patients, but their effectiveness remains unproved. An exception is yoga, which has been shown to reduce pain and improve grip strength among patients with CTS.

Surgery   Carpal tunnel release is one of the most common surgical procedures in the United States. Generally recommended if symptoms last for 6 months, surgery involves severing the band of tissue around the wrist to reduce pressure on the median nerve. Surgery is done under local anesthesia and does not require an overnight hospital stay. Many patients require surgery on both hands.

Open release surgery, the traditional procedure used to correct CTS, consists of making an incision up to 2 inches in the wrist and then cutting the carpal ligament to enlarge the carpal tunnel. The procedure is generally done under local anesthesia on an outpatient basis, unless there are unusual medical considerations. Endoscopic surgery may allow faster functional recovery and less postoperative discomfort than traditional open release surgery.

Although symptoms may be relieved immediately after surgery, full recovery from carpal tunnel surgery can take months. Some patients can have infection, nerve damage, stiffness, and pain at the scar. Occasionally the wrist loses strength because the carpal ligament is cut. Patients should undergo physical therapy after surgery to restore wrist strength. Some patients may need to adjust job duties or even change jobs after recovery from surgery. Recurrence of CTS following treatment is rare. The majority of patients recover completely.

Prevention   At the workplace, workers can do on-the-job conditioning, perform stretching exercises, take frequent rest breaks, wear splints to keep wrists straight, and use correct posture and wrist position. Wearing fingerless gloves can help keep hands warm and flexible. Workstations, tools and tool handles, and tasks can be redesigned to enable the worker's wrist to maintain a natural position during work. Jobs can be rotated among workers. Employers can develop programs in ergonomics, the process of adapting workplace conditions and job demands to the capabilities of workers. However, research has not conclusively shown that these workplace changes prevent the occurrence of CTS.

Comprehension Questions

Match the clinical descriptions [42.1–42.3] with the correct diagnosis [A–E]. Choose an answer only once.

    A. C 5 radiculopathy
    B. Brachial plexopathy
    C. Focal myositis
    D. Median mononeuropathy
    E. Motor neuron disease

[42.1] A 42 year old man presents with a radiating pain down his right shoulder to his elbow with numbness and tingling in the lateral ventral aspect of his right forearm and palm. Examination reveals decreased sensation of lateral should, anterior arm and forearm as well as an absent biceps reflex on the right.

[42.2] A 53 year old woman presents with numbness and pain in her hands which often awaken her from sleep. She has noticed decrease ability to pick up small items, such as a penny or paper clip. Her examination reveals decreased sensation on the thenar surface of both hands, right greater than left. She also has decreased sensation of digits II and III of both hands. There is small degree of muscle atrophy of the right thenar muscle.

[42.3] A 65 year old woman with history of left breast cancer status-post a mastectomy and lymph node irradiation presents with painless weakness and numbness of her left shoulder and arm muscles, and decreased ability to open or close her left hand. Examination reveals muscle atrophy and muscle twitches of the left hand intrinsic muscles, biceps, deltoids and scapular muscles. The biceps and brachioradialis reflexes are absent.

Answers

[42.1] **A.** C 5 Radiculopathy. Radiating pain in presence of symptoms and signs that extends beyond one single nerve but is consistent with one or two nerve roots.

[42.2] **B.** Median mononeuropathy. Bilateral pain, numbness, and weakness in distribution of median nerve.

[42.3] **B.** Brachial Plexopathy. Muscle weakness, atrophy, and sensory deficit in distribution of >1 nerve (median, ulnar, radial, musculocutaneous) and >1 nerve root (C4-C7) suggests brachial plexopathy. History of prior radiation is a risk factor for this condition.

CLINICAL PEARLS

❖ Carpal tunnel syndrome involves compression of the median nerve at the wrist and involves the thumb, index and middle finger.

❖ Nonsurgical treatment of CTS includes immobilization of the wrist during sleep and minimizing activity of the affected hand.

❖ Surgical therapy of CTS involves releasing the carpal ligament, which can be approached endoscopically.

❖ Contrary to common belief, chronic use of a computer keyboard is not the main cause of CTS.

❖ Tarsal tunnel syndrome is analogous to, but far less common than CTS and is caused by pressure of the nerve passing through the tarsal tunnel of the ankle. It is treated similarly.

REFERENCES

Bongers FJ, Schellevis FG, van den Bosch WJ, et al. Carpal tunnel syndrome in general practice (1987 and 2001): incidence and the role of occupational and non-occupational factors. ANZ J Surg 2006 Dec;76(12):1131–1132.

Furman MB, Simon J, Puttlitz KM, et al. Cervical disk disease. Available at: http://www.emedicine.com/PMR/topic25.htm.

National Institute of Neurological Disorders and Stroke. Carpal tunnel syndrome fact sheet. Available at: http://www.ninds.nih.gov/disorders/carpal_tunnel/detail_carpal_tunnel.htm.

Stapleton MJ. Occupation and carpal tunnel syndrome. Br J Gen Pract 2007 Jan; 57(534):36–39.

Wilder-Smith EP, Seet RC, Lim EC. Diagnosing carpal tunnel syndrome—clinical criteria and ancillary tests. Nat Clin Pract Neurol 2006 Jul;2(7):366–374.

A 21-year-old college student presents with a 4 week history of frequent falls and difficulty jogging. This athletic woman states she noticed that she was frequently tripping when walking and falling when jogging. She often "stubs" her right toe and misses steps when climbing stairs. She is quite distressed because of concerns that she will not be able to function as catcher on the intercollegiate softball team. Her past medical history is not significant. On physical examination, her general examination is normal. Her neurologic examination is significant for decreased ankle dorsiflexion and eversion of her right foot. There is mild muscle atrophy and visible muscle "twitches" of the lateral lower right leg muscles not seen on the right. The sensory examination shows decreased sensation to light touch and pin prick of the lateral aspect of her lower right leg and foot. The patient has normal coordination and normal reflexes.

◆ **What is the most likely diagnosis?**

◆ **What is the next diagnostic step?**

◆ **What is the next step in therapy?**

ANSWERS TO CASE 43: Foot Drop

Summary: This is a case of right foot drop in a young, athletic woman. Abnormal examination findings are limited to her right distal lower extremity, which includes inability to raise her right foot against gravity or to evert it laterally.

◆ **Most likely diagnosis:** Peroneal palsy

◆ **Next diagnostic step:** Electromyography of muscle and nerve conduction study of peripheral nerve and nerve roots

◆ **Next step in therapy:** Ankle-foot orthotic evaluation and rehabilitation; possible surgical repair

Analysis

Objectives

1. Know diagnostic approach to isolated foot drop.
2. Be familiar with the causes of isolated foot drop.
3. Be familiar with the management of isolated foot drop.

Considerations

The clinical presentation of this case is straightforward for an isolated nerve palsy resulting in a foot drop. The common peroneal nerve (L4–5) innervates the muscles (superficial and deep peroneus muscles) of the lower foot and ankle that mediate flexion of the foot above gravity (foot/toes raised above the ground) and lateral deviation of the foot outward. Isolated foot drop is often caused by pathology associated with the common peroneal nerve and its branches or of the muscles, directly. However, the presence of an isolated group of weakened muscles and a sensory deficit that follows the distribution of a single nerve points toward to the involvement of a single nerve, mononeuropathy, as the cause. Nevertheless, other clinical conditions can also present with foot drop including sciatic neuropathy, lumbar plexopathy, or lumbar radiculopathy, muscular dystrophies, and motor neuron disease and require a thorough evaluation to rule them out.

APPROACH TO FOOT DROP

Definitions

Fasciculation: Small, local, involuntary muscle contraction (twitching) visible under the skin arising from the spontaneous discharge of a bundle of skeletal muscle fibers.

Denervation: Loss of nerve supply from either motor neuron, nerve root, or peripheral nerve injury or insult.

Compressive neuropathy: Neuropathy caused by compression. Compression can occur as a result of trauma, inflammation or entrapment. The most common type of compression neuropathy is carpal tunnel syndrome or median nerve entrapment.

Clinical Approach

"Foot drop" is a simple description for a potentially complex problem. Foot drop is associated with a variety of conditions such as dorsiflexor injuries, peripheral nerve injuries, stroke, neuropathies, drug toxicities, or diabetes. The causes of foot drop include neurologic, muscular, and anatomic. These causes can overlap. Treatment is variable and is directed at the specific cause. Foot drop can be defined as a significant weakness of ankle and toe dorsiflexion. The foot and ankle dorsiflexors include the tibialis anterior, extensor hallucis longus, and extensor digitorum longus. These muscles help the body clear the foot during swing phase of walking and on heel strike. Such weakness often results in a steppage gait, because the patient tends to walk with an exaggerated flexion of the hip and knee to prevent the toes from catching on the ground during swing phase of walking, resulting in the foot slapping the ground. As stated, foot drop can result if there is injury to the dorsiflexors or to any point along the neural pathways that supply them, from the motor neuron to the nerve-muscle junction.

Foot drop can be observed with direct injury to the dorsiflexors. A few cases of rupture of the tibialis anterior tendon leading to foot drop have been reported. This subcutaneous tendon rupture usually follows a minor trauma with the foot in plantar flexion.

Compartment syndromes can also lead to foot drop as a result of progressive edema, or hemorrhage in the muscles of the anterior compartment of the lower leg, often associated with strenuous activity in unconditioned individuals.

Sciatic nerve lesions, lumbosacral plexopathy, lumbar radiculopathy, motor neuron disease, myopathy, or parasagittal cortical or subcortical cerebral lesions also can manifest as foot drop. The latter lesions are often differentiated by involvement of other muscle groups or extremities through clinical and electrodiagnostic examinations.

Peroneal neuropathy is caused by compression at the fibular head and is the most common compressive neuropathy in the lower extremity, likely because it is susceptible to injury along its course. The sciatic nerve is made up of nerve fiber bundles that make up the common peroneal and tibial nerve. These nerves branch off right above the posterior knee to innervate the anterior/lateral and posterior compartments of the lower leg and foot, respectively. As part of the sciatic nerve, the common peroneal nerve is relatively isolated from the tibial nerve. Therefore, trauma to the sciatic nerve might only affect one of its divisions. Also, the peroneal nerve is larger and has less protective connective tissue, making the peroneal nerve more susceptible to trauma. In addition, the peroneal nerve has fewer autonomic fibers, so in any injury, motor and sensory fibers bear the brunt of the trauma. The peroneal nerve runs a more superficial course, especially at the fibular neck, making it vulnerable to direct insult, such as during surgical procedures or compression due to boots or knee braces.

Diagnosis

Workup of foot drop proceeds according to the suspected cause. In instances where a cause is readily identified, such as trauma, no specific diagnostic laboratory studies are required. A spontaneous unilateral foot drop in a previously healthy patient as presented in this case requires further investigation into metabolic causes, including diabetes, alcohol abuse, and exposure to toxins.

Imaging Studies

If foot drop is posttraumatic, plain films of the tibia/fibula and ankle are appropriate to uncover any bony injury. In the absence of trauma, when anatomic dysfunction (e.g., Charcot joint) is suspected, plain films of the foot and ankle provide useful information.

If a tumor or a compressive mass lesion to the peroneal nerve is being investigated, magnetic resonance neurography (MRN) can be used. MRN has made it possible to produce high-resolution images of peripheral nerves, as well as associated intraneural and extraneural lesions when compared to standard MRI.

Electrodiagnostic Tests

Electromyography and nerve conduction studies are useful in differentiating among the various causes. This study can confirm the type of neuropathy, establish the site of the lesion, estimate extent of injury, and predict a prognosis. Sequential studies are useful to monitor recovery of acute lesions.

Treatment

Treatment of foot drop is directed to its etiology. If foot drop is not amenable to surgery, an ankle-foot orthosis (AFO) often is used. The specific purpose of an AFO is to provide toe dorsiflexion during the swing phase, medial and/or lateral stability at the ankle during stance.

Foot drop caused by direct trauma to the dorsiflexors generally requires surgical repair. When nerve insult is the cause of foot drop, treatment is directed at restoring nerve continuity, either by direct repair or removal of the insult. If foot drop is secondary to lumbar disc herniation (a finding in 1.2–4%

of patients with this condition), consider discectomy. Gait training and stretching through a rehabilitation program should be incorporated whether surgery is indicated or not.

Prognosis

In a peripheral compressive neuropathy, recovery can be expected in up to 3 months, as long as further compression is avoided. A partial peroneal nerve palsy following total knee replacement has a uniformly good prognosis. A variable amount of recovery is seen with a complete postoperative palsy. Follow-up EMG and nerve conduction studies can be useful to assess recovery. A partial palsy recovers faster because of local sprouting. Complete axon loss reinnervates by proximal-to-distal axonal growth only, usually proceeding at 1 mm per day. Therefore, injuries of a nerve close to its target muscle also have a more favorable outcome. In a nerve root compressive neuropathy, one study concluded that severe motor weakness of longer than 6 months duration, a negative straight leg raising test, and old age were considered poor prognostic factors for recovery of dorsiflexion.

When there is direct injury to the peroneal nerve, a more favorable outcome is noted with sharp versus blunt trauma. A traction or stretch injury to the nerve has an intermediate outcome. When nerve grafting is used, functional recovery depends on the severity of injury, and therefore, the length of graft used. Good functional recovery in grafts longer than 12 cm is rarely seen.

Comprehension Questions

[43.1] A 14-year-boy has recently begun playing ice hockey as the goalie for 3 weeks. Two weeks after frequent practice and games, he began experiencing bilateral foot weakness resulting in frequent tripping of feet. His examination reveals mild to moderate bilateral foot drop and weakness with eversion of his feet, in addition to tenderness along the upper lateral leg below the knee, which he attributes to wearing shin protectors that he wears during games. Which of the following is the likely site of disease?

A. Sciatic nerve as it exits the sciatic notch below the buttocks
B. Peroneal nerve at the head of the fibula bone
C. Posterior tibial nerve in the calves
D. Lumbar nerve root in the spinal column

[43.2] What nerve roots are likely to be associated with the condition in question [43.1]?

A. L2–3
B. L3–4
C. L4–5
D. L5–S1

[43.3] Which of the following is the best method of assessing the damage in the condition of question [43.3]?

    A. MRI of the spine
    B. CT scan of the spine
    C. Radiograph of the lower leg
    D. Electromyelography

Answers

[43.1] **B.** The patient has isolated weakness of dorsiflexion and eversion of both feet and a history of wearing sports equipment associated with compression of the peroneal nerve as it wraps around the head of the fibula in the lower leg.

[43.2] **C.** The nerve roots associated with the peroneal nerve is L4–5.

[43.3] **D.** EMG is the best modality to assess damage and recovery of the peripheral nerve.

CLINICAL PEARLS

❖ An isolated foot drop can be the initial or predominant manifestation of an inherited demyelinating polyneuropathy, hereditary neuropathy with liability to pressure palsies.

❖ Certain muscular dystrophies affect distal muscles, resulting in foot drop, including myotonic dystrophy, Duchenne and Becker muscular dystrophy.

❖ Amyotrophic lateral sclerosis or Lou Gehrig disease can present with an isolated foot drop caused by motor neuron degeneration.

REFERENCES

Anselmi SJ. Common peroneal nerve compression. J Am Podiatr Med Assoc 2006 Sep-Oct;96(5):413–417.
Gilchrist RV, Bhagia SM, Lenrow DA, et al. Painless foot drop: an atypical etiology of a common presentation. Pain Physician 2002 Oct;5(4):419–421.
Nercessian OA, Ugwonali OF, Park S. Peroneal nerve palsy after total knee arthroplasty. J Arthroplasty 2005 Dec;20(8):1068–1073.

An 8-year-old boy is brought into the emergency room by his mother after he awoke from sleep with right-mouth tingling followed by 1 minute of right facial twitching and drooling. During this spell, he had difficulty speaking. His mother says that when he was 1 year old he had an episode of generalized shaking while ill with a viral gastroenteritis with a fever of 38.9°C (102°F). On further questioning, she recalls that on one occasion when he was 4 years old, he awoke having urinated in his bed and bitten his tongue, and was lethargic for half a day. The family history is significant for childhood seizures in his father, who grew out of them by the time he was 13 years old. The patient has otherwise developed normally, scoring A's in the gifted and talented school program. He has not had any recent fevers or head trauma. On examination, he appears slightly tired but otherwise back to his baseline. His temperature is 36.7°C (98°F); heart rate, 80 beats/min; respiration rate, 18 breaths/min; and blood pressure, 90/60 mmHg. His examination is normal with appropriate comprehension and good fluency, normal funduscopic examination without papilledema, no residual facial paresthesia, and no focal weakness or numbness. His reflexes are normoactive, and his gait is steady. He has no skin lesions. He has no evidence of head trauma, and his neck is soft and supple. His heart, lung, and abdominal examinations are unremarkable.

◆ **What is the most likely diagnosis?**

◆ **What is the next diagnostic step?**

◆ **What is the next step in therapy?**

ANSWERS TO CASE 44: New Onset Seizure, Child

Summary: An 8-year-old healthy boy presents to the ER with a nocturnal episode of facial twitching and speech arrest. He has a history of a similar nocturnal event when he was 4 years old, and a seizure during a fever when he was 1 year old. His father had childhood seizures. The patient's development has been normal. His examination is unremarkable.

◆ **Most likely diagnosis:** Pediatric seizure disorder, history of febrile seizure

◆ **Next diagnostic step:** Rule out status epilepticus, electroencephalograph (EEG), MRI

◆ **Next step in therapy:** Observation in most cases

Analysis

Objectives

1. Understand appropriate terminology to accurately describe seizures.
2. Understand common causes of seizures by age and epileptic syndromes of childhood.
3. Know a diagnostic and treatment approach to new onset seizure in the pediatric population based on historical and examination findings.

Considerations

In the presented case, this 8-year-old boy experienced a characteristic nocturnal seizure with right facial twitching and drooling. His consciousness was preserved. Before 5 years of age, patients can also have secondary generalization, with spread from the facial twitching to involve whole body tonic-clonic activity with incontinence, tongue-biting, and postictal confusion. The patient also has a history of a febrile seizure and family history of childhood seizures, therefore this presentation is highly suggestive of benign rolandic epilepsy, which has an autosomal dominant pattern of inheritance (see Case 49).

However, new onset seizures in the pediatric population can be associated with a variety of acquired or inherited conditions that require practical approach to diagnosis and management.

APPROACH TO NEW ONSET CHILDHOOD SEIZURE

Definitions

Seizure: Single event characterized by abnormal excessive synchronized discharge of cortical neurons. Between 7–10% of people will have a seizure at some point in their lives.

Epilepsy: The tendency to have recurrent seizures with stereotyped cognitive or physical manifestations. The lifetime risk of epilepsy is 3%. Epileptic syndromes can be categorized broadly into generalized epilepsies and localization-related epilepsies.

Generalized epilepsy: Recurrent seizures that arise from both cerebral hemispheres at once because of an inherited predisposition. These include absence seizures, tonic-clonic seizures, atonic seizures, and myoclonic seizures. They occur suddenly without auras or other focal symptoms.

Localization-related epilepsy: Recurrent focal seizures that arise from a single unilateral brain region or multiple discrete areas in the brain. **Idiopathic** causes have a known genetic basis and include autosomal dominant benign rolandic epilepsy and temporal lobe epilepsy, whereas **symptomatic** causes involve acquired pathologies such as strokes, neoplasms, and congenital malformations. **Cryptogenic** causes are associated with clinical, mental, and developmental retardation with no obvious structural lesion.

Simple partial seizure: Focal seizure with no impairment of consciousness. Auras such as odd smell or taste are simple partial seizures.

Complex partial seizure: Focal seizure with impairment of consciousness during or after the event. Both simple and complex partial seizures can spread to produce secondary generalized tonic-clonic seizures with urinary incontinence, tongue-biting, and postictal confusion.

Status epilepticus: A neurologic emergency in which a seizure persists or recurs for 30 minutes without return to baseline mentation. Some authorities believe that seizure activity is unlikely to stop after 5–10 minutes and should be treated sooner to avoid injury.

Clinical Approach

Common Causes of Pediatric Seizures

From the neonatal period until 3 years of age, the most common cause of seizures is prenatal injury, followed in order of decreasing occurrence by perinatal injury, metabolic defects, congenital malformations, CNS infections, and postnatal trauma. In children between 3 and 20 years of age, genetic predisposition is the most common cause, followed by infections, trauma, congenital malformations, and metabolic defects. The four most common hereditary epilepsies are febrile convulsions, benign rolandic epilepsy, childhood absence epilepsy, and juvenile myoclonic epilepsy. The first three syndromes resolve spontaneously. Febrile seizures are very common, occurring in 3–5% of children between 6 months and 3 years of age during illness with high fevers, and should disappear by 5 years of age. Absence epilepsy is a generalized epilepsy characterized by brief staring spells with behavioral arrest, and EEG pattern of generalized 3 Hz spike-and-wave discharges provoked by hyperventilation. Juvenile myoclonic epilepsy involves myoclonic seizures that occur shortly after awakening and generalized tonic-clonic seizures that are triggered by sleep deprivation, and responds well to antiepileptic treatment with valproic acid.

Diagnostic Evaluation of a New Onset Seizure in a Child

The **first priority** in any seizure patient is to determine that active seizures have stopped. **Status epilepticus** is defined as **a seizure lasting longer than 30 minutes or multiple seizures in succession without return to baseline alertness;** this is a neurologic emergency because of the potential to cause permanent brain injury and complications such as hypoxia and autonomic instability. A patient may not be overtly convulsing, but still have impaired mentation with subtle focal twitching in a condition called **nonconvulsive status epilepticus,** which carries similar morbidity. When status epilepticus is suspected, the ABC (airway protection, breathing, and circulation) measures should be mobilized, and antiepileptic medications should be expeditiously administered, beginning with benzodiazepines and phenytoin. STAT chemistries should be checked for correctible metabolic abnormalities such as hypoglycemia and hypocalcemia, as well as other tests as indicated such as toxicology. When status epilepticus has been ruled out or addressed, it will be important to obtain an accurate history and examination of the child to rule out head trauma, infection, developmental abnormalities, and focal neurologic deficits. These atypical features should alert the physician to a symptomatic epilepsy that can be caused by focal etiologies such as stroke, neoplasm, infection, and congenital malformations. Historical description of the seizure can also help to differentiate this patient's localization-related symptomatology from a generalized epilepsy such as absence seizures, which involve staring spells, or primary generalized tonic-clonic seizures.

The EEG can clarify any question of nonconvulsive status epilepticus in somnolent patients, and is recommended after all first childhood seizures for seizure classification. Up to 50% of epilepsy patients will have a normal first EEG. MRI should be performed particularly with an abnormal developmental history or physical examination. If the history and examination suggests infection, a lumbar puncture should be performed and empiric antibiotics initiated promptly. In the neonate with seizures and a suspected metabolic abnormality, serum ammonia, and serum and urine organic acids should be sent.

The patient should be admitted for further monitoring and treatment if altered mental status or focal deficits are slow to resolve, if seizures or a malignant underlying etiology persists, or if there are abnormal findings such as fevers and papilledema. A neurologist should be consulted to assist with diagnosis, therapy, family counseling, and follow-up.

Treatment

Transferral to the intensive care unit for intubation and **continuous EEG and cardiovascular monitoring is necessary when status epilepticus fails to respond to benzodiazepines and phenytoin, and requires further suppression with midazolam or phenobarbital.** For new onset seizures, treatment should be directed at the underlying etiology. Between 20–70% of people with a first unprovoked generalized tonic-clonic seizure will never have a second seizure, so **initiation of antiepileptic agents is usually postponed until the second seizure** or unless there is a high suspicion that epilepsy will ensue. These higher-risk patients are those with focal neurologic deficits, mental retardation, or MRI or EEG abnormalities. **Primary generalized epilepsies** such as **absence seizures** respond better to **valproate and ethosuximide**, while **localization-related epilepsies** should be treated with medications such as **phenytoin or carbamazepine**. Benign rolandic epilepsy has infrequent seizures and can do fine with mere observation. Should the seizures worsen, a medication for partial seizures can be instituted. The patient's parents should be counseled about the importance of not leaving the child in the tub or pool alone, or unmonitored where a seizure can put the child in danger. Teenage patients should be forbidden to drive until they have been seizure-free for at least 6 months.

Comprehension Questions

Match the following etiologies (A-E) to the clinical situation [44.1] to [44.4]:

    A. Symptomatic seizure
    B. Cryptogenic seizure
    C. Primary generalized epilepsy
    D. Localization-related epilepsy
    E. Simple partial seizure

[44.1] A 7-year-old boy is brought to clinic by his mother after complaining of smelling a foul odor.

[44.2] An 8-year-old girl develops seizures. She has dysmorphic facies and is in special education. Her MRI and EEG are normal.

[44.3] A 5-year-old girl is noted by her teacher to have sudden staring spells with blinking while in class.

[44.4] A 3-year-old boy is brought for multiple episodes of right arm stiffening followed by generalized shaking. He is found on MRI to have a left parietal brain tumor.

Answers

[44.1] **E.** Auras are simple partial seizures.

[44.2] **B.** The etiology of a cryptogenic seizure might not be well established for a particular patient, but it is clear that underlying abnormalities exist.

[44.3] **C.** Absence seizures are a form of primary generalized epilepsy and respond well to ethosuximide.

[44.4] **A and D.** The partial seizures with secondary generalization are symptomatic from an identified lesion and will likely continue to recur without antiepileptic therapy.

CLINICAL PEARLS

❖ A new onset seizure often does not progress to epilepsy and can be followed for recurrence before considering the initiation of an antiepileptic agent.

❖ Status epilepticus is a neurologic emergency and can be the presentation of a patient's first seizure. It does not necessarily signify an increased risk for epilepsy.

❖ Persisting altered mental status can be the only manifestation of nonconvulsive status epilepticus, and there should be a low threshold for treating with benzodiazepines or phenytoin while awaiting EEG confirmation.

❖ The history with an accurate description of the seizure and epilepsy will usually provide the highest diagnostic and prognostic yield out of all diagnostic tests available.

❖ Primary generalized epilepsies have the best prognosis.

❖ Benign rolandic epilepsy, febrile seizures, absence seizures, and juvenile myoclonic epilepsy are the four most common inherited epilepsies, and patients will "grow out of" the first three.

❖ Broad spectrum antiepileptic drugs such as valproate are better for treating generalized epilepsy, whereas narrow spectrum drugs such as phenytoin and carbamazepine are more suited for localization related epilepsy.

REFERENCES

Fenichel GM. Clinical pediatric neurology: a signs and symptoms approach, 5th ed. Philadelphia, PA: Saunders; 2005.
Guerrini R. Epilepsy in children. Lancet 2006 Feb 11;367(9509):499–524.

A 22-month-old female is brought to the emergency room (ER) after a 5-minute convulsion at home witnessed by her parents. The child was well until 1 day ago when she developed rhinorrhea, cough, decreased appetite, and increased fussiness. This morning the patient's mother took the child's tympanic membrane temperature and found it to be 39.3°C (102.7°F). Approximately 15 minutes later the patient's father heard a "gurgling" noise coming from the child's room and found the child unresponsive, foaming at the mouth, with "jerking movements" of all four extremities. Both parents estimate that the motor activity persisted for approximately 5 minutes although both report that it "seemed much longer." On examination the patient is sleepy but can be aroused. Her examination is significant only for crusting of the nares and an erythematous oropharynx without exudate. There is no nuchal rigidity or focal findings on her neurologic examination. Her rectal temperature is now 39.5°C (103.2°F), her pulse 110 beats/min, with unlabored breathing at 16 breaths/min and an oxygen saturation of 99%. The child is the product of a full-term uncomplicated pregnancy and went home on day 2 of life. She has had no other significant medical problems. By history she is developmentally on track with an eight-word vocabulary, a normal toddler gait, appropriate fine motor skills, and no hint of developmental regression. There is no history of seizures in the family nor neurologic events except for a stroke in the patient's maternal grandmother at age 78 years.

◆ **What is the most likely diagnosis?**

◆ **What is the next diagnostic step?**

◆ **What is the next step in therapy?**

ANSWERS TO CASE 45: Febrile Seizures

Summary: A 22-month-old previously healthy neurodevelopmentally normal female with a 1-day history of upper respiratory symptoms developed a fever this morning followed by a 5-minute generalized convulsion. Now in the ER, she is febrile and somewhat obtunded but without other significant physical findings.

◆ **Most likely diagnosis:** Simple febrile seizure

◆ **Next diagnostic step:** Evaluation for fever source (such as a nasal wash for viral studies and a complete blood count [CBC])

◆ **Next step in therapy:** Symptomatic treatment of fever (antipyretics)

Analysis

Objectives

1. Understand the difference between provoked and unprovoked seizures as well as between a seizure and epilepsy.
2. Know the criteria for a simple febrile seizure and the definition of a complex febrile seizure.
3. Be aware of the relationship between febrile seizures and the development of epilepsy.
4. Know when a seizure in the context of a fever necessitates further workup or treatment and when reassurance is all that is needed.

Considerations

This 22-month-old child developed a generalized convulsion in association with a fever and is now postictally obtunded without any focal findings on neurologic examination. Since the seizure is now over, attention should first be turned to finding a source for the child's fever. Given the patient's nasal discharge and lack of other symptoms it is most likely caused by a viral upper respiratory infection. If the patient was tachypneic then consideration would have to be given to pneumonia. There is no evidence to suggest a central nervous system infection, neither by history nor on examination. Clearly seizures can occur in association with meningoencephalitis but are rarely the sole manifestation of such a serious infection. Of course, if any clinical suspicion for CNS infection exists, then a lumbar puncture (LP) must be performed to obtain cerebrospinal fluid (CSF) for analysis. In particular, children younger that 12 months presenting with fever and a seizure can have only minimal additional signs of meningitis and an LP should be performed. After 18 months of age, however, an LP can safely be reserved for patients with nuchal rigidity or other suggestive findings on history and examination.

APPROACH TO SEIZURES WITH FEVER

Febrile seizures are common, most are simple, and usually have a benign course; they are, however, a diagnosis of exclusion. In order to be considered a **simple** febrile seizure, a convulsive event must meet certain criteria: (1) patient age between 3 months and 5 years, (2) a generalized seizure without focal elements, (3) a seizure lasting less than 15 minutes, (4) associated with a fever (38.5°C [101°F]) that is not caused by a CNS infection, and (5) occurs only once in a 24-hour period. If the seizure is focal in nature, lasts longer than 15 minutes, or recurs within 24 hours then it is considered to be a **complex** febrile seizure. Febrile seizures, either simple or complex, are a type of *acute symptomatic* or *provoked* seizure just like acute traumatic seizures or alcohol withdrawal convulsions. In fact, febrile seizures are the most common type of provoked seizure—occurring in up to 5 percent of all children in the United States. It is important to understand the difference between epilepsy and an acute symptomatic (provoked) seizure. The former indicates that a patient has had two or more unprovoked seizures separated by at least 24 hours. The later refers to convulsions that occur immediately in response to a precipitating event (such as fever, ischemia, anoxia, or trauma).

Febrile seizures most commonly occur **within the first 24 hours** of an illness with fever and it is not at all unusual for them to be the first manifestation of illness. The underlying illness is more commonly viral than bacterial and may be due to a large number of different causative agents. However, certain viral agents—particularly **human herpesvirus 6**—do seem to be disproportionately associated with febrile convulsions for unknown reasons. There are also familial genetic syndromes that can include febrile seizures as part of the phenotype—particularly the generalized epilepsy with febrile seizures plus (GEFS+) syndromes. In this heterogeneous disorder patients in a given family can have typical febrile seizures or febrile seizures persisting beyond 5 years of age as well as various forms of generalized epilepsy typically beginning in childhood. Significant phenotypic variability is the rule in GEFS+. Mutations in the gene coding for voltage-gated sodium channel subunits (alpha-1, alpha-2, and beta-1) as well as the gamma-2 subunit of the GABA(A) receptor have been found to underlie some of these cases. Furthermore, several genetic loci have been identified which appear to increase the likelihood of febrile seizures without leading to subsequent epilepsy.

For patients who have experienced a **single simple febrile seizure**, the **overall risk of at least one recurrence is approximately 30%.** If the seizure occurred prior to 12 months of age then the risk increases to 50%, and if the seizure occurred after age 3 then the risk is closer to 20%. This might be caused, in part, by the fact that febrile seizures are an age-dependent phenomenon occurring before the age of 5 years. In addition to the age at which the first seizure occurred, the duration of fever and degree of fever appear to be related to recurrence risk. The longer the duration of the fever and the higher the degree of the fever associated with the first febrile convulsion, the lower the risk of recurrence. As might be expected, a family history of febrile seizures also increases the risk of recurrence. **Half of all recurrences occur within 6 months, and 90% will occur within 24 months.**

The relationship between febrile seizures and the subsequent development of afebrile unprovoked seizures (epilepsy) is somewhat complex. Examined retrospectively, approximately 15% of children with epilepsy have a history of febrile seizures earlier in life. However, of all children who experience febrile seizures, only 2 to 4 percent will develop epilepsy—a two- to fourfold increase over the baseline incidence of epilepsy (approximately 1% in the United States). Stated conversely, 96 to 98% of patients with febrile seizures will not develop epilepsy— which is one reason that physicians generally can be quite reassuring in talking to the parents of a child who experiences a simple febrile seizure. Factors that are known to increase the risk of later epilepsy include: (1) preexistent neurodevelopmental problems (such as cerebral palsy or developmental delay), (2) complex febrile seizures, (3) family history of epilepsy, and (4) febrile seizures early in life or associated with mild fevers. Temporal lobe epilepsy (TLE) is the most common type of epilepsy in adults, and there has been significant debate regarding the role that febrile seizures might play in the etiology of TLE. On the one hand, it could be that frequent febrile seizures damage the temporal lobe and lead to epilepsy. On the other hand, the temporal lobe might already be abnormal thereby increasing the patient's susceptibility to febrile seizures. There is data from clinical and animal research to support both of these contentions.

Treatment and Prophylaxis

Although the vast majority of febrile seizures last less than 15 minutes, approximately 5 percent will last 30 minutes or more (febrile status epilepticus). Management of such patients is a medical emergency because **prolonged seizures can cause significant neurologic injury.** As with any acute life-threatening emergency, initial attention must be paid to the patient's **airway, breathing, and circulation**. Subsequent management proceeds as with status epilepticus of any cause: parenteral benzodiazepines followed by phenobarbital. Attention should also be paid to controlling the patient's fever by removing clothing, using a cooling blanket, and administering antipyretics.

As described above, the majority of febrile seizures do not recur, and the vast majority of cases are not associated with development of epilepsy. In other words, most simple febrile seizures can safely be seen as a benign age-limited event. However, they are truly terrifying events for the patient and the patient's family, and a small percentage of patients do develop afebrile seizures. Given these factors, it is not surprising that prophylaxis of febrile seizures has been a longstanding controversy in pediatric neurology. There have been two approaches to prevention: daily medication regimens and intermittent prophylaxis. Although the **daily administration of phenobarbital and valproic acid is effective in reducing the occurrence of febrile seizures**, their **frequent side effects** makes their use in this context difficult to justify. **Intermittent prophylaxis**, giving antipyretics or anticonvulsants only during a febrile illness, decreases the frequency of such side effects. Parents are generally able to anticipate the onset of a febrile illness, although at times the seizure can seem to be the first manifestation. The simplest approach is to treat children with **antipyretics** during an illness, yet this does not seem to reduce the risk of seizures. Treatment with rectal or oral preparations of diazepam during a febrile illness, however, does reduce the risk of recurrence in children who have already had a febrile seizure. Additionally, a rectal diazepam gel (Diastat) can be used to abort a convulsion at home once it has begun. It is not clear, however, whether or not prevention of febrile seizures has any long-term impact on neurodevelopmental outcome.

Comprehension Questions

[45.1] Which of the following would qualify a febrile seizure as *complex*?

A. Loss of consciousness
B. Duration of 14 minutes
C. Focal onset
D. Association with a fever of 38.6°C (101.5°F)
E. Age of 4 years

[45.2] Which of the following has been shown to be effective in preventing the recurrence of febrile seizures with an acceptable side-effect profile?

A. Daily oral phenobarbital
B. Oral valproic acid during febrile illnesses
C. Fever reduction with antipyretics
D. Rectal diazepam
E. Daily phenytoin

[45.3] Which of the following is true regarding the relationship between febrile seizures and the development of subsequent epilepsy?

A. Patients who experience a febrile convulsion are at a high risk of developing epilepsy
B. Patients who have their first febrile seizure older than age 3 are at greater risk of epilepsy than those with a first event younger than 12 months of age
C. Preventing febrile seizures clearly reduces the risk of epilepsy
D. Of patients with a febrile seizure, 96–98% will not develop epilepsy
E. Only patients with a complex febrile seizure develop epilepsy

[45.4] Which of the following patients should have a lumbar puncture?

A. A 3-year-old previously healthy boy now in the ER after a 10-minute generalized seizure in association with a 39.1°C (102.5°F) temperature caused by a viral respiratory illness
B. A 9-month-old girl presenting after a 5-minute generalized seizure in association with a 38.6°C (101.5°F) fever
C. A 7-year-old boy with known epilepsy who has a typical seizure while ill with gastroenteritis
D. A 30-month-old boy now in the ER with his third simple febrile seizure in 6 months

Answers

[45.1] **C.** A febrile seizure is considered complex if it lasts longer that 15 minutes, is focal, or recurs within 24 hours.

[45.2] **D.** Although daily treatment with phenobarbital or valproic acid reduces recurrence, it is associated with significant side effects. Treatment with oral or rectal diazepam during febrile illness is both effective and better tolerated.

[45.3] **D.** Although the risk of epilepsy can double from 1% (population base-line incidence) to 2% or even quadruple to 4%, that still means that 96–98% of patients will never develop epilepsy.

[45.4] **B.** Children younger than 12 months of age can present with minimal or only subtle signs of CNS infections. Of course, an LP should be per-formed in any patient in whom a CNS infection is clinically suspected.

CLINICAL PEARLS

❖ It is critical to differentiate simple from complex febrile seizures—duration greater than 15 minutes, focal, or recurrence in 24 hours are complex.

❖ Treating children with daily phenobarbital to prevent febrile seizures is associated with poorer performance on cognitive tests.

❖ An EEG is not useful in the acute evaluation of simple febrile seizures, because epileptiform abnormalities are present for up to 2 weeks after a seizure regardless of cause.

❖ The peak age of incidence for febrile seizures is approximately 18 months.

❖ The overall risk of recurrence of a simple febrile seizure is 30%.

REFERENCES

Audenaert D, Van Broeckhoven C, De Jonghe P. Genes and loci involved in febrile seizures and related epilepsy syndromes. Human Mutat 2006;27(5):391–401.

Nakayama J, Aranami T. Molecular genetics of febrile seizures. Epilepsy Res 2006;70S:S190–S198.

Rosman NP. Febrile seizures. In: Pellock J, Dodson W, Bourgeois B, eds. Pediatric epilepsy: diagnosis and therapy. New York: Demos Medical Publishing; 2001:163–175.

A 13-year-old right-hand dominant girl has increasingly frequent headaches over the past year. She has "always" had headaches, but they became more bothersome approximately 3 years ago in association with onset of menses, and decreased sleep. Her typical headache begins with a sense of slowed thinking and malaise followed soon after by a throbbing pain over the left side of her head, the right side of her head or, at times, over her forehead. The pain increases to its maximum severity of 8 to 9 out of 10 over the course of approximately 1 hour and will last for "many hours" if untreated. The patient reports that even light touch over the affected part of her head causes pain, and she is sensitive to bright lights and loud sounds. She typically feels nauseous and will occasionally have emesis. Acetaminophen and ibuprofen seem to help, but the best pain relief comes with sleeping in a dark room. After the pain resolves, she feels cognitively slow and "out of sorts" for up to a full day. Over the past year, however, the frequency of such attacks has increased to once every 2 to 3 weeks leading to frequent missed days in school and a drop in school performance. They seem to be associated with menses or poor sleep. Her physical examination and neurologic examination are completely normal. She consistently has had motion sickness "for as long as she can remember." Neurodevelopmentally she met all milestones. The patient's mother had "bad headaches" as a teenager and young adult and she has a maternal aunt who was diagnosed with migraines at approximately 20 years of age. No other neurologic diseases are noted in the family.

◆ **What is the most likely diagnosis?**

◆ **What is the next diagnostic step?**

◆ **What is the next step in therapy?**

ANSWERS TO CASE 46: Pediatric Headache

Summary: This 13-year-old right-handed healthy girl presents with a history of recurrent hemicranial headaches that are throbbing with moderate to moderately severe pain in a crescendo-decrescendo pattern associated with nausea and occasional emesis. She also reports photophobia and phonophobia. The headaches will last for many hours untreated, are improved somewhat with low doses of acetaminophen, and resolve if the patient can get to sleep. There is a brief prodrome of malaise and a more prolonged postdrome of cognitive dulling. The only noted triggers are sleep deprivation and strong odors, and she has noted an association with her menstrual cycle. Her neurologic examination is completely normal, and her family history is significant for two people with probable migraines.

◆ **Most likely diagnosis:** Migraine without aura (*common migraine*).

◆ **Next diagnostic step:** No diagnostic workup necessary at this point.

◆ **Next step in therapy:** Trial of appropriately dosed nonsteroidal antiinflammatory drugs (NSAIDs) followed by a trial of triptans if necessary. Consider prophylactic therapy given headache frequency.

Analysis

Objectives

1. Understand the difference between primary and secondary headaches.
2. Know the clinical criteria for pediatric migraine headaches.
3. Understand the role of neuroimaging in evaluating headaches.
4. Know the different options available for acute abortive therapy for pediatric migraines.
5. Recognize when daily prophylactic therapy is warranted in migraine treatment and what possible options exist.

Considerations

This otherwise healthy and neurodevelopmentally normal 13-year-old girl is brought in for evaluation of frequent headaches. Because she is currently headache-free with a normal neurologic examination, attention can be turned to classifying her headache disorder, which will aid in dictating any necessary workup and intervention. A primary headache is one in which the head pain itself is the principal clinical entity, and there is no other underlying causative disorder. Tension-type headaches and migraine headaches would be common examples of such conditions. Secondary headaches, conversely, are headaches caused by another underlying disorder such as intracranial hemorrhage, central nervous system infection, temporomandibular joint pain, or substance abuse. In general, secondary headaches are defined by the underlying principal problem and require a more extensive and prompt evaluation. Primary headaches, however, are generally defined by their clinical symptoms and can require no workup if clinical criteria are met. The history in this scenario is classic for migraine with the unilateral aspect, throbbing, aura, family history, and triggers.

APPROACH TO PEDIATRIC HEADACHE

Head pain in children and adults can be divided into primary and secondary headaches. It can also be useful to consider the pattern of the patient's headaches: (1) **acute recurrent**—episodic head pain with pain-free intervals in between, (2) **chronic progressive**—gradually worsening head pain with no pain-free intervals, (3) **chronic daily** headache—a persistent headache that neither worsens nor remits, and (4) a **mixed headache**—a chronic daily headache with episodic exacerbations. **Chronic progressive headaches raise the possibility of increasing intracranial pressure** and require further evaluation with neuroimaging. Chronic daily headaches can be a secondary headache caused by cerebral venous sinus thrombosis, or can arise from a primary headache disorder. This condition as well as mixed headaches can require referral to a headache specialist.

In 2004, the International Headache Society defined the criteria for pediatric migraine:

- A. Headache attack lasting 1 to 72 hours
- B. Headache has at least two of the following four features:
    - (1) Either bilateral or unilateral (frontal/temporal) location
    - (2) Pulsating quality
    - (3) Moderate to severe intensity
    - (4) Aggravated by routine physical activities
- C. At least one of the following accompanies headache:
    - (1) Nausea and/or vomiting
    - (2) Photophobia and phonophobia (can be inferred from their behavior)
- D. Five or more attacks fulfilling the above criteria

The mean age of onset for pediatric migraine is approximately 7 years of age for boys and 11 years of age for girls. With regards to prevalence, 8–23% of children meet criteria for migraines in the second decade of life making such primary headaches a very common problem. Although migraines can be seen in children as young as 3 years of age, the prevalence is less than 3%. This is likely an underestimate, however, given the difficulty of making the diagnosis in very young children. Migraines commonly "run in families" and have a significant genetic component although only relatively rare migraine syndromes have been directly linked to a single gene mutation. Many cases of familial hemiplegic migraine, for example, have been linked to a mutation in the CACNA1A gene that encodes a voltage gated P/Q-type calcium channel. One interesting association with migraine is that many patients report having motion sickness (i.e., "carsickness") as children. Although this clinical finding is useful if present, its absence in no way diminishes the possibility of migraine.

As in adults, migraines in children often begin with a prodromal premonitory phase with neurologic or constitutional symptoms lasting for hours or days before the headache. These "warning signs" can slowly increase over time or remain constant. Some patients develop an aura prior to the onset of pain that consists of a stereotyped focal symptom usually preceding the headache by no more than an hour. Visual auras are the most common type and can involve a variety of visual aberrations such as scotomata, flashes, or geometric forms. Motor, sensory, and cognitive auras can also be seen. The pattern of the pain is typically crescendo in onset and decrescendo in offset and is certainly not maximal from the beginning. As the pain continues the patient often develops cutaneous allodynia, which means that normally non-noxious stimulation is perceived as painful during the headache. Associated elements such as nausea, photophobia, phonophobia, vertigo, and nasal congestion are common. Following the headache, most patients experience a post-dromal phase with symptoms such as difficulty concentrating, particular food cravings, and fatigue. Triggers commonly associated with migraine headaches include strong smells, particularly if noxious, exercise, sleep deprivation, missing meals, and mild head trauma. Many patients associate certain foods with the onset of their migraines, but this can at times be difficult to distinguish between food-cravings occurring during the prodromal phase. Women with migraines are more likely to experience headaches around the time of menses.

Evaluation

A careful history and physical examination are the most important aspects of the evaluation. When the history is unequivocally consistent with migraine and the neurologic examination is completely normal, no further workup is needed. In particular, neuroimaging is unnecessary, and the yield is low. However, an abnormal neurologic examination, or worrisome feature on history necessitates an MRI scan. Although most parents fear the presence of a brain tumor, more than 98% of patients with intracranial masses have abnormalities on their neurologic examination. It is important that the neurologic examination include an assessment of head circumference, visualization of the optic discs, assessment of nuchal rigidity, and palpation of the sinuses in order to carefully screen for underlying causes. Electroencephalography (EEG) is not routinely indicated in the evaluation of headaches. Patients with epilepsy often have postictal headaches, but it would be quite unusual for the headache to be the primary presenting complaint. Lumbar puncture is essential if head pain is thought to be caused by a CNS infection and is part of the evaluation of subarachnoid hemorrhage (if a CT scan is unrevealing). It has no routine role in the evaluation of primary headache disorders, however.

Treatment and Management

Treatment of migraine focuses on two concepts: **acute pain relief (abortive therapy) and headache prevention (prophylactic therapy).** There are an ever-increasing number of available medications that can be used for abortive therapy with few controlled trials to help guide decision making. Perhaps the best studied medications are ibuprofen and acetaminophen and both have been shown to be safe and effective in children. Many patients will already have tried such medications prior to coming to see their doctor, but they often have been underdosed or given the medication late in the headache, which renders it as much less effective. In such patients, it is worth a trial of adequately dosed ibuprofen (10 mg/kg) or acetaminophen (15 mg/kg) given as soon as possible after the onset of the pain. If these medications prove ineffective, then a trial of 5-hydroxytryptamine receptor agonists (the *triptans*) is indicated. These agents are available in a variety of formulations and also differ from one another in terms of half-life. At present, the best pediatric data supports the use of **sumatriptan nasal spray as an abortive agent in children.** Oral formulations and subcutaneous injections have not been subjected to adequate trials in children at this point.

For patients with frequent migraines (e.g., two or more a month) or particularly long-lasting or disabling migraines, daily prophylactic medications can be considered with the treatment goal being to decrease headache frequency. Compliance with a daily medication is a requirement. Sometimes, avoidance of triggers can significantly diminish headache frequency obviating the need for prophylactic medications. Simple lifestyle modification, such as keeping to a regular schedule of eating and sleeping and avoiding triggers, can significantly decrease their headache burden. Should medication be necessary, several classes of pharmacologic agents are used as prophylactic treatments: beta-blockers, tricyclic antidepressants, antihistamines, calcium channel blockers, and anticonvulsants. As is the case with abortive therapies, much better data exists for the use of prophylactic medications in adults. Cyproheptadine has long been used in younger children for this purpose, but supportive data is based on retrospective non-blinded trials. Similarly, amitriptyline is somewhat sedating although generally well tolerated, but its efficacy has only been shown in retrospective studies. The use of anticonvulsants, particularly topiramate, for migraine prophylaxis is increasing in both adult and pediatric patients. Although good quality studies have supported its use in adults, there have yet to be adequate clinical trials in children.

Comprehension Questions

[46.1] Which of the following would be classified as a secondary headache?

    A. Migraine with aura

    B. Cluster headaches

    C. Subarachnoid hemorrhage

    D. Migraine without aura

    E. Tension-type headaches

[46.2] Which of the following is a criteria for pediatric migraine?

    A. A visual aura preceding the onset of head pain

    B. Pain improved by physical activity

    C. Moderate to severe intensity of head pain

    D. A family history of migraine

    E. Response to nonsteroidal antiinflammatory medication

[46.3] Which of the following patients should have neuroimaging as part of the evaluation of their headache?

    A. An 18-year-old girl who was found unconscious at home and is now in the emergency room with the worst headache of her life

    B. A 14-year-old boy with acute recurrent attacks of moderate intensity throbbing hemicranial pain associated with nausea and photophobia

    C. A 12-year-old straight-A student who is healthy and neurodevelopmentally normal, but who complains of mild squeezing head pain when he is studying for tests

    D. A 17-year-old boy who develops a moderate global headache one day after he decides to quit drinking coffee "cold turkey"

[46.4] Which of the following is the best initial choice for abortive therapy for a child with migraines?

    A. Topiramate

    B. Naproxen

    C. Rizatriptan

    D. Ibuprofen

    E. Amitriptyline

Answers

[46.1] **C.** A headache caused by a subarachnoid hemorrhage would be classified as a secondary headache disorder. All of the other listed possibilities are primary headaches.

[46.2] **C.** To meet criteria, the patient must have had five or more headaches with certain characteristics including moderate to severe pain. A family history of migraines, while common and helpful, is not required for the diagnosis.

[46.3] **A.** This history is very concerning for a subarachnoid hemorrhage and requires an emergent CT scan.

[46.4] **D.** A trial of ibuprofen at an adequate dose (10 mg/kg) would be the best choice.

CLINICAL PEARLS

❖ Having migraine headaches doubles the chance that a patient will have epilepsy, and having epilepsy doubles a patient's chance of having migraines.

❖ It is not uncommon for patients with migraines to experience vertigo in association with their headaches. If associated without headache, it is termed a *migraine equivalent*.

❖ Although migraine headaches are classically described as unilateral (*hemicranial*), this is actually only true in approximately 60% of all headaches. It is quite common for migraines to be bifrontal.

❖ Asking what the patient does during a headache is a key clinical question. Patients with migraines generally report wanting to lay still in a darkened room and wanting to go to sleep. Although not all migraine headaches are severe, headaches which do not interrupt a patient's activities are unlikely to be migrainous.

REFERENCES

Damen L, Bruijn J, Verhagen A, et al. Symptomatic treatment of migraine in children: a systematic review of medication trials. Pediatrics 2005;116:295–302.

Lewis, D. Headaches in children and adolescents. Am Fam Physician 2002;65: 625–632.

Lewis D, Ashwal S, Hershey A, et al. Practice parameter: pharmacological treatment of migraine headache in children and adolescents: Report of the American Academy of Neurology Quality Standards Subcommittee and the Practice Committee of the Child Neurology Society. Neurology 2004;63:2215–2224.

Young W, Silberstein S. Migraine: spectrum of symptoms and diagnosis. Continuum 2006;12(6):67–86.

A 3-year-old boy is brought to his pediatrician to be evaluated for difficulty walking and clumsiness. According to his parents, the patient began walking at the age of 18 months, but in the past year he has begun to fall more frequently and has difficulty getting up from the floor; often supporting himself with his hands along the length of his legs. Birth and developmental history until symptom onset are reportedly normal. There is no contributing family history.

On physical examination the young boy has significant muscle weakness of his hip flexors, knee extensors, deltoids, and biceps muscles. His calves are large, and he walks on his toes during ambulation. Laboratory studies reveal an elevated serum creatine kinase (CK) level of greater than 900. Electromyography of his muscles reveals a myopathy. Nerve conduction studies reveal relative normal nerve function.

◆ **What is the most likely diagnosis?**

◆ **What is the next diagnostic step?**

◆ **What is the next step in therapy?**

ANSWERS TO CASE 47: Duchenne Muscular Dystrophy

Summary: A 3-year-old boy presents with regression of motor milestones with gait instability. His examination is significant for proximal muscle weakness, toe walking, and calf enlargement. Diagnostic studies are significant for a primary muscle disorder with myopathic changes on electrodiagnostic testing and significantly elevated levels of a muscle enzyme, creatinine kinase.

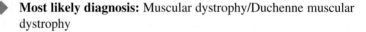 **Most likely diagnosis:** Muscular dystrophy/Duchenne muscular dystrophy

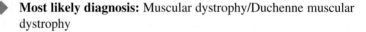 **Next diagnostic step:** Skeletal muscle biopsy

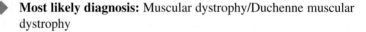 **Next step in therapy:** Supportive management of mobility and monitoring of cardiac and respiratory function

Analysis

Objectives

1. Know the clinical presentation of the most common child hood onset muscular dystrophy.
2. Be familiar with the diagnostic workup of muscular dystrophies.
3. Be familiar with the treatment and management of Duchenne muscular dystrophy.

Considerations

The regression of motor milestones in a previously healthy male toddler is suggestive of a neuromuscular disorder in the absence of delays in other developmental milestones. The diagnostic studies are supportive of a primary muscle disorder. An important consideration in this case is the clinical presentation. The toddler has proximal muscle weakness resulting in gait instability (toe walking) and inability to rise from a sitting position or from a fall; often requiring the child to push on his knees to upright himself. The electromyographic and nerve conduction studies reveal a muscle problem. The elevated muscle enzyme, creatinine kinase, supports a destructive process. Thus, the clinical consideration is of a primary myopathy, either acquired or inherited. In this case, the toddler presents with regression of motor milestones, enlarged calves, and an elevated creatinine kinase, and no family history. Although not completely specific, the presentation is highly suggestive of Duchenne muscular dystrophy, the most common form of muscular dystrophy (MD). It is caused by the absence of dystrophin, a protein involved in maintaining the integrity of muscle. The most distinctive feature of Duchenne MD (DMD) is a progressive proximal MD with characteristic enlargement (pseudohypertrophy) of the calves. The bulbar (extraocular) muscles are spared, but the myocardium is affected. There is massive elevation of CK levels in the blood, myopathic changes by electromyography, and myofiber degeneration with fibrosis and fatty infiltration on muscle biopsy. DMD has an X-linked inheritance pattern, affecting only males. In the absence of a family history, a patient is unlikely to be diagnosed younger than the age of 2 or 3 years. Most boys with DMD walk alone at a later age than average. Parents usually worry something unusual in the way the child walks, due to frequent falling or difficulty rising from the ground or going up steps. The serum creatinine kinase level is always at least five times the upper limit of normal and makes the diagnosis of DMD probable. However, the diagnosis is confirmed by muscle biopsy and/or genetic testing.

APPROACH TO DUCHENNE/BECKER MUSCULAR DYSTROPHY

Definitions

Myopathy: Disorders in which the primary symptom is muscle weakness because of dysfunction of muscle fiber.

Creatinine kinase: An enzyme found primarily in the heart and skeletal muscles, and to a lesser extent in the brain. Significant injury to any of these structures will lead to a measurable increase in serum CK levels.

Muscular dystrophy: Inherited disease characterized by progressive weakness and degeneration of the skeletal muscles that control movement.

X-linked inheritance: Inherited disease passed from mother to son because of a genetic abnormality on the X chromosome.

Dystrophin protein: Rod-shaped protein, and a vital part of a protein complex that connects the cytoskeleton of a muscle fiber to the surrounding extracellular matrix through the cell membrane. Its gene is the longest known to date and accounts for 0.1% of the human genome.

Clinical Approach

Clinical Features and Epidemiology

Dystrophin-associated MDs are the most common types of inherited muscular dystrophy and are characterized by rapid progression of muscle degeneration that occurs early in life. The severe form occurs earlier and is called Duchenne, and the milder form, which can occur later, is called Becker MD (BMD). Both are caused by the same genetic mutation and follow an X-linked inheritance pattern, affecting mainly males—an estimated 1 in 3500 boys worldwide. Symptoms usually appear younger than age 6, but can appear as early as infancy. Patients present with progressive muscle weakness of the legs and pelvis, which is associated with a loss of muscle mass or muscle atrophy. Muscle weakness occurs in the arms, neck, and other areas, but it is usually not as severe or with as early an onset as the muscles of the lower extremities. Calf muscles initially grow larger because of replacement of muscle tissue with fat and connective tissue, a condition called pseudohypertrophy. With progressive weakness, muscle contractures occur in the hips, knees, and ankles. Thus, the muscles are unusable because the muscle fibers shorten and fibrosis (scarring) occurs in connective tissue. By age 10 years, braces might be required for walking, and by age 12 years, most patients are confined to a wheelchair. Bones develop abnormally, causing skeletal deformities of the spine (scoliosis) and other areas.

Muscular weakness and skeletal deformities contribute to respiratory or breathing problems, leading to frequent infections and often requiring assisted ventilation. **Cardiac muscle is also commonly affected**, leading to cardiomyopathy and in almost all cases leading to congestive heart failure and arrhythmias. Intellectual impairment can occur, but it is not inevitable and does not worsen as the disorder progresses. Death usually occurs by 25 years of age, typically from respiratory (lung) disorders.

BMD is very similar to DMD and is caused by a mutation of the dystrophin gene on the X chromosome, however, BMD progresses at a much slower rate. It occurs in approximately 3–6 in 100,000 male births. Symptoms usually appear in males at approximately age 12 years, but can sometimes begin later. The average age of becoming unable to walk is 25–30 years. Women rarely develop symptoms. Muscle weakness is slowly progressive, causing difficulty with running, hopping, jumping, and eventually, walking. Patients may be able to walk well into adulthood, but it is associated with instability and frequent falls. Similar to DMD, patients experience respiratory weakness, skeletal deformities, and muscle contractures and pseudohypertrophy of calf muscles. **Heart disease is also commonly associated, but heart failure is rare.**

Etiology and Pathogenesis

The particular gene mutation that causes Duchenne and Becker muscular dystrophies (DBMD) is found on the X chromosome and results in loss of a functional muscle protein, dystrophin. A functional copy of the gene is needed for normal muscle function. In females, one functional copy is usually enough to compensate, and a female with a *DBMD* mutation usually has few or no symptoms. Most boys with *DBMD* inherited the mutation from their mother. However, in about 30% of the patients with *DBMD,* it is a result of a new mutation. In these cases, it is unlikely that future children will also have *DBMD.*

Dystrophin is considered a key structural element in the muscle fiber, and the stabilization of the muscle plasma membrane, and possibly has a role of signaling (Fig. 47–1). Mechanically induced damage through muscle contractions puts a high stress on fragile membranes that could eventually lead to loss of regulatory processes leading to cell death. Altered regeneration, inflammation, impaired vessel response, and fibrosis are probably later events that take part in the muscular dystrophy.

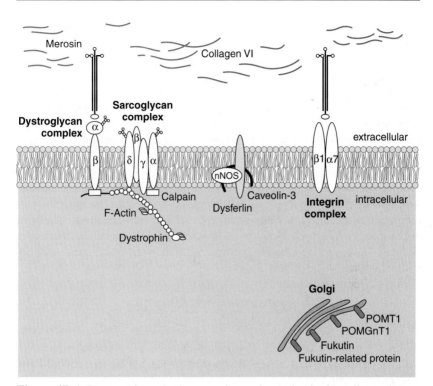

Figure 47–1. Dystrophin and other sarcolemmal proteins in the cell membrane. (*With permission from Kasper DL, Braunwal E, Fauci A, et al. Harrison's principles of internal medicine, 16th ed. New York: McGraw-Hill; 2004: Fig. 368–1.*)

Diagnosis

The diagnosis of DMD and BMD depends on obtaining a complete medical and family history and documentation of muscle weakness and pseudohypertrophy on physical examination. Diagnostic tests include measurement of a muscle enzyme, creatinine kinase, in the blood. Because of the release of CK from damaged muscles, high blood levels of CK in DMD is often at least five times as high as the maximum for unaffected people. It is sometimes 50 to 100 times as high. In addition, electrodiagnostic studies of nerve and muscle function (electromyography and nerve conduction studies) will confirm abnormal muscle function (myopathy) and the pattern or distribution of muscle dysfunction, in the absence of a peripheral nerve disorder. Muscle biopsy is often diagnostic of the disease with confirmation of muscle pathology and a loss or decrease of the dystrophin protein.

DNA from a person with DMD or BMD can be tested to see if the genetic defect is present. If so, testing for that defect can be offered to other family members. It is used to determine probabilities of carrier status and also for prenatal diagnosis but should not be the sole basis for diagnosis as standard DNA analysis might not reveal the gene defect in a patient.

Treatment and Management

Treatment is aimed at control of symptoms to maximize the quality of life. Modalities can include physical therapy, respiratory therapy, speech therapy, orthopedic appliances used for support, and corrective orthopedic surgery. Drug therapy includes corticosteroids to slow muscle degeneration, anticonvulsants to control seizures and some muscle activity, immunosuppressants to delay some damage to dying muscle cells, and antibiotics to fight respiratory infections. Some individuals can benefit from occupational therapy and assistive technology. Some patients might need assisted ventilation to treat respiratory muscle weakness and a pacemaker for cardiac abnormalities. Therefore, patients require multispecialty care from neurologists, rehabilitative services, pulmonologists, and cardiologists.

Comprehension Questions

[47.1] A young child is brought into the pediatric neurologist's office because of progressive weakness. The neurologist is contemplating a diagnosis between Becker and Duchenne muscular dystrophies. Which of the following statements is most accurate regarding these two conditions?

A. BMD differs from DMD because of later onset and different inheritance pattern

B. BMD is similar to DMD because of a shared genetic mutation and inheritance pattern

C. Mothers of BMD and DMD patients are often symptomatic in late adulthood

D. BMD is a more rapidly progressive form of DMD

[47.2] A 32-year-old woman is 32 weeks pregnant, and is a known carrier for DMD. She asks what the ramifications are for her unborn child. Which of the following statements is most accurate?

A. 25% of her daughters will be affected with the disease

B. 50% percent of her daughters will be carriers

C. 75% of her sons will be affected with the disease

D. 100% of sons will either be carriers or inherit the disease

[47.3] Which of the following diagnostic tests is supportive in diagnosing DMD/BMD?

A. Serum creatinine kinase

B. Echocardiogram

C. Pulmonary lung function tests

D. MRI of the brain and spine

Answers

[47.1] **B.** BMD is very similar to DMD and because of a mutation of the dystrophin gene on the X chromosome with a male specific inheritance pattern, however, BMD progresses at a much slower rate.

[47.2] **B.** Because males have only one X chromosome, a male carrying a copy with a dystrophin gene mutation will have the condition. Because females have two copies of the X chromosome, a female can have one copy with a *DBMD* mutation and one functional copy. Thus a mother who is a carrier has a 50% chance passing the mutation to her sons or daughters. Of those children, 50% of the boys will have the disease, and 50% of the girls will be carriers.

[47.3] **A.** CK in DMD is often at least five times as high as the maximum for unaffected people. Because it is a primary skeletal muscle disorder, the other mentioned tests are of limited value.

CLINICAL PEARLS

❖ Duchenne and Becker muscular dystrophy are X-linked. When the woman is a carrier for the dystrophin mutation, half of her sons will have the disease, and half of her daughters will be carriers.

❖ Behavioral studies have shown that DMD boys have a cognitive impairment and a lower IQ (average 85) because of mutant dystrophin in neurons.

❖ Corticosteroids can be beneficial in the treatment of DMD and can be offered as a treatment option.

❖ Elevated creatinine kinase levels is very typical for DMD.

REFERENCES

Deconinck N, Dan B. Pathophysiology of Duchenne muscular dystrophy: current hypotheses. Pediatr Neurol 2007 Jan;36(1):1–7.

Kakulas BA. The differential diagnosis of the human dystrophinopathies and related disorders. Curr Opin Neurol 1996 Oct;9(5):380–388.

Kalra V. Muscular dystrophies. Indian J Pediatr 2000 Dec;67(12):923–928.

Neuromuscular Disease Center. Home page. Available at: http://www.neuro.wustl. edu/neuromuscular/.

Mayo Clinic. Muscular dystrophy. Available at: http://www.mayoclinic.com/ health/ muscular-dystrophy/DS00200/DSECTION=3.

An 8-year-old boy is brought to the neurologist's office on the recommendation of the allergist. His parents complain that their son is constantly clearing his throat and coughing, repetitive jerking hand movement and dystonic neck posturing. These symptoms started approximately 1 year ago. The child has a socially disturbing habit of constantly touching his genital region and recently has been having difficulty paying attention at school. The child had a normal birth and development with no recent illnesses. He suffered from night terrors when he was 4 years old and still occasionally exhibits sleepwalking. Family history is remarkable for his older brother with attention-deficit disorder (ADD). On examination, the patient is a quiet, cooperative boy in no apparent distress. He admits to the stated behavior and reports that he has an overwhelming desire to clear his throat, which he is unable to suppress. When reminded of this behavior, he started to manifest it despite an obvious attempt to control it. He exhibits multiple repetitive stereotyped jerking movements of his hand and shoulder as well as twisting movement of his neck. He states that he is aware of these movements and can control them for a short period of time with mounting tension, which results in an inevitable release with more exaggerated behavior. The child manifested an unusual insight into his behavior and appeared to be highly intelligent and motivated. He is embarrassed by his habit of touching his genitals but cannot resist an urge and instead attempts to cover it up by adjusting his clothing.

◆ **What is the most likely diagnosis?**

◆ **What is the next diagnostic step?**

◆ **What is the next step in therapy?**

ANSWER TO CASE 48: Tourette Syndrome

Summary: An 8-year-old boy with a 12-month history of motor and phonic tics accompanied by obsessive-compulsive behavior that affects his performance in school.

◆ **Most likely diagnosis:** Tourette syndrome with concurrent obsessive-compulsive disorder (OCD).

◆ **Next diagnostic step:** Tourette syndrome is purely a clinical diagnosis and does not require any additional testing.

◆ **Next step in therapy:** Education of parents, teachers, community. Pharmacologic therapy if indicated.

Analysis

Objectives

1. Know the diagnostic criteria for Tourette syndrome and its comorbidities.
2. Know etiology of tics other than Tourette syndrome.
3. Understand management of tics and accompanied behavioral symptoms.

Considerations

This 8-year-old boy has been noted to have phonic and motor tics. He has obsessive-compulsive tendencies and is having performance issues in school. His examination is otherwise unremarkable. This boy most likely has Tourette syndrome. Tics are the clinical hallmark of Tourette syndrome. Tics are brief and episodic movements or sounds induced by internal stimuli that are only temporarily suppressible. Of note, the tics associated with Tourette syndrome are often **suggestible**; discussing the tics leads to an irrepressible manifestation despite attempts to control them. A full evaluation including physical examination, assessment for illicit drugs, mental status examination, and neurologic examination are important. The most important aspect of therapy is education, as it can be very distressing for both child and parents.

APPROACH TO SUSPECTED TOURETTE SYNDROME

Definitions

Tics: Brief and episodic movements or sounds induced by internal stimuli that are only temporary suppressible.

Autistic spectrum disorders: Impaired social interactions, poorly developed language, and frequent cognitive impairment.

Obsessions and compulsions: *Obsessions* are intense and often intrusive thoughts, which compel patients to perform mostly meaningless, time-consuming, and sometimes embarrassing rituals or *compulsions*.

Clinical Approach

Although Tourette syndrome is the most common cause of childhood-onset tics, there are many other neurologic and psychiatric disorders that exhibit tics as part of its presentation. The differential is based on other accompanied symptoms. Autistic spectrum disorders usually manifest by impaired social interactions, poorly developed language, and frequent cognitive impairment. Although symptoms of Tourette syndrome and OCD can lead to certain self-imposed social isolation, children with Tourette syndrome have excellent insight into their condition and can interact fully with the environment in which they are accepted. There is usually no cognitive or intellectual deficits associated with Tourette syndrome. Such progressive neurodegenerative disorders as neuroacanthocytosis and Huntington disease can often present with tics but rapidly develop other hyperkinetic movements that differentiate them from Tourette syndrome.

Tourette syndrome is a neuropsychiatric disorder characterized by motor and phonic tics usually starting in childhood and often accompanied by poor impulse control, OCD, and attention-deficit/hyperactivity disorder (ADHD) (Jankovic, 1987; Feigin and Clarke, 1998). The cause of TS is unknown, but it appears to be inherited in many cases.

Tics are the clinical hallmark of TS. Tics are brief and episodic movements or sounds induced by internal stimuli that are only temporarily suppressible. It is often difficult to differentiate tics from compulsive movements, which are also semivoluntary, but instead induced by unwanted feeling or compulsion. For example, in our patient touching of genitalia is probably not a tic, but a compulsion, but throat clearing, coughing, and hand jerking are simple phonic and motor tics.

Tics are divided into **simple** and **complex.** Simple motor tics involve single groups of muscles, causing jerk-like movement in cases of clonic tics, or briefly sustained posture in cases of dystonic or tonic tics. Simple clonic tics include blinking, head or limb jerking, and nose twitching. Simple dystonic tics include oculogyric deviation, bruxism, blepharospasm, and torticollis-like posturing. Most common tonic tics include tensing of abdominal and other muscles.

Simple phonic tics include coughing, sniffing, throat clearing, and grunting among others.

Complex motor tics include coordinated movements, which involve multiple muscles and often resemble normal movements. They vary from head shaking to touching and hitting. Complex tics should be considered a compulsion if it is preceded by obsessive thought, anxiety, or fear. Complex tics are often camouflaged by incorporating them into seemingly planned and purposeful movement.

Some patients become experts at those so-called *parakinesias*, confusing the clinical picture. Complex phonic tics include linguistically meaningful verbalizations. Although rare, but notoriously associated with Tourette syndrome, is shouting obscenities or profanities called **coprolalia.** More common, however, is repetition of someone else's or one's own words or sentences (**echo-** or **palilalia**).

In contrast to most other hyperkinetic movement disorders, tics are episodic, repetitive and often stereotypic, being mistaken for mannerisms. Tics wax and wane and vary in frequency and intensity. They are unpredictable and often change distribution. Most patients report an ability to suppress tics with mental effort at the expense of mounting inner tension with eventual explosive release in the more appropriate environment. Despite common belief, suppressibility is not unique to tics. Tics are often exacerbated by stress, fatigue, or exposure to heat. The unique feature of tics is suggestibility. No other movement disorders have this feature. Also in contrast to other hyperkinetic movements, motor and phonic tics can persist during all stages of sleep (Jankovic 1984).

In addition to tics, patients with Tourette syndrome exhibit multiple behavioral symptoms including ADHD and OCD. Both, like Tourette syndrome, are clinically diagnosed, and no tests or imaging is required. Those comorbidities often interfere with learning and social activities more than tics. It is essential to recognize and treat those symptoms to help an affected child.

It is important to elucidate family history of ADHD and OCD, which are now well accepted as part of the spectrum of neurobehavioral symptoms of Tourette syndrome. In our case, a family history of ADD in his older brother, and obsessive-compulsive behavior (OCB) in father, add to the diagnostic certainty of Tourette syndrome in this patient. *Obsessions* are intense and often intrusive thoughts, which compel patients to perform mostly meaningless, time-consuming, and sometimes embarrassing rituals or *compulsions*. In contrast to primary OCD, in Tourette syndrome symptoms rarely relate to hygiene and compulsive cleaning. They more commonly involved symmetry, requiring constant rearrangement; forced touching; fear of harming self or family; and overwhelming desire to do things "right" (in a very strict predetermined way). One of the most distressing symptoms of Tourette syndrome is a self-injurious behavior, which varies from minor skin damage by biting or scratching, to life-threatening injuries. These irresistible urges are not tics, but obsessions followed by a compulsive injurious behavior.

Treatment

The first and most important step in the management of Tourette syndrome is education of the patient and caregivers, which in their turn should educate teachers, coaches, and principals. Most Tourette syndrome patients do not need medications, but require reassurance and help in arranging the most productive environment for the child at school and at home.

However, if education and behavioral modification are not enough, medications can be considered to improve the child's performance and facilitate social interactions. Most physicians attempt to treat tics, however, priority should be given not to the most visible, but to the most disturbing symptoms, which are often related to the child's ADHD or OCD. Tics should be treated if they interfere with school or work, cause embarrassment, and disturb others to a degree that patient avoids social interactions. The most effective pharmacologic agents for tic suppression are dopamine receptor blocking agents. Haloperidol (Haldol) and pimozide (Orap) are the only neuroleptics that are approved by the FDA for the treatment of Tourette syndrome. Typical neuroleptics such as Haldol, despite being effective, are rarely used as first-line therapy because of the side effects. Most feared side effects of the long-term neuroleptic therapy are tardive dyskinesia and hepatotoxicity. That is why most specialists use so-called *atypical neuroleptics* such as fluphenazine (Prolixin) and pimozide as the first-line pharmacotherapy because they reportedly have lower incidence of tardive dyskinesia as well as less sedation.

In addition to dopamine receptor blockers, dopamine depleter, tetrabenazine, was found to be effective in treatment of tics. Unfortunately, it is not available in the United States. The second line of tic therapy includes clonazepam, naltrexone, and even botulinum toxin injections for the specific, well defined tic. Botulinum toxin injections were found to be beneficial also in the treatment of phonic tics including coprolalia (Jankovic, 1994). Unfortunately the benefit from injection lasts on average 3–4 months, and then the patient needs to be reinjected.

Often tics do not present a major concern to the patient, but behavioral symptoms that do not respond to more conservative approach of behavioral modification and classroom adjustments require pharmacotherapy. The most effective agents for the treatment of ADHD are CNS stimulants, such as methylphenidate (Ritalin), dextroamphetamine (Dexedrine), pemoline (Cylert) and many others. The problem is that according to some reports CNS stimulants can exacerbate or precipitate tics in up to 25% of patients (Robertson, 1992). If this is the case, alpha-2 agonists and tricyclic antidepressants can be used instead of stimulants. However, obsessive compulsive behavior responds well to the combination of cognitive-behavioral psychotherapy and selective serotonin reuptake inhibitors (SSRIs), including fluoxetine (Prozac), sertraline (Zoloft), and many others (Hensiek and Trimble, 2002).

Recently, there have been reports of successful treatment of severe drug-resistant tics and OCD with deep brain stimulation. Studies are ongoing, and it remains to be seen if this aggressive therapy will be justified in treatment of the symptoms of Tourette syndrome.

In this case, the child and parents were informed of the diagnosis but chose not to start pharmacotherapy. The patient's teachers were also informed, and they modified his class environment. He improved in his school performance, and within a year his tics became less pronounced and less bothersome to the patient and his immediate family.

Comprehension Questions

[48.1] Which of the following behavioral abnormalities are associated with Tourette syndrome?

A. Attention-deficit disorder
B. Schizophrenia
C. Trichotillomania
D. Autism

[48.2] Which of the following statements is correct regarding Tourette syndrome?

A. Motor and vocal tics remit during sleep
B. Tics in Tourette syndrome are suggestible by talking about it or demonstrating it.
C. Tics and compulsions mean the same thing in Tourette syndrome
D. Risk of Tourette syndrome is associated with vaccinations as an infant

[48.3] A 12-year-old boy has been recently diagnosed with Tourette syndrome. Medications are being contemplated to help to control the symptoms. Which of the following is most likely to be prescribed?

A. Haloperidol
B. Dopamine blocking agents
C. Anticholinergic agents
D. Tricyclic antidepressant

Answers

[48.1] **A.** In addition to tics, patients with Tourette syndrome exhibit multiple behavioral symptoms including ADHD and OCD.

[48.2] **B.** The tics are a characteristic aspect of Tourette syndrome and can be brought on by talking about it.

[48.3] **B.** Dopamine blocking agents are commonly prescribed as first-line therapy for Tourette syndrome. Although haloperidol is sometimes used for this condition, it is used rarely because of side effects.

CLINICAL PEARLS

❖ Tourette syndrome is a sensory-motor disorder: the sensory component is necessary for the correct diagnosis.
❖ Most tics are suggestible and at least temporarily suppressible.
❖ Poor impulse control, ADHD, and obsessive compulsive behavior are often more debilitating than tics.
❖ Treat tics only if they interfere with school, work, or social activities.
❖ Patients with Tourette syndrome almost always have excellent insight into their disease even very early in life.

REFERENCES

Feigin A, Clarke H. Tourette's syndrome: update and review of the literature. Neurologist 1998;4:188–195.

Hensiek AE, Trimble MR. Relevance of new psychotropic drugs for the neurologist. J Neurol Neurosurg Psychiatry 2002;72:33, 281–285.

Jankovic J. The neurology of tics. In: Marsden CD, Fahn S, eds. Movement disorders 2. London: Butterworths Scientific; 1987:383–405.

Jankovic J. Botulinum toxin in the treatment of dystonic tics. Mov Disord 1994 May;9(3):347–349.

Jankovic J, Glaze DG, Frost JD. Effects of tetrabenazine on tics and sleep of Gilles de la Tourette's syndrome. Neurology 1984;34(5):688–692.

Robertson M, Eapen V. Pharmacologic controversy of CNS stimulants in Gilles de la Tourette's syndrome. Clin Neuropharmacol 1992;15(5):408–425.

A right-hand dominant 7-year-old boy is brought to the emergency room (ER) after having had an unusual spell at night. He came into his parent's room looking very frightened, making gurgling noises but unable to speak, with twitching noted over the right side of his face. After approximately 30 seconds he fell to the ground and had a 2-minute generalized tonic-clonic event. Immediately afterwards he was drowsy and confused but now is completely back to his normal baseline. His vital signs are within the range of normal for his age, and his physical examination, including a detailed neurologic examination, are normal. He has never experienced any similar events, and there is no history of febrile seizures, central nervous system infections, significant head trauma, headaches, developmental or behavioral problems, or changes in personality. He was born at 38 weeks of gestation after an uneventful pregnancy and went home on the second day of life. He has not been febrile nor had any recent illnesses. The child's father states that he had similar episodes as a child.

◆ **What is the most likely diagnosis?**

◆ **What is the next diagnostic step?**

◆ **What is the next step in therapy?**

ANSWERS TO CASE 49: Benign Rolandic Epilepsy

Summary: This previously healthy and neurodevelopmentally normal 7-year-old boy is brought to the ER after a nocturnal spell involving speech arrest and hemifacial clonus followed by an apparent secondarily generalized tonic-clonic convulsion. Although postictally confused, he is now back to his normal baseline. His examination is unremarkable, and there is nothing of note regarding his birth history, past medical history, or developmental history. Family history is significant for similar episodes in his father when he was a child.

◆ **Most likely diagnosis:** Benign rolandic epilepsy

◆ **Next diagnostic step:** Perform an electroencephalograph (EEG) as an outpatient

◆ **Next step in therapy:** Reassurance as well as monitoring for subsequent events

Analysis

Objectives

1. Understand the difference between partial, generalized, and secondarily generalized seizures.
2. Know the clinical characteristics of benign rolandic epilepsy (BRE) as well as other benign focal epilepsies of childhood.
3. Be aware of long-term prognosis of BRE and considerations in deciding on treatment.
4. Know when focal seizures in childhood require further workup and how to proceed with such an evaluation.

Considerations

This 7-year-old boy experienced a nocturnal seizure with secondary generalization and not associated with any obvious provocation. The most common focal epilepsy of childhood, BRE, has no known etiology, and is localization-related epilepsy because it is highly heritable, although the mode of inheritance remains unclear. BRE typically has its onset between 3 and 13 years of age. Generally, the seizures stop before patients turn 20 years of age, and about two-thirds of patients will have only one or very few seizures. The typical seizure presentation with BRE begins with sensorimotor manifestations on one side of the face and mouth. Unilateral oral paresthesias as well as facial clonic and/or tonic activity are common. Speech arrest, which can be seen regardless of whether the seizure involves the dominant or nondominant hemisphere, and hypersalivation are also frequently reported. Most of the seizure activity is at night, occurring soon after falling asleep or on awakening. The EEG is particularly helpful in making the diagnosis of BRE. Although the patient in this case has returned to baseline, the age of the patient, the presentation, and a family history of similar episodes in his father is highly suggestive of BRE (see also Case 44).

APPROACH TO BENIGN ROLANDIC SEIZURES

Regarding an initial classification, seizures are considered generalized if they involve both cerebral hemispheres at onset. Partial seizures, also referred to as focal or as localization-related, begin in one part of one hemisphere. Partial seizures can be further categorized into those that do not impair consciousness—simple partial seizures—and those that do impair consciousness—complex partial seizures. It is not uncommon for partial seizures to spread and involve a greater cortical region as the seizure progresses. If this abnormal activity spreads to involve the contralateral hemisphere then the seizure is said to be secondarily generalized. This would appear to be what happened in the case under consideration because the child initially had focal manifestations (speech arrest and right hemifacial clonus) followed by generalized motor activity (a generalized tonic-clonic seizure).

A partial seizure is by definition a manifestation of a focal physiologic abnormality in the cortex. Oftentimes this will be associated with an anatomic abnormality able to be seen with an MRI scan. Examples of common causes of such a lesion would be trauma, stroke, infection, tumor, or a congenital malformation of cortical development. If an anatomical substrate is seen in association with the region of seizure onset (the seizure focus) in a patient with epilepsy, then the disorder is classified as *symptomatic*. Alternatively, a seizure focus can exist without any obvious finding on neuroimaging. In this case, the disorder would be considered *cryptogenic* (indicating that the cause *remains hidden*). The third category of epilepsies is *idiopathic*, which refers to conditions in which there is a known or presumed genetic etiology. The most common focal epilepsy of childhood, BRE, is an example of an idiopathic localization-related epilepsy as it is highly heritable although the mode of inheritance remains unclear.

The behavioral manifestations, or *semiology*, of focal seizures reflect the normal function of the region of the brain from which they arise. For example, an occipital lobe focus can produce visual manifestations whereas a focus in the primary motor cortex can generate contralateral tonic and/or clonic activity. In this patient, his speech arrest and right hemi-facial clonus suggests a seizure focus near the facial aspect of the left motor strip as well as the nearby regions responsible for expressive language. This would be consistent with a *peri-rolandic* location involving the lateral aspect of the left hemisphere near the central sulcus (formerly referred to as the *rolandic fissure*). Information about seizure presentation is combined with the findings of MRI and electroencephalography in an attempt to localize the focal abnormality.

BRE, which also is referred to as *benign epilepsy with centrotemporal spikes*, is an age-dependent epilepsy syndrome with onset between 3 and 13 years. Essentially all patients will cease having their habitual seizures by 20 years of age, which is one reason that the condition is labeled *benign*. Another reason for this is that approximately two-thirds of patients will have only one or very few seizures, which is important when considering whether or not to begin anticonvulsant therapy. The typical seizure of BRE begins with sensorimotor manifestations on one side of the face and mouth. Unilateral oral paresthesias as well as facial clonic and/or tonic activity are common. Speech arrest, which can be seen regardless of whether the seizure involves the dominant or nondominant hemisphere, and hypersalivation are also frequently reported. Some variability in seizure symptomatology between seizures can be seen for any given patient with some having two distinct seizure types. Approximately 75% of seizures are nocturnal, occurring soon after falling asleep or on awakening. The remainder of patients have nocturnal and daytime seizures or, more rarely, only events during waking hours.

Obtaining an EEG is particularly helpful in making the diagnosis of BRE because several characteristic features can be seen interictally. If a period of sleep is captured during the recording session, then approximately 30% of patients with BRE will have sharp waves seen arising from the centrotemporal region. Although beyond the scope of this review, there are other features, such as a *frontal dipole* and a *prepotential*, which aid in identifying these sharp waves as consistent with BRE. If both the history and the EEG are consistent with BRE then no further diagnostic workup needs to be undertaken. If the history is consistent, but the EEG is unrevealing then it can be worth obtaining another EEG to see if diagnostic abnormal activity is captured. Certainly if there are focal features on neurologic examination, concerning aspects to the history (such as developmental regression), or abnormalities on EEG that are not consistent with BRE then neuroimaging with an MRI should be strongly considered. Interestingly, not all patients with EEG abnormalities consistent with BRE actually have seizures. In fact, only 10% of patients with centrotemporal sharp waves of the BRE type ever experience one or more clinical seizures.

Once the diagnosis is made, consideration must turn to treatment. Most patients experience only one or very few seizures, and all patients eventually outgrow BRE. Also, although this is a matter of some debate, there is no evidence that the typical and infrequent seizures of BRE are harmful to the developing nervous system. Given these factors, as well as the side effects of anticonvulsants, many neurologists recommend withholding treatment until a patient has experienced three or more seizures. Clearly this is a decision that must be tailored to the individual patient in careful consultation with the child and the child's parents. If treatment is initiated, then most all of the anticonvulsants have shown some efficacy against the seizures of BRE and usually at relatively low dosages. Oxcarbazepine and gabapentin are frequently used as first-line agents. The diagnosis of BRE must be reconsidered in patients who do not respond to treatment, whose seizures persist into adulthood, or in those who have very frequent or otherwise atypical seizures.

Comprehension Questions

[49.1] A third-year medical student observes a seizure occurring in one of the neurology ward patients and determines that it was a "simple partial" seizure. The student would be correct if:

A. It involves the movement of only one limb
B. It is easily described by observers
C. It is focal and normal consciousness is preserved
D. It is focal and consciousness is altered but not completely lost
E. It is focal and very brief

[49.2] Which of the following is typical of the seizures seen in patients with BRE?

A. Occur mostly during the daytime
B. Are generalized from the outset
C. Primarily involve the lower extremities
D. Recur frequently
E. Often begin in the face or mouth

[49.3] A 5-year-old boy with epilepsy has partial seizures arising from the left frontal lobe. An MRI of his brain reveals a large area of gliosis in the left dorsolateral frontal lobe consistent with an old stroke. This patient's epilepsy would be classified as:

A. Idiopathic generalized
B. Cryptogenic localization-related
C. Idiopathic localization-related
D. Symptomatic localization-related
E. Acute symptomatic

[49.4] A 9-year-old girl is brought to the clinic with a history entirely consistent with the diagnosis of BRE. An EEG is obtained that reveals the centrotemporal sharp waves characteristic of this disorder. The patient has had one witnessed seizure 2 weeks ago and had one unwitnessed event 1 year ago, which may have been a seizure. The child's parents are not very interested in beginning daily anticonvulsant medication. Which of the following would be the best course of treatment for this patient?

A. Strongly encourage the parents to begin a low dose of daily valproic acid
B. Prescribe prophylactic diazepam in case of febrile illness
C. Reassure the family and encourage "watchful waiting" to see if further seizures occur
D. Obtain an MRI prior to making any treatment recommendations
E. Recommend twice-daily dosing of oxcarbazepine

Answers

[49.1] **C.** A simple partial seizure is a focal seizure that does not alter the patient's level of consciousness.

[49.2] **E.** The seizures of BRE are usually nocturnal, infrequent, begin with orofacial involvement, and can secondarily generalize.

[49.3] **D.** The patient has an anatomic abnormality (an area of glial scarring) visible on MRI at the area of seizure onset and therefore has symptomatic localization-related (partial) epilepsy. These are not acute symptomatic seizures as described because there is no provoking factor present. Instead, they are a chronic sequelae of a remote event.

[49.4] **C.** In the context of typical BRE with infrequent seizures "watchful waiting" is the most prudent approach. An MRI is unnecessary in this patient at this time.

CLINICAL PEARLS

❖ Although BRE is the most common focal epilepsy of childhood, the most common focal epilepsy in adults is temporal lobe epilepsy.

❖ A small subset of patients have been described with *malignant rolandic epilepsy* in which the seizures look similar to those of BRE but are frequent, difficult to treat, and do not remit by 16 years of age. It is likely that these patients have a different syndrome rather than a severe form of BRE.

❖ Approximately 50% of patients with BRE are not treated with anticonvulsants because of the generally infrequent nature of the seizures.

❖ A somewhat similar but much less frequent idiopathic localization-related epilepsy syndrome is benign epilepsy of childhood with occipital paroxysms. Seizures in these patients begin with visual symptoms followed by psychomotor, sensorimotor, or migraine-like phenomena. EEG reveals occipital spikes that go away with eye opening.

REFERENCES

Arunkumar G, Kotagal P, Rothner D. Localization-related epilepsies: simple partial seizures, complex partial seizures, benign focal epilepsy of childhood, and epilepsia partialis continua. In: Pellock J, Dodson W, Bourgeois B, eds. Pediatric epilepsy: diagnosis and therapy. Demos Medical Publishing: New York; 2001:243–264.

Camfield P, Camfield C. Epileptic syndromes in childhood: Clinical features, outcomes, and treatment. Epilepsia 2002;43(suppl 3):27–32.

Loiseau P. Idiopathic and benign partial epilepsies. In: Wyllie E, ed. The treatment of epilepsy: principles and practice. Philadelphia, PA: Lippincott Williams and Wilkins; 2001:475–484.

Willmore LJ. Treatment of benign epilepsy syndromes throughout life. Epilepsia 2001;42(suppl 8):6–9.

A 13-month-old baby boy is brought to the clinic by his pregnant mother after he experienced a seizure. He has had recurrent seizures since 6 months of age, and generalized spasms as an infant. She expresses concern that he has not been sitting up by himself yet and has always been a weak baby. He has not been feeding well and lately has had a wet cough with low-grade fevers. Developmentally, he has not said his first word, compared to his older sister who was able to say three words as well as "Mama" and "Dada" by the same age. His birth history is significant for intrauterine growth retardation and reduced fetal movements. After birth he underwent surgery for cryptorchidism. On examination, his head circumference is small for his age. General examination reveals a high forehead with vertical wrinkling, bitemporal hollowing, widely spaced eyes with epicanthal folds, flattened ears, short nose with upturned nares, prominent nasal folds, a flat midface with a round philtrum and upper lip, and a small chin. He is tachycardic, and his chest sounds are diminished in the right lower lobe. A back examination reveals a sacral dimple. Neurologically, he has generalized hypotonia and is unable to support himself when sitting up.

◆ **What is the most likely diagnosis?**

◆ **What is the next diagnostic step?**

◆ **What is the next step in therapy?**

ANSWERS TO CASE 50: Lissencephaly

Summary: A 13-month-old baby boy is brought by his mother for recurrent seizures with a history of infantile spasms. He has severe mental retardation and motor developmental delays as well as poor feeding. His past history is significant for intrauterine growth retardation and cryptorchidism. On examination, he has microcephaly, craniofacial dysmorphisms including hypertelorism with epicanthal folds, short nose with upturned nares, and micrognathia, tachycardia, a sacral dimple, and generalized hypotonia.

◆   **Most likely diagnosis:** Miller-Dieker syndrome or lissencephaly type 1

◆   **Next diagnostic step:** Brain MRI

◆   **Next step in therapy:** Symptomatic management of seizures and poor feeding/ swallowing, genetic counseling

Analysis

Objectives

1. Know the clinical features and epidemiology of Miller-Dieker syndrome.
2. Understand the differential diagnosis of lissencephaly.
3. Understand the management of lissencephaly patients and their families.

Considerations

The 13-month-old child in the case is a typical case of Miller-Dieker syndrome. Severe mental retardation, recurrent seizures, and infantile spasms are typical. Refractory epilepsy presents during the first 6 months of life in 75% of affected children, with infantile spasms beginning shortly after birth in 80%. Overall, more than 90% of these patients will develop seizures. Mental retardation and developmental delay are severe, with most cases not capable of progressing beyond the 3- to 6-month level of milestones. Distinct craniofacial dysmorphic features as described for our patient, generalized hypotonia that progresses to opisthotonos and spasticity with age, contractures, clinodactyly, cryptorchidism, omphaloceles (an abdominal wall defect), cardiac and renal abnormalities are all phenotypic. Feeding and swallowing problems often result in poor weight gain and aspiration pneumonia. Past history will often reveal a gestation complicated by polyhydramnios, intrauterine growth retardation, and decreased fetal movements.

APPROACH TO LISSENCEPHALY

Definitions

Lissencephaly: *Smooth brain* genetic malformation of the cerebral cortex in which abnormal neuronal migration during early neural development results in smooth cerebral surfaces with absent (agyria) or decreased (pachygyria) convolutions.

Miller-Dieker syndrome: A severe lissencephaly phenotype secondary to deletion on chromosome 17p13.3 with agyria and characteristic dysmorphic features.

Isolated lissencephaly sequence: Milder phenotype compared to Miller-Dieker syndrome, with pachygyria and mild or absent dysmorphic features because of autosomal dominant mutations in the LIS 1 gene on chromosome 17p13.3 or X-linked mutations in the doublecortin (DCX) gene on chromosome Xq22.3. Pachygyria caused by LIS 1 mutations is posterior-predominant on neuroimaging whereas anterior-predominant pachygyria is more typical of DCX mutations.

Infantile spasms: Dramatic repetitive bouts of rapid neck flexion, arm extension, hip and knee flexion, and abdominal flexion, often with arousal from sleep. The mother might describe them as unprovoked startle responses or colicky spells as a result of abdominal pain, although there is no crying typical of colic. Typical presentation occurs between 3 and 8 months of age.

Hypertelorism: Abnormally increased distance between the eyes.

Epicanthal fold: Skin fold of the upper eyelid (from the nose to the medial side of the eyebrow) covering the medial corner (medial canthus) of the eye.

Clinodactyly: Congenital condition where the little finger is curved toward the ring finger.

Opisthotonus: Severe hyperextension of the back caused by spasm of the muscles along the spinal column.

Clinical Approach

Epidemiology and Differential Diagnosis

Lissencephaly is a set of rare brain disorders where the whole or parts of the surface of the brain appear smooth. The word lissencephaly is derived from the Greek lissos meaning smooth and *encephalos* meaning brain. The human brain normally has a convoluted surface. In lissencephaly these convolutions are completely or partially absent from the brain, or areas of it, have a smooth appearance. The convolutions are also called *gyri* and their absence is known as *agyria* (without gyri). In some cases convolutions are present, but thicker and reduced in number, and the term *pachygyria* (broad gyri) is used. The diagnosis is usually made with the help of a CT scan or MRI scan of the brain.

With lissencephaly, the early brain development is normal until month 3 or 4 of development, when the brain fails to progress normally. Different types of lissencephaly have different causes. **Miller-Dieker syndrome** has been reported to occur in 11.7 per million live births. This severe form is estimated to be the cause of almost one-third of patients with identified lissencephaly. It is caused by a chromosome deletion resulting in monosomy of chromosome 17p13.3 with the LIS1 gene. The main differential diagnosis is isolated lissencephaly sequence, which has a milder phenotype and is caused by a smaller mutation in the LIS1 gene with an autosomal dominant pattern of inheritance, or the DCX gene, with X-linked transmission.

Both Miller-Dieker syndrome and isolated lissencephaly sequence are considered classical lissencephalies or lissencephaly type 1. The differential diagnosis also includes other migrational defect syndromes that present with seizures, mental retardation, and lissencephaly, including lissencephaly with cerebellar hypoplasia (AR, RELN gene on 7q22) and lissencephaly with abnormal genitalia (X-linked, ARX on Xp22.13). Related syndromes that present with similar clinical presentations but different neuroimaging findings include subcortical band heterotopia (LIS1 or DCX), polymicrogyria, bilateral periventricular nodular heterotopia, and schizencephaly.

Diagnosis

An accurate diagnosis is important for two reasons. First, if the condition is genetic and has been inherited, it will allow parents to understand the risk for future pregnancies and also whether other children in the same family are also *carriers* for the faulty gene. Second, it is useful for parents of children with lissencephaly to meet other parents and children with the same condition so they can learn from each others' experience.

A diagnosis of lissencephaly or pachygyria is not a full diagnoses, and the cause cannot be determined without a more detailed evaluation from a neurologist, pediatrician, or geneticist. Neuroimaging is very important in the evaluation and diagnosis. An MRI scan is almost always superior for detailing the brain malformation especially for conditions such as polymicrogyria where CT scans do not provide the resolution required. Similarly, these conditions are so rare many neuroradiologists might never have seen a scan like this before or might not have adjusted the MRI scanner correctly to detail some of the small malformations that occur. In these instances it is important to be referred to specialists where the expertise exists.

The management of the Miller-Dieker lissencephaly patient is supportive, centering around the three major complications: epilepsy, poor feeding, and spasticity. Improved symptomatic therapy has lengthened the life expectancy of these patients from a few years to the early teens. The use of steroids (prednisone) and adrenocorticotropic hormone (ACTH) is an accepted treatment for infantile spasms, but may or may not be successful. Seizures will return following treatment with steroids and are often intractable. Multiple anticonvulsants are often required with vigilance for life-threatening status epilepticus. Poor feeding and swallowing predispose to malnutrition and aspiration pneumonia; a feeding tube and gastrostomy in the long-term can help reduce these comorbidities. Hypotonia in the early years progresses to spasticity and contractures that, if untreated, can result in severe pain and discomfort, as well as immobility and complications such as falls, atelectasis, and decubitus ulcers. Frequent stretching physical therapies, braces, and muscle relaxants can slow the development of spasticity and contractures, whereas special wheelchairs and mattresses can reduce problems arising from immobility. Lissencephaly patients can also have congenital cardiac and renal abnormalities that must be closely monitored and managed.

As in the case of this patient's family, genetic counseling plays an important role because of concern for a hereditary syndrome. The recurrence risk for Miller-Dieker syndrome is very low, because most cases are caused by a de novo chromosomal deletion. However, recurrence risk can be as high as 33% if a familial reciprocal translocation is determined. The workup can begin with a fluorescent in situ hybridization (FISH) analysis for the 17p13.3 deletion, and a genetics specialist can be consulted. Prenatal testing is possible through fetal chromosome analysis by karyotyping, FISH, chorionic villus sampling, or amniocentesis. Imaging for cerebral gyral malformations is more sensitive beyond 28 weeks of gestation.

Comprehension Questions

[50.1] A 14-month-old baby is diagnosed as having Miller-Dieker syndrome. Which of the following would be most likely noted on physical examination?

A. Macrocephaly
B. Motor delay
C. Ambiguous genitalia
E. Abnormal X chromosome studies

[50.2] Which of the following is one of most common sequela of Miller-Dieker syndrome?

A. Epilepsy
B. Respiratory Failure
C. Hypotonia
D. Rhabdomyolysis

[50.3] A 2-month-old infant is noted to draw up his legs and tighten his abdomen after feeding with formula. There seems to be no abnormal seizure activity. The developmental milestones seem to be normal. Which of the following is the most likely diagnosis?

A. Infantile spasms
B. Intestinal colic
C. Lissencephaly, early onset
D. Noonan syndrome

Answers

[50.1] **B.** Motor delay, seizures, microcephaly are the hallmarks of this Miller-Dieker syndrome.

[50.2] **A.** The management of the Miller-Dieker lissencephaly patient is supportive, centering around the three major complications: epilepsy, poor feeding, and spasticity.

[50.3] **B.** This infant is normal in every way except drawing up of his legs and tightening of the abdomen after feeding, which is most likely intestinal colic.

CLINICAL PEARLS

❖ Lissencephaly should be considered in the differential diagnosis of a child presenting with mental retardation, motor delay, infantile spasms, and characteristic craniofacial dysmorphic features including microcephaly, short nose with upturned nares, and micrognathia

❖ Brain MRI and consultation with a pediatric neurologist are important steps in the work-up of lissencephaly.

❖ Treatment of lissencephaly patients should focus on symptomatic therapy for complications including epilepsy, poor feeding, and spasticity.

❖ Genetic counseling is an important part of the care of lissencephaly patients and their families.

REFERENCES

Dobyns WB, Curry CJ, Hoyme HE, et al. Clinical and molecular diagnosis of Miller-Dieker syndrome. Am J Hum Genet 1991 Mar;48(3):584–594.

Guerrini R, Marini C. Genetic malformations of cortical development. Exp Brain Res 2006 May 25;173:322–333.

Lissencephaly Contact Group. About lissencephaly. Available at: http://www.lissencephaly.org.uk/aboutliss/index.htm.

Pilz D. Miller-Dieker syndrome. Orphanet encyclopedia. Available at: http://www.orpha.net/data/patho/GB/uk-MDS.pdf. Last updated September 2003.

Radiology.com. CT scan files—lissencephaly type 1. Available at: http://www.radiologyworld.com/Ctscan-lissen.htm.

Tulane University. Lissencephaly type 2. Available at: http://www.mcl.tulane.edu/classware/pathology/medical_pathology/neuropathology/congenitalq.htm.

A 28-month-old male is brought to the doctor's office because he "isn't talking like other kids his age." He was the product of an uncomplicated pregnancy and delivery at term. Although not a particularly warm or cuddly child, the patient's parents did not notice anything unusual in the first year of life. At 16 months, the child had not yet articulated any words although he was noted to babble occasionally and showed no affection to his parents or siblings. He was easily upset, particularly by changes from his usual routine, and soothed himself by rocking back and forth or slowly spinning in a circle. At presentation, the child had not developed any spoken words, and his temperament remained irritable and isolative. His parents state that he hardly ever makes eye contact, and if forced by others, he becomes upset. On examination, he is an active and healthy appearing toddler who is wandering around the office, ignoring the doctor and his parents, paying attention only to the books, which he rhythmically pulls off the shelf without playfulness. When his mother tries to keep him from doing so the little boy screams, looks up to the ceiling, flaps his arms, and then retreats to the corner and rocks back and forth. He has a normal toddler gait but seems somewhat uncoordinated for his age when reaching for and grasping objects. There are no noted dysmorphic features, and his skin examination is normal. Developmental history in the family is normal. The child's two older siblings are healthy and neurodevelopmentally normal. The child has physically been healthy, has never been hospitalized, and has never had surgery. His immunizations are up to date.

◆ **What is the most likely diagnosis?**

◆ **What is the next diagnostic step?**

◆ **What is the next step in therapy?**

ANSWERS TO CASE 51: Autism

Summary: This physically healthy 28-month-old boy is presents with delayed language development, abnormal social interactions, and unusual behaviors. He is physically healthy, and there is nothing of note in his prenatal, medical, surgical, or family histories. His examination is significant only for demonstrating the deficits and behaviors reported by the parents.

◆ **Most likely diagnosis:** Autism

◆ **Next diagnostic step:** Audiological evaluation

◆ **Next step in therapy:** Educational intervention and behavioral modification

Analysis

Objectives

1. Understand the difference between developmental delay and developmental regression.
2. Know the four domains of development and how to assess them clinically.
3. Remember the importance of evaluating hearing in evaluating a language delay.
4. Know the cardinal features of autism.

Clinical Considerations

This 28-month-old boy is brought to the office with concerns about his development and his behavior. Clinically, the most important first step is to carefully distinguish between developmental delay and developmental regression. Delay implies that the child is making progress, although at a rate slower than that considered to be normal. This is generally because of a static process and can lead to an eventual diagnosis of mental retardation. Developmental regression, conversely, implies that the child is now losing previously attained skills and raises the possibility of a progressive neurodegenerative process. Distinguishing between delay and regression can be clinically difficult, at times. For example, children can inconsistently demonstrate a new developmental skill leading to the impression that it has been lost. **True developmental regression is a *red flag*, which necessitates an expedited search for a progressive disorder of the nervous system.** In this patient, however, there is no hint of developmental regression but instead a picture of developmental delay.

Evaluation of problems with development is facilitated by assessing four distinct developmental aspects: gross motor skills, fine motor skills, personal-social interactions, and language capabilities. An isolated language deficit, for example, can be caused by hearing impairment alone, while global developmental delay (involving all four domains) is more likely to be caused by a significant in utero, perinatal, or genetic disturbance. A delay in gross motor skills arising prior to 1 year of age strongly suggests the diagnosis of cerebral palsy. Assessing which developmental spheres are impacted is facilitated by the use of the Denver Developmental Screening Test (DDST), and confirmed with more sophisticated psychometric measures that are available, either for use in the office or on referral to a pediatric neuropsychologist.

Applying such an approach to his patient reveals that although the child is meeting gross motor milestones appropriately, he is slightly behind in fine motor skills and disproportionately significantly delayed in the language and personal-social domains. With respect to language, children begin babbling by approximately 6 months of age, articulate one word by approximately 1 year of life, and by 2 years of age are able to combine two words to form rudimentary sentences as well as follow simple verbal commands. This patient, at age 28 months, is therefore significantly delayed given that he is only able to babble and does not seem to follow commands. Although most newborns are screened for hearing problems in the newborn nursery (using a neurophysiologic test called *Auditory Brainstem Evoked Responses*), clinicians must be sure that hearing is normal when faced with a language delay. This patient, however, has delays in more than just the language domain. By parental report and based on observations, he also has significant problems with social reciprocity. He is not affectionate toward his parents and is unable to maintain eye contact. At times he seems to treat people in the same detached way that he treats other objects around him. Although solitary play is a normal developmental stage, this child has never progressed to including any type of social play, which is certainly abnormal at his age. Furthermore, he has a variety of odd and idiosyncratic behaviors. For example, he is fascinated with removing books from shelves but does so in a mechanical way rather than a playful one. Also, he uses repetitive behaviors such as rocking, slowly spinning, or rapidly flapping his hands in order to soothe himself when upset rather than seeking comfort from his caretakers. These repetitive stereotyped self-stimulating behaviors are referred to as stereotypies and are commonly seen in children with autism or autistic spectrum disorders. Taken together, this child's clinical condition appears to meet criteria for autism.

APPROACH TO AUTISM

Definitions

Autism spectrum disorder (ASD) or pervasive developmental disorder (PDD): Disorders characterized by varying degrees of impairment in communication skills, social interactions, and restricted, repetitive, and stereotyped patterns of behavior.

Asperger syndrome: One of five neurobiologic PDDs and is characterized by deficiencies in social and communication skills, normal to above normal intelligence, and standard language development.

Developmental delay: Developmental delay occurs when children have not reached these milestones by the expected time period for all five areas of development or just one (cognitive, language and speech, social and emotional, fine motor, and gross motor).

Clinical Approach

Autism is a condition toward the more severe end of a spectrum of neurobehavioral disorders that involve deficits in communication, social interactions, and behavior. The diagnosis is made clinically according to criteria detailed in the *Diagnostic and Statistical Manual of Mental Disorders, fourth edition, text revision* (DSM-IV-TR). First, with regards to social deficits, a patient must have at least two of the following:

1. Marked impairment in the use of multiple nonverbal behaviors such as eye-to-eye gaze, facial expression, body posture, and gestures necessary to regulate social interaction
2. Failure to develop peer relationships
3. Lack of spontaneous seeking to share enjoyment, interests, or achievement with other people
4. Lack of social or emotional reciprocity

Second, in terms of communication skills, a patient must have at least one of the following:

1. Delay in, or total lack of, the development of spoken language
2. In individuals with adequate speech, marked impairment in the ability to initiate or sustain a conversation with others
3. Stereotyped and repetitive use of language or idiosyncratic language
4. Lack of varied, spontaneous make-believe play or social imitative play

Finally, regarding behavioral criteria, the patient must demonstrate at least one of the following:

1. Encompassing preoccupation with one or more stereotyped and restricted patterns of interest that is abnormal either in intensity or focus
2. Apparently inflexible adherence to specific, nonfunctional routines or rituals
3. Stereotyped and repetitive motor mannerisms
4. Persistent preoccupation with parts of objects rather than the whole

Furthermore, six of the above symptoms (in any category) must be evident in the child prior to 3 years of age. If findings suggestive of autism are obtained by history or on a developmental screening examination, then the patient should be referred for more detailed evaluation by a clinician familiar with the formal diagnosis of autism.

In addition to autism, there are other conditions along this disease continuum (referred to as *ASD*). It affects an estimated 3.4 of every 1000 children ages 3–10 years although rates vary depending on reports. The ASDs can often be reliably detected by the age of 3 years, and in some cases as early as 18 months.

Children with normal language but with restricted interests, abnormal behaviors, and poorly developed social interaction can have Asperger syndrome. At times these children are difficult to distinguish from high functioning children with autism (those with an IQ in the average range). Patients who develop autistic symptoms older than age 3 years are less impaired than typical autistic patients, or those who otherwise have atypical features can be diagnosed with PDD not otherwise specified (PDD-NOS). ASDs are more common in boys than in girls (4:1) and have an overall prevalence rate of approximately 60 per 10,000 people. The most frequently encountered type of ASD is PDD-NOS, followed by autistic disorder, with Asperger syndrome being the least common subtype.

Although the cause of the ASD is unknown, increasing evidence points to its being an underlying pathophysiologic process ongoing long before the developmental delays become evident and likely present from birth. Although multiple brain regions are likely to be involved in such a complex disorder, it appears as though the frontal lobe and the amygdala are significantly involved. This makes sense given the frontal lobe's involvement in regulating emotion, and behavior, as well as the role of the amygdala in mediating the response to stress. Recently there has been a flurry of research investigating a possible link between routine childhood vaccinations containing the preservative thimerosal and autism. Although large epidemiologic studies have failed to support this linkage, it remains a significant concern in the minds of many parents and might need to be addressed directly with them.

Management

Perhaps the most important aspect of management in patients with autism is a well-designed appropriately structured educational environment. Given that autism is a developmental disorder, it is vital to begin such interventions early to maximize the development of the child's potential. Additionally, behavioral interventions can be very helpful both for the patient as well as for the family and caretakers. Pharmacologic interventions are, at times, employed although there currently are not many large clinical trials to support this. Smaller studies have suggested that the use of selective serotonin reuptake inhibitors and atypical antipsychotic medication can have some benefit. It should be noted that no medication currently has an indication from the FDA for use in treating the symptoms of autism. It is not surprising, therefore, that many complementary and alternative treatments have been promoted for these patients: mercury chelation therapy, intravenous secretin treatments, and a host of supplements. Parents should be asked about the use of such therapies and counseled about their potential dangers.

Prognosis

The disease usually is nonprogressive, although occasionally, as an affected child grows, additional deficits can be evident. Although less affected individuals can develop improvement in social relationships, the outlook for those children that are significantly affected is poor. The degree of language impairment and intelligence ability usually predict outcome of eventual function; a child that has not learned to speak by 5 years of age usually will not gain communicative ability.

Comprehension Questions

[51.1] Of the following patients referred for developmental problems, which would be the most clinically concerning?

    A. A 3-year-old child who has never learned to speak

    B. A 5-year-old child who has moderate delays in all four developmental domains

    C. A 2-year-old child with cerebral palsy and epilepsy

    D. A 30-month-old child who was speaking normally for age but now has no intelligible words

    E. A 4-year-old child who has always been clumsy

[51.2] The Denver Developmental Screening Test is best described as a:

    A. Comprehensive evaluation of all developmental spheres

    B. An unnecessary tool with modern neuroimaging techniques such as MRI

    C. A quick method for picking up potential developmental problems in an office practice

    D. A well standardized tool for diagnosing autism

    E. A test of expressive and receptive language skills

[51.3] Which of the following is most important in the diagnosis of autistic disorder?

    A. A family history of autism

    B. Atrophy of the frontal lobe on MRI

    C. Development of symptoms before 5 years of age

    D. Normal language function

    E. Abnormal social reciprocity

[51.4] Of the following interventions, what would be the most important for a child recently diagnosed with autism?

    A. Prescribing a moderate dose of an atypical antipsychotic drug such as risperidone

    B. Making sure that the child gets no further immunizations

    C. Enrolling the child in a highly structured educational program

    D. Getting the child involved in highly social activities such as team sports

    E. Daily multivitamin therapy

Answers

[51.1] **D.** Any sign of developmental regression (such as the loss of expressive language skills) is very concerning.

[51.2 **C.** The Denver Developmental Screening Test is useful to pick up potential developmental problems that can then be further evaluated using more in-depth techniques.

[51.3] **E.** Abnormal social reciprocity, along with abnormalities in communication and behavior, is a key feature of autistic disorders. At present autism is a clinical diagnosis without useful findings on ancillary tests such as MRI or EEG.

[51.4] **C.** Children with autism benefit from a very structured educational environment designed to teach skills in a concrete way. Although medication can be helpful in some patients, there are no large-scale trials at present to support their usage.

CLINICAL PEARLS

❖ Although developmental regression is a *red flag,* it is not uncommon to see some language regression as autistic symptoms become evident late in the second year of life.

❖ Often children with autism will develop a vocabulary with a few words at an apparently appropriate age and then lose the use of those words by 2 years of age. This *autistic regression* is seen in approximately 25% of patients.

❖ More than 25% of children with autism develop epilepsy, which is a striking increase from the rate of 1% in the general population. Patients with lower IQs are at higher risk of developing epilepsy.

❖ Although language and communication problems do not show up until the second year of life in patients with classic autism, parents often report that these children seem different from early in the first year of life.

❖ Although cerebral palsy and mental retardation can coexist, they are different diagnoses.

REFERENCES

American Psychiatric Association. Diagnostic and statistical manual of mental disorders, 4th ed. Text revision. Washington, DC: American Psychiatric Association; 2000.

Barbaresi W, Katusic S, Voigt R. Autism—a review of the state or the science for pediatric primary health care clinicians. Arch Pediatr Adolesc Med 2006;160: 1167–1175.

Fenichel G. Clinical pediatric neurology: a signs and symptoms approach, 3rd ed. Philadelphia, PA: WB Saunders; 1997:118–152.

Sugden S, Corbett B. Autism—presentation, diagnosis, and management. Continuum 2006:12(5):47–59.

A 43-year-old right-handed woman presents to the office with hearing loss, facial paralysis, and headache. Her history began 1 month ago with a sudden decrease in hearing in her right ear. One week prior to this visit she began to notice weakness of the right face, which has now progressed to complete paralysis. Over the last 3 months she has had intermittent right occipital headache, and clumsiness and imbalance if she turns quickly. She denies any change in her voice or difficulty with swallowing or swallowing difficulty. Her past medical history is unremarkable. She is not on any medications except birth control pills. Her physical examination shows a 43-year-old woman that has an obvious right facial paralysis. Her pulse is 62 beats/min; blood pressure, 118/62 mmHg; and temperature, 36.7°C (98.6°F). The head and face have no lesions. Her voice is normal, but her speech is slightly distorted because of the facial paralysis. Her extra-ocular movements are normal. Her eye grounds do not show any papilledema. Her ears have normal tympanic membranes. The Weber tuning fork lateralizes to the left ear. Air conduction is louder than bone conduction in both ears. There is no neck lymphadenopathy or other masses. There are no cerebellar signs. The remaining physical examination, including the neurologic examination, is normal. An audiogram shows a mild sensorineural hearing loss in the right ear; the left ear has normal hearing. An auditory brainstem response (ABR) is abnormal for the right ear; it is normal for the left ear.

◆ **What is the most likely neuroanatomic etiology and diagnosis?**

◆ **What is the next diagnostic step?**

ANSWERS TO CASE 52: Meningioma of the Acoustic Nerve

Summary: A 43-year-old woman has a history of headache, hearing loss, and facial paralysis.

◆ **Neuroanatomic Etiology and Diagnosis:** Cerebellopontine angle tumor, with the most common tumors being acoustic neuroma and meningioma

◆ **Next diagnostic step:** MRI with gadolinium

Analysis

Objectives

1. Learn the most common tumors that occur in the cerebellopontine angle.
2. Learn the most common imaging features of these tumors.
3. Learn the available treatment options for these tumors.

Considerations

This 43-year-old woman has symptoms of hearing loss, facial paralysis, and headache. She also has symptoms of imbalance and disequilibrium. The most common cause of facial nerve paralysis is Bell palsy; however, this patient also has hearing loss, balance issues, and headache, which point to a central rather than peripheral disorder. **Patients that present with the combination of hearing loss and facial paralysis demand evaluation by diagnostic imaging.** This patient's symptoms strongly suggest an abnormality in the cerebellopontine angle. Modern imaging techniques have revolutionized the evaluation of this area. MRI with contrast can readily differentiate the various pathologic processes that occur in this area (Table 52-1).

Table 52–1

MRI CHARACTERISTICS OF COMMON PATHOLOGY IN THE
CEREBELLOPONTINE ANGLE

Tumor Type	T1 Appearance*	T2 Appearance*	Gadolinium Enhancement	Special Features
Schwannoma	Isointense	Intermediate	++++	Can be cystic, inside or centered on the IAC
Meningioma	Isointense or slightly hypointense	Hyperintense to hypointense	+++	Dural tail, eccentric to the IAC, can have calcification
Epidermoid	Hypointense	Isointense	None	Internal stranding
Glomus tumor (Paraganglioma)	Hypointense	Isointense	+++	"salt and pepper appearance"
Arachnoid cyst	Hypointense	Hyperintense	None	Homogenous contents
Lipoma	Hyperintense	Hypointense	None	Intensity disappears with fat suppression
Cholesterol cysts	Hyperintense	Hyperintense	None	Located within the petrous apex

IAC, internal auditory canal.
*Intensity relative to brain.
+ Minimal enhancement.
+++ moderate enhancement.
++++ Maximal enhancement.

APPROACH TO CEREBELLOPONTINE ANGLE TUMORS

Definitions

Acoustic neuroma: A benign tumor that rises from Schwann cells on the vestibular nerve also called vestibular schwannoma. This is the most common tumor found in the cerebellopontine angle.

Auditory brainstem response (ABR): An electrical evoked hearing test. In this test, electrodes are placed on each ear lobe and on the forehead. A stimulus sound (either a click or tone burst) is delivered into the test ear at a specified loudness; an attached computer captures the electrical brain activity that results from this stimulus and filters out background noise.

Bell palsy: Idiopathic facial weakness.

Cerebellopontine angle: The anatomic space between the cerebellum, pons, and temporal bone. This space contains cranial nerves V through XI.

Conductive hearing loss: A form of hearing loss that results from a defect in the sound collecting mechanism of the ear. These structures include the ear canal, tympanic membrane, middle ear, and the ossicles.

Epidermoid tumor: A benign tumor composed of squamous epithelial elements thought to arise from congenital rests.

Glomus tumor: The common name for paraganglioma. This highly vascular tumor arises from neuroepithelial cells. These tumors are further named by the structures that they arise from: glomus tympanicum (middle ear), glomus jugulare (jugular vein), glomus vagale (vagus nerve), and carotid body tumor (carotid artery). A rule of *10%* is associated with this tumor: approximately 10% of these tumors produce a catecholamine-like substance, approximately10% of these tumors are bilateral, approximately10% are familial, and approximately 10% are malignant (i.e., potential to metastasize).

Meningioma: Common benign extra-axial tumors of the coverings of the brain. The cell of origin is probably from arachnoid villi. Several histologic subtypes are described: syncytial, transitional, fibroblastic, angioblastic, and malignant.

Sensorineural hearing loss: A form of hearing loss that results from an abnormality in the cochlea or auditory nerve.

Clinical Approach

Meningiomas

Meningiomas are usually benign tumors, of mesodermic origin, attached to the dura. They commonly are located along the sagittal sinus, over the cerebral convexities, and in the cerebellar-pontine angle. Grossly, they are gray, sharply demarcated, and firm. Microscopically, the cells are uniform with round or elongated nuclei, and a characteristic tendency to whorl around each other. Meningiomas tend to affect women more than men in the middle age. The typical clinical presentation is the slow onset of a neurologic deficit or a focal seizure; an unexpected finding on a brain imaging is also a common presentation. MRI usually reveals a dural-based mass with dense homogeneous contrast enhancement. Surgical therapy is optimal, and complete resection is curative. For lesions not amenable to surgery, local or stereotactic radiotherapy can ameliorate symptoms. Small asymptomatic lesions in older patients can be observed.

Rarely, meningiomas can be more aggressive and have malignant potential; these tumors tend to have higher mitosis and cellular and nuclear atypia. Surgical therapy followed by radiotherapy should be used in these instances.

Approach to Facial Paralysis

Facial paralysis is a relatively common disorder. In its most common presentation, facial paralysis occurs as a sudden sporadic cranial mononeuropathy. It is not associated with hearing loss; rather, it might be associated with hyperacusis. This form of facial paralysis, also called Bell palsy, is not associated with middle ear disease, parotid tumor, Lyme disease or any other known cause of facial paralysis. Essentially, Bell palsy is a diagnosis of exclusion. Generally, a pointed history and detailed physical examination will eliminate most of the differential diagnosis. Likewise, the various causes of hearing loss can be eliminated by a careful physical examination. Disease processes, such as otitis media, cholesteatoma, and otosclerosis, can be eliminated by careful history and physical examination with tuning fork tests. However, to know the type and degree of hearing loss, an audiogram is necessary.

Although it requires patient cooperation, the audiogram will give the clinician a very accurate measure of the patient's hearing level. The audiogram can distinguish between sensorineural and conductive hearing loss. Occasionally, patients have mixed hearing loss, or a combination of conductive and sensorineural losses in a single ear. Furthermore, the audiogram can give a clue regarding the presence of *retrocochlear* hearing loss or hearing loss caused by diseases proximal to the cochlea. Tests that might indicate retrocochlear pathology include speech discrimination, acoustic reflexes, and reflex decay.

Diagnosis

Sensorineural hearing loss can be further evaluated by **auditory brainstem response (ABR).** This test measures the electrical activity within the auditory pathway; and as such, this test helps to evaluate retrocochlear causes of hearing loss. The ABR has five waves that are numbered I through V, and these are correlated to major neural connections in the auditory pathway. These waves have expected morphologies and occur at predictable latencies. Waves that are absent or delayed are indicative of pathology at that point in the auditory pathway. The interwave latencies (such as I to III, III to V, or I to V) can be compared to the opposite side or to standard norms. Abnormalities on ABR need to be further evaluated by imaging studies.

MRI provides excellent definition of the structures within the posterior fossa. **Gadolinium contrast** allows additional differentiation of various pathologies. Additionally, newer technology, such as fat suppression and diffusion weighted imaging can help to identify pathology (Fig. 52–1). The MRI appearances of the most common tumors in the posterior fossa are indicated in the Table 52–1.

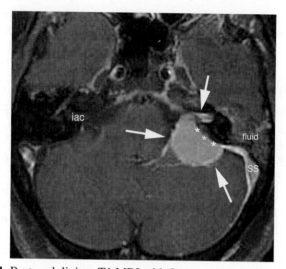

Figure 52–1. Post-gadolinium T1 MRI with fat suppression. Cerebellopontine angle meningioma. (*With permission from Fischbein NJ, Ong KC, Radiology. In: Lalwani A. Current Diagnosis and Treatment in Otolaryngology Head & Neck Surgery, New York: McGraw-Hill; 2004, p 158.*)

Although MRI with gadolinium contrast gives excellent resolution for brain, nerve and soft tissues, CT scanning is necessary for bony imaging. Often, both imaging modalities are combined to understand the full extent of the disease process within the skull base.

Treatment

A treatment plan must be created once a tumor in the cerebellopontine angle is diagnosed. Many factors must be considered when approaching these tumors. The patient's age, overall health status, tumor size and location, degree of hearing loss, and other neurologic signs are all factors to be taken into account. The various available treatment options must be discussed with the patient; the final decision of treatment course must be decided between the patient and the physician.

At least **three options** should be considered in managing tumors in the posterior fossa: **observation and serial imaging, stereotactic radiosurgery, or conventional surgery**. Some of these options might be unavailable or unwise for certain tumor types or tumor size. Clearly, the patient that has a large tumor that is producing brainstem compression or obstructive hydrocephalus should not be observed over time and serially imaged. These findings demand immediate attention.

Surgery can provide several benefits to the patient. Removal of tumor allows for final pathologic diagnosis, might correct neurologic deficits, and might prevent further complications caused by continued tumor growth. These benefits can come at a price of new neurologic deficits, meningitis, infection, stroke, or even death. The patient's underlying health status must be considered because these surgical procedures are often lengthy. Patients with low overall health status might not tolerate such a procedure.

A relatively new (although more than 20 years experience) type of therapy involves the use of **directed, focus radiation beam to the tumor**. Several different proprietary devices have been developed to destroy or at least prevent growth of these types of tumors. The experience with stereotactic radiotherapy is probably greatest with **acoustic neuroma**, because that tumor is the **most common mass found in the cerebellopontine angle**. Stereotactic radiotherapy has been found to be very effective at managing small to medium sized tumors (up to 3 cm). In these tumors, the complication rate for stereotactic radiotherapy is at least as low as that from conventional surgery; and with this type of therapy, a long hospital stay or recovery period is not required. The disadvantage with stereotactic radiotherapy is the potential for continued growth, and this growth does occur in a significant number of patients. Unfortunately, surgery following stereotactic radiotherapy is technically more difficult, and surgical results are not as good as from surgery alone.

Stereotactic radiotherapy does have limitations. It is not useful for certain tumor types (meningiomas and epidermoids). Of course, stereotactic radiotherapy cannot provide pathologic specimens for study, and it should never be used when the pathologic diagnosis is in doubt.

Comprehension Questions

[52.1] A 45-year-old painter is found to have ataxia. An MRI scan shows a tumor of the cerebellopontine angle. What is the most likely tumor in the location?

   A. Epidermoid tumor
   B. Paraganglioma
   C. Meningioma
   D. Acoustic neuroma
   E. Lipoma

[52.2] What is the best test to evaluate unilateral sensorineural hearing loss?

   A. Otoacoustic emissions
   B. Auditory brainstem response
   C. MRI of the internal auditory canals with gadolinium
   D. Electronystagmography
   E. Detailed physical examination

[52.3] What is the most common cause of unilateral facial paralysis?

   A. Idiopathic
   B. Otitis media
   C. Parotid malignancy
   D. Acoustic neuroma
   E. Lyme disease

Answers

[52.1] **D.** By far, the most common tumor in the cerebellopontine angle is the acoustic neuroma.

[52. 2] **C.** Although ABR is used to evaluate unilateral sensorineural hearing loss, its limitation is a lack of specificity for diagnosis. Otoacoustic emissions can measure the degree of hearing loss, but it cannot shed light on a pathologic cause. Electronystagmography is a test that measures the vestibular ocular reflex. Detailed physical examination is an important prerequisite before any diagnostic tests are ordered. Only MRI with contrast enhancement can elucidate the cause of unilateral sensorineural hearing loss.

[52.3] **A.** The most common form of facial paralysis is idiopathic. It is also called Bell palsy. Recent evidence suggests that the cause of Bell palsy is probably recrudescence of herpes simplex virus. Every patient should have a careful examination to rule out other causes of facial paralysis, such as those diagnoses listed. Where indicated, this examination might require an audiogram or MRI imaging.

CLINICAL PEARLS

❖ Idiopathic facial paralysis (also called Bell palsy) is the most common cause of unilateral facial weakness.

❖ Bell palsy is a diagnosis of exclusion, and patients with facial paralysis require a careful otologic and cranial nerve examination.

❖ Patients that present with a complaint related to one cranial nerve require evaluation of all cranial nerves.

❖ Acoustic neuromas are the most common tumor of the cerebellopontine angle.

❖ Unilateral sensorineural hearing loss should be further evaluated by MRI with gadolinium contrast.

REFERENCES

Fan G, Curtin H. Imaging of the lateral skull base. In: Jackler R, Brackmann D, eds. Neurotology, 2nd ed. Philadelphia, PA: Elsevier; 2004, pp 383–418.
Lo W, Hovsepian M. Imaging of the cerebellopontine angle. In: Jackler R, Brackmann D, eds. Neurotology, 2nd ed. Philadelphia, PA: Elsevier; 2005. pp 349–382.

A 59-year-old retired bartender presents with the complaint of headaches and difficulty concentrating over the past 6 weeks. He has been healthy all of his life and presents yearly for an annual checkup. He describes the headaches as occurring primarily over the right frontal temporal region and describes it as "dull" in nature. He has experienced occasional nausea but no vomiting with the headaches. Additionally, he has had difficulty focusing and concentrating on tasks at hand, such as reading the newspaper or playing cards. His wife states that he has been more irritable, moody, and "not himself" for 1 month. There is no history of alcohol abuse or exposure to toxins. He admits to a 30-pack-a-year smoking history. The review of systems is significant for weight loss and productive cough.

His examination reveals that he is afebrile with a blood pressure of 124/72 mmHg and a heart rate of 78 beats/min. His general examination is normal. He is oriented to person, time, location, and situation, although he becomes upset during the examination. Cranial nerve and sensory examination findings are unremarkable. Motor strength testing is normal except for questionable weakness in the left finger extensors. The deep tendon reflexes are normal except for a Babinski sign present on the left. With ambulation, he has less arm swing on the left than the right.

◆ **What is the most likely diagnosis?**

◆ **What is the next diagnostic step?**

◆ **What is the next step in therapy?**

ANSWERS TO 53: Metastatic Brain Tumor

Summary: A 59-year-old healthy man presents with a 6-week history of right frontal temporal headaches associated with difficulty concentrating, weight loss, and coughing. His headaches are often associated with nausea and are dull in nature. His wife reports personality changes and the patient himself recognizes mood disturbances. His examination is notable for decreased arm swing on the left, questionable weakness of the left finger extensors, and a left Babinski sign.

◆ **Most likely diagnosis:** Metastatic brain tumor affecting the right cerebral hemisphere.

◆ **Next diagnostic step:** MRI of the brain with and without gadolinium and chest x-ray.

◆ **Next step in therapy:** Corticosteroids and anticonvulsants are started immediately while waiting for surgical evaluation.

Analysis

Objectives

1. Know the clinical presentation and diagnostic approach to metastatic brain tumor.
2. Be familiar with the differential diagnosis of metastatic brain tumor.
3. Describe the treatment for metastatic brain tumor.

Considerations

This 59-year-old otherwise healthy man presents with unilateral dull headaches associated with nausea and personality changes. Additionally there is a history of difficulty concentrating, weight loss, and cough. His physical examination suggests mild left-sided weakness most likely from a right hemispheric lesion given the left Babinski sign. Based on the history and examination the most likely diagnosis is a right hemispheric mass lesion. Taking it one step further the history of weight loss and cough are concerning for a lung cancer. With this in mind, metastatic lung cancer should be considered. A chest x-ray will reveal that he has a large right upper-lobe mass lesion highly suggestive of lung cancer. An MRI of the brain will show a right frontal temporal well-circumscribed lesion at the gray-white junction with hemorrhage and surrounding edema. Evidence of midline shift or impending herniation should be evaluated. Corticosteroids such as dexamethasone should be started as this reduces edema and capillary permeability. Prophylaxis with anticonvulsants in individuals with metastatic tumors that have not experienced a seizure is controversial. Approximately 40% of patients with metastatic brain tumors will experience a seizure. Only 20% of patients with metastatic brain tumors present with seizures. In this particular case the patient has a hemorrhage, which is known to be epileptogenic. Most physicians would begin anticonvulsants. Caution should be taken in patients who are receiving both anticonvulsants and corticosteroids as the latter can significantly reduce anticonvulsant levels. Neurosurgical consultation should be obtained as should an oncology consultation.

APPROACH TO METASTATIC BRAIN TUMORS

Definitions

Metastatic brain tumors: Tumors that arise from metastasis of systemic neoplasm to the brain parenchyma.

Babinski sign: Extension of the big toe followed by abduction of the other toes when the lateral sole of the foot is stimulated. It is performed by stroking the foot at the heel and moving the stimulus toward the toes. It is a sensitive and reliable sign of cortical spinal tract disease. It is also known as the plantar reflex.

Midline shift: Movement of a cerebral hemisphere to the opposite side secondary to intracranial swelling. This can cause compression of the lateral ventricles and contribute to further elevated intracranial pressure.

Herniation: Downward displacement of the cerebral hemisphere from increased intracranial pressure.

Clinical Approach

Metastatic brain tumors can arise from primary systemic cancers that spread to the leptomeninges, brain parenchyma, calvaria, or dura. **Brain metastases are 10 times more common than primary brain tumors.** In the United States roughly 150,000 new cases per year of metastatic brain tumors are reported. Men have a slightly higher incidence than females at a ratio of 1.4:1. Approximately 66% of metastatic brain tumors go to the parenchyma with almost 50% of these being a solitary lesion. The most common tumors that metastasize to the brain are listed in the Table 53–1, with lung cancer being most common.

Table 53–1
METASTATIC TUMOR AND FREQUENCY

Tumor Type	Cases (%)
Lung cancer	50%
Breast cancer	20%
Melanoma	10%
Unknown primary	10%
Others: thyroid and sarcoma	Unknown

Tumors metastasize to the brain most commonly by entering the systemic circulation known as hematogenous spread. The distribution of tumor parallels blood flow to the brain with approximately **82% metastasizing supratentorially**, 15% spreading to the cerebellum, and 3% affecting the brain stem. **Metastatic brain tumors are commonly located at the gray-white junction and arterial border zones**, locations that have narrowed blood vessels that can trap tumor cells.

Clinical features of metastatic brain disease are varied and can depend on location. Neurologic symptoms occur from direct tumor infiltration, hemorrhage, edema, or even hydrocephalus. Table 53–2 illustrates the most common clinical features of brain metastases.

The differential diagnosis for metastatic brain tumors includes brain abscess, demyelinating diseases, radiation necrosis, cerebral vascular accidents, intracranial bleed, and primary brain tumors. **Approximately 60% of those without any known primary tumor that present with brain metastasis have a primary lung cancer.**

The clinical evaluation in patients with unknown primary cancer is focused and includes an MRI of the brain with gadolinium. **Gadolinium or contrast is critical as it will show enhancement around the lesions.** Given the fact that lung cancer is the most common type to metastasis to brain, a chest x-ray followed by a CT scan of the chest should be performed. If these studies are

Table 53–2
CLINICAL FEATURES OF BRAIN TUMORS

Clinical Features	Patients Presenting with Features (%)
Headaches dull and associated with nausea **Visual disturbances** including blurred vision; unilateral on side of tumor and more commonly associated with posterior fossa metastases	45–50%
Cognitive impairment including personality changes, mood and memory problems	33%
New onset seizure; more frequently associated with frontal, temporal or multiple metastases	10–20%
Stroke-like syndrome	5–10%
Papilledema	10% (at time of presentation)
Other nonspecific neurologic findings	20–40%

unrevealing, than an abdominal or pelvic CT scan should be performed. Careful attention should be placed to the prostate, testicles, breasts, and rectum during clinical examination. A guaiac examination should be performed to evaluate for occult blood. This will help evaluate for gastrointestinal cancers.

Unfortunately an MRI of the brain cannot diagnose the type of tumor in patients with unknown primary malignancy. One exception is malignant melanoma, which has been shown to be hyperintense on T1-weighted images and hypointense on T2-weighted images. **A brain biopsy can be necessary if a primary tumor cannot be found.** Patients with signs of severe increased intracranial pressure can benefit from surgery.

Treatment with corticosteroids such as dexamethasone is important in reducing intracranial pressure and edema. Commonly a dose of 10 mg of dexamethasone, either orally or intravenously, followed by 4 mg every 6 hours is given. As previously discussed, it is controversial as to whether or not anticonvulsants are necessary in patients who have not experienced seizures. However those individuals that have presented or developed a seizure warrant anticonvulsant therapy.

The decision as to whether or not patients should undergo surgery is dependent on the number of brain metastases, location, the size, the likelihood of response to treatment, and the patient's overall health status. The most important factor when considering surgery is the tumor burden located outside the brain. **Improved survival** and quality of life has been shown in patients with **single lesions** when they have been treated with whole brain radiotherapy and surgery. Those that do better following this treatment are individuals that present at a younger age, absence of extracranial disease, and increased time to developing brain metastasis. **Radiation therapy** has been shown to decrease the mortality from neurologic dysfunction. The most common regimen is given over a period of 2 weeks using 30 Gy in 10 fractions. Radiation therapy improves neurologic symptoms in 50% to 93% of patients. Complications from radiotherapy include brain necrosis, brain atrophy, cognitive deterioration, leukoencephalopathy, and neuroendocrine dysfunction. Stereotactic radiation via the gamma knife, linear particle accelerators, or charged particles can also be used. This has been found to decrease toxicity to healthy tissue and minimize side effects. Stereotactic radiation is often used in tumors that are surgically inaccessible; complications from stereotactic radiation include seizures, headaches, nausea, hemorrhage, and radiation necrosis. For the most part chemotherapy is not used for brain metastasis.

Favorable prognostic factors include being less than 60 years of age, two or less brain metastasis, good baseline function, and accessible to surgical resection. Individuals with single brain metastasis who receive all brain radiation plus surgery have a median survival of 10 to 16 months. Patients who have metastasis to infratentorial regions of the brain carry a worse prognosis than those with supratentorial metastasis.

Comprehension Questions

[53.1] A 56-year-old man who is complaining of confusion and motor deficits is noted to have multiple lesions to the brain. A metastatic tumor is suspected. Which of the following is the most common tumor causing brain metastasis?

A. Breast
B. Melanoma
C. Renal
D. Lung
E. Thyroid

[53.2] A 50-year-old man is noted to have some symptoms suggestive of a brain tumor. Which of the following is the most commonly found symptom for brain tumors?

A. Seizures
B. Headaches
C. Papilledema
D. Personality changes
E. Ataxia

[53.3] A 45-year-old man with a history of smoking presents after experiencing a generalized tonic-clonic seizure. He has been experiencing dull left-sided headaches over the past 2 months. His examination reveals hyper-reflexia on the right with mild weakness of the right iliopsoas and finger extensor muscles. The MRI of the brain shows a large 7 cm × 10 cm lesion over the left frontal region with associated midline shift. A chest x-ray shows a left lower lobe mass. What is the next step?

A. Consult neurosurgery for immediate brain biopsy and debulking
B. Start dexamethasone at a dose of 10 mg followed by 4 mg every 6 hours. Concomitantly begin an anticonvulsant medication
C. Start dexamethasone at a dose of 100 mg followed by 4 mg every 6 hours and hold off on starting anticonvulsant medication
D. Consult the oncology service to assist you in deciding on chemotherapy
E. Start whole brain radiation therapy

Answers

[53.1] **D.** Lung cancer is the most common tumor metastasizing to brain, accounting for approximately 50% of all cases.

[53.2] **B.** Headache is the most commonly found symptom associated with brain tumors and is found in approximately half of cases.

[53.3] **B.** Patients with brain metastasis that present with seizures should be started on anticonvulsant therapy in addition to dexamethasone. In this particular case there is associated midline shift that warrants immediate medical management.

CLINICAL PEARLS

❖ Metastatic malignancies account for the majority of brain tumors in adults.

❖ Enhancing brain lesions on MRI that are located at the gray-white junction are likely to be metastatic brain tumors.

❖ Most metastatic MRI brain lesions are nonspecific. Melanoma is an exception, being consistently hyperintense on T1-weighted images and hypointense on T2-weighted images.

❖ Patients that present with new onset headaches, personality changes, and mood disorders need to be evaluated for brain tumors.

REFERENCES

Kaye AH, Laws ER. Brain tumors, an encyclopedic approach, 2nd ed. Philadelphia, PA: Churchill Livingstone; 2001.

Dorland's Illustrated Medical Dictionary, 27th ed. Philadelphia, PA: WB Saunders; 1988.

Nathoo N, Toms SA, Barnett GH. Metastases to the brain: current management. Expert Rev Neurother 2004;4:4, 633–640. Online publication updated: July 1, 2004.

Sawaya R, Ligon BL, Bindal RK. Management of metastatic brain tumors. Ann Surg Oncol 1994;1(2):169–178.

SECTION III

Listing of Cases

Listing by Case Number

Listing by Disorder (Alphabetical)

LISTING BY CASE NUMBER

LISTING BY DISORDER (ALPHABETICAL)

❖ INDEX